NEUROMODULATION TECHNIQUES FOR THE SPINE

Other books in this series

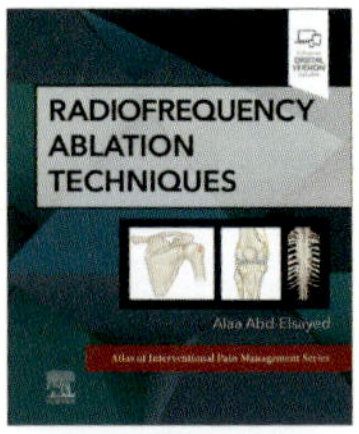

Alaa Abd-Elsayed, Radiofrequency Ablation Techniques, 1e
ISBN: 9780323870634

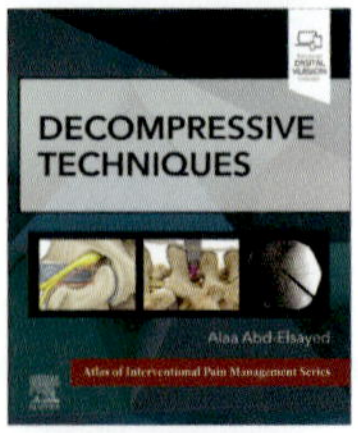

Alaa Abd-Elsayed, Decompressive Techniques, 1e
ISBN : 9780323877510

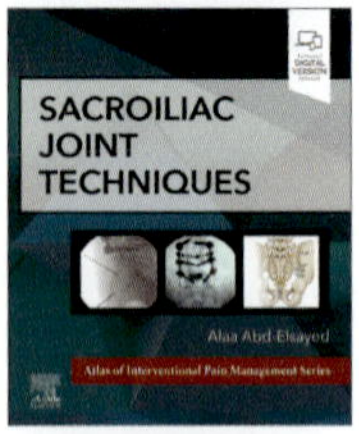

Alaa Abd-Elsayed, Sacroiliac Joint Techniques, 1e
ISBN: 9780323877541

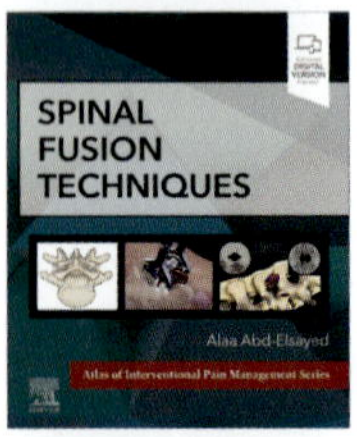

Alaa Abd-Elsayed, Spinal Fusion Techniques, 1e
ISBN: 9780323882231

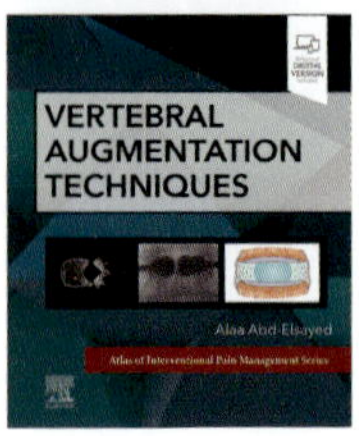

Alaa Abd-Elsayed, Vertebral Augmentation Techniques, 1e
ISBN: 9780323882262

NEUROMODULATION TECHNIQUES FOR THE SPINE

Atlas of Interventional Pain Management Series

Alaa Abd-Elsayed, MD, MPH, CPE, FASA

Medical Director, UW Health Pain Services
Medical Director, UW Pain Clinic
Division Chief, Chronic Pain Management
Department of Anesthesiology
University of Wisconsin
Madison, Wisconsin
United States

ELSEVIER

Elsevier
1600 John F. Kennedy Blvd.
Ste 1800
Philadelphia, PA 19103-2899

Neuromodulation Techniques for the Spine:
Atlas of Interventional Pain Management Series

ISBN: 978-0-323-87584-4

Senior Content Development Manager: Somodatta Roy Choudhury
Executive Content Strategist: Michael Houston
Senior Content Development Specialist: Akanksha Marwah
Publishing Services Manager: Shereen Jameel
Project Manager: Maria Shalini
Senior Designer: Patrick C. Ferguson
Marketing Manager: Kate Bresnahan

Printed in India

Last digit is the print number: 9 8 7 6 5 4 3 2 1

Dedication

*I would like to dedicate this book to my parents, my wife,
and my two beautiful kids Maro and George.*

Contributors

Cristina Abad Salom, MD
Interventional pain physician
Pain medicine
Pain Unit in Hospital Quirónsalud Madrid, Spain

Alaa Abd-Elsayed, MD, MPH, CPE, FASA
Medical Director, UW Health Pain Services
Medical Director, UW Pain Clinic
Division Chief, Chronic Pain Management
Department of Anesthesiology
University of Wisconsin
Madison, Wisconsin
United States

David Abejón González, MD, PhD
Unit Pain
Hospital Universitario Quironsalud Madrid
Madrid, Spain

Rohit Aiyer
Interventional Pain Physician
Richmond Interventional Pain Management
2066 Richmond Avenue
Staten Island, New York
United States

Nomen Azeem, MD, FAAPMR
Founder & CEO
Florida Spine & Pain Specialists
Assistant Professor of Pain Medicine,
University of South Florida-Department of Neurology
Tampa, Florida
United States

Caitlin Bakke, BS
Univeristy of St. Thomas
Des Moines University College of Osteopathic Medicine Nura Pain Clinics

Amy Commers, PharmD
Pharmacy Director
Nura Pain Clinics,
Minneapolis
Minnesota,
United States

William T. Daprano
Department of Physical Medicine & Rehabilitation
University of Central Florida College of Medicine
Orlando, Florida
United States

Raymon S. Dhall
Department of Anesthesiology, Perioperative Care & Pain Medicine
NYU Langone Health
New York, New York
United States

Andrew J. Duarte, MD
Pain Medicine Fellow
Department of Neurology
USF Morsani College of Medicine
Tampa, Florida
United States

Alyson M. Engle, MD
Assistant Professor
Division of Pain Medicine
Department of Anesthesiology
Northwestern University Feinberg School of Medicine
Chicago, IL, United States

Kenneth J. Fiala, BS
University of Wisconsin-Madison School of Medicine and Public Health Department of Anesthesiology
Madison, Wisconsin
United States

Michael Alan Fishman, MD, MBA
Interventional Pain Physician
Director of Research
Center for Interventional Pain and Spine
Lancaster, Pennsylvania
United States

Chris Gilligan, MD, MBA
Associate Chief Medical Officer
Brigham & Women's Hospital
Director, Brigham & Women's Spine Center
Assistant Professor of Anaesthesia
Harvard Medical School
Boston, Massachusetts
United States

Amitabh Gulati, MD, FIPP, CIPS, ASRA-PMUC
Director of Chronic Pain
Memorial Sloan Kettering Cancer Center New York, New York
United States

Behnum Habibi, MD
Assistant Professor
Chief of Pain Management
Department of Physical Medicine and Rehabilitation
Lewis Katz School of Medicine at Temple University

Joseph Hanna, MD
Senior Staff Physician
Henry Ford Health
Detroit, Michigan
United States

Terence Hillery, MD
Pain Medicine Physician
MetroHealth/ Case Western Reserve University
Cleveland, Ohio
United States

Nasir Hussain, MD, MSc
Assistant Professor
Anesthesiology
The Ohio State University Wexner Medical Center
Columbus, Ohio
United States

Navdeep S. Jassal, MD
EXCEL Pain and Spine
Assistant Clinical Professor
Neurology/Pain
University of South Florida
Tampa, Florida
United States

Ashley Katsarakes, BA
Clinical Research Coordinator
Research
Center for Interventional Pain and Spine
Lancaster, Pennsylvania
United States

Chong Kim, MD
Professor
Department of Physical Medicine and Rehabilitation
MetroHealth System/Case Western Reserve University School of Medicine
Cleveland, Ohio
United States

Wendell Bradley Lake, MD
Assistant Professor
Neurosurgery
University of Wisconsin Hospitals and Clinics
Madison, Wisconsin
United States

Nathanael Leo, MD
Clinical Assistant Professor Dept. of Anesthesiology, Perioperative Care and Pain Medicine NYU Langone Health NYU School of Medicine, New York, United States

Tariq Malik, MD
Associate Professor
Anesthesia and Critical Care
University of Chicago
Chicago, Illinois
United States

Mark N. Malinowski, DO
Interventional Pain Physician
Interventional Pain Management
OhioHealth/Grant Medical Center
Columbus, Ohio
United States

Joshua M. Martens, BS
University of Wisconsin-Madison School of Medicine and Public Health Department of Anesthesiology
Madison, Wisconsin
United States

Nicholas Mata, MD
Physician
All Star Pain Management
Annapolis, Maryland
United States

Neel Mehta, MD
Medical Director
Anesthesiology
Weill Cornell Medicine
New York, New York
United States

Weston Nadherny, MD
Physical Medicine and Rehabilitation
MetroHealth/Case Western Reserve University
Cleveland, Ohio
United States

Lakshmi Akhila Nerusu, MD
Anesthesiology
The Ohio State University
Columbus, OH
United States

Shiv Patel, MD
Staff Physician
Pain Medicine
Precision Spine Care
Longview, TX
United States

Kailash Pendem, MD
Department of Physical Medicine & Rehabilitation University of Florida College of Medicine Gainesville,
Florida
United States

Neal Rakesh, MD, MSE
Department of Anesthesia and Critical Care
Memorial Sloan Kettering Cancer Center
New York, New York
United States

Ramsey Saad, MD
Henry Ford Health
Detroit, Michigan
United States

Ashley Scherer, MS
Clinical Research Coordinator
Center for Interventional Pain and Spine
Lancaster, Pennsylvania
United States

David M. Schultz, MD
CEO,
Nura Pain Clinics, Minneapolis Adjunct
Professor
Department of Anesthesiology University of Minnesota
Minnesota
United States

Nabil Sibai, MD
Henry Ford Health
Detroit, Michigan
United States

R. Scott Stayner, MD, PhD
Surgery Center Medical Director
Nura Pain Clinics Minneapolis, MN,
United States

Gustaf Van Acker, MD, PHD
Assistant Professor
Physical Medicine and Rehabilitation
Case Western Reserve University/MetroHealth Medical Center
Cleveland, Ohio
United States

Shashank Vodapally, DO
Department of Physical Medicine and Rehabilitation
Michigan State University
Sparrow Hospital and McLaren Hospital
Lansing, Michigan
United States

Sayed Emal Wahezi, MD
Program Director,
Pain Medicine Fellowship
Professor of Physical Medicine and Rehabilitation
Professor of Anesthesiology
Professor of Orthopedic Surgery
Montefiore Medical Center, Bronx New York
United States

Lindsay Kate Wanner, BA
Clinical Research Coordinator
Center for Interventional Pain and Spine
Lancaster, Pennsylvania
United States

Steven Zhou, MD
Anesthesiology
The Ohio State University Wexner Medical Center
Columbus, Ohio
United States

Xiaoying Zhu, MD, PhD
Associate Professor
Anesthesiology
University of Virginia
Charlottesville, Virginia
United States

Preface

The use of electrical stimulation (Neuromodulation) as a treatment for conditions associated with significant pain was first reported in the 19th century. Since then, the technology has continued to develop at an accelerated pace as technique improvements and clinical applications expand the range of patients that might benefit from this therapeutic modality.

Examples of technological advances include new devices, generators, wireless systems, wave forms, and stimulation targets.

This text is one in an atlas book series that focuses on the deployment of minimally invasive pain procedures and was written by experts in the field with significant clinical experience. Through considerable author effort, this text contains the most up to date and experience-based information/guidance relevant to device specifics and procedural guidance. Detailed figures accompany the text and provide additional insight to improve procedural technique and success.

This book provides readers the totality of information relevant to spinal cord stimulation, medial branch nerve stimulation, dorsal root ganglion stimulation, and intrathecal drug delivery systems. For each device, readers will gain an appreciation for patient selection, perioperative management considerations, and detailed technique descriptions that are augmented with numerous anatomy and fluoroscopy images.

This book is one that will be valued by trainees, physicians at all levels of expertise, advanced pain practitioners, nurses, and all other healthcare team members involved in the management of pain mitigation devices.

I would like to thank all authors for their time and significant effort required to produce these impactful and high quality chapters.

I would like also to thank the publisher for their support which has facilitated this book becoming the modern guide for neuromodulation.

Alaa Abd-Elsayed, MD, MPH, CPE, FASA

Contents

Chapter 1

History of Neuromodulation

Terence Hillery, Nicholas Mata, and Chong Kim

Chapter Outline

Introduction

When the first-century Roman physician Scribonious Largus recommended a torpedo, an electrical fish, be placed in a pool of sea water beneath a patient suffering from gout "until his whole foot and leg up to the knee is numb," he made one of the earliest recorded prescriptions for electricity.[1] While the use of electricity in medical treatment has grown dramatically in sophistication and scale, early contributions to the field were often made by amateurs. The American polymath Benjamin Franklin recorded treating painful conditions in several patients with static electrical currents, though in a 1747 letter to his parents, he admitted that he was apprehensive "meddling in the Dr's sphere."[2,3] In the late 18th century, Luigi Galvani hypothesized that "animal electricity" intrinsic within frog legs was responsible for the muscle twitch he stimulated with direct current.[4] Defending the competing hypothesis of the time, Alessandro Volta invented the first battery to demonstrate that frog muscle instead conducted extrinsic electrical current.[5]

These advances in the understanding of electricity laid the foundation for more rigorous study of the human nervous system in the 19th century. In 1822, Francois Magendie, building on the work of Charles Bell, described the sensory and motor division of the dorsal and ventral roots of the spinal cord.[6] A reported negative finding on the electrical excitability of the central nervous system by Jean Pierre Flourens in 1824 led to decades of silence on the topic until Eduard Hitzig and Gustav Fritsch demonstrated, in 1870, that direct current stimulation of the motor cortex in dogs produced leg movement.[7] Just a few years later, Roberts Bartholow demonstrated the same finding on a patient whose cerebral cortex was exposed after debridement of skull osteomyelitis, an experiment that generated controversy at the time.[8] Victor Horsley (Fig. 1.1) reported using an alternating current electrode to guide tumor resection in an 1886 surgery.[9]

An understanding had been reached that the nervous system was fundamentally electrical, mappable, and amenable to human intervention, however crudely. Perhaps surprisingly, it was 19th-century quacks who created the first mass-market electric medical devices, which they marketed as panaceas. One device, the Electreat, patented by Charles W. Kent in 1919, claimed to cure "headache, rheumatism, neuralgia,

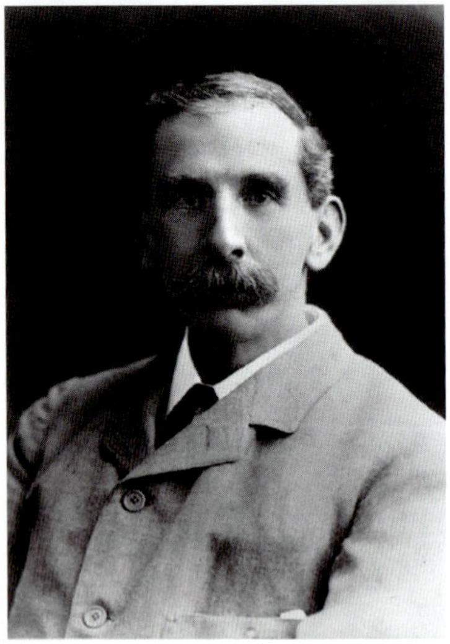

Fig. 1.1 Victor Horsley, an early leader in neurological surgery. (From Paget S. *Sir Victor Horsley: A Study of His Life and Work*. Harcourt, Brace & Howe;1920.)

pains of any kind."[10] While Kent was later sued by the newly formed US Food and Drug Administration (FDA),[11] the Electreat endured to bridge the gap to the modern era of electrical medical devices. Norm Shealy used the device, which functioned similarly to a modern transcutaneous electrical nerve stimulation (TENS) unit, to guide patient selection for early spinal cord stimulation (SCS) trials.[12]

The remainder of this chapter will examine milestones in the history of neuromodulation, defined by Philip Gildenberg as "chronic therapeutic electrical stimulation of the central nervous system or special nerves with an implanted stimulating device."[13]

Gate Theory

The advancement of gate theory by Ronald Melzack and Patrick D. Wall in 1965 revolutionized scientific understanding of pain. In the early 1960s, Melzack and Wall argued in support of Pattern Theory, which held that disparate somatic signals underwent computation at multiple ascending sites in the central nervous system (CNS), culminating in firing patterns experienced by an individual as pain.[14] A prior study of the histology of herpes zoster lesions had found that allodynic areas showed a relative paucity of large sensory fibers relative to small fibers.[15] This finding, combined with a growing understanding of spinal neurophysiology and Szentagothai's detailed neuroanatomic evidence,[16] inspired the hypothesis that Melzack and Wall called the Gate Theory (Fig. 1.2). This posited that prolonged large sensory fiber activation, through intermediary interneurons (termed *substantia gelatinosa* and *T cells*), inhibited or "closed the gate" on the sensory signals from small sensory fibers.[17] In this elegant theory, Melzack and Wall hinted at an explanation for the anesthetic effect of therapies as disparate as electrical torpedo fish and the Electreat.

Wall and collaborator William Sweet, Chair of Neurosurgery at Massachusetts General Hospital, provided initial support for the theory in humans by

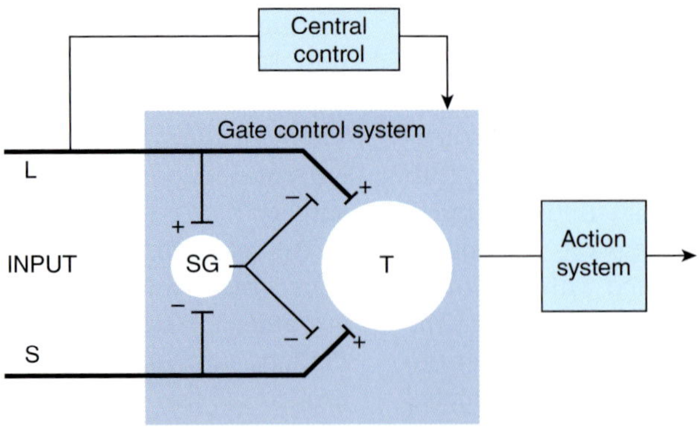

Fig. 1.2 This diagram illustrates the key principles of gate theory, namely, that large sensory fibers (L) can overwhelm the input of small sensory fibers (S) in ascending neural pathways. ***SG*, Substantia gelatinosa; *T*, T cell.** (From Melzack R, Wall PD. Pain mechanisms: a new theory. *Science*. 1965;150(3699):971-979.)

stimulating their own infraorbital nerves, in effect, creating the first peripheral nerve stimulator.[18] This work was well known to Norm Shealy, who had completed a fellowship under Dr. Sweet.[19] In 1967, Shealy, then new to the neurosurgery faculty at Western Reserve Medical School (now Case Western Reserve University), recruited graduate student J. Thomas Mortimer to develop treatments based on gate theory. Shealy reasoned that human anatomy was favorable to direct application of gate theory on the spinal cord, as the large-diameter sensory fibers mainly ran through the dorsal columns, easily accessible via laminectomy and conveniently distant from tracts transiting small-diameter sensory and motor fibers. This held the theoretical advantage of stimulating large sensory fibers, felt by patients as paresthesias, to inhibit small sensory fiber activation, felt by patients as pain, in the distribution of multiple peripheral nerves.[19]

In 1967, Shealy, now Chief of Neurosurgery at The Gunderson Clinic in Lacrosse, Wisconsin, surgically implanted the first dorsal column stimulator in a 70-year-old man suffering from cancer pain.[20] The device, a modified cardiac pacemaker designed by Mortimer, used a single bipolar Vitallium lead sutured inside the dura. In this initial trial, the patient achieved significant pain relief, though he died a few days later from complications of his cancer.

Mortimer set out to address some of the flaws in the initial design, including the need to access subcutaneous jacks with needles to power the device. Here, he was again able to draw on revolutionary developments in cardiac pacemakers. While some primitive devices were produced as early as the 1920s, modern cardiac pacemakers were born in the 1950s with the development of transvenous pacing. The units, developed separately in the 1950s by John Hopps, Paul Zoll, and others, proved reliable but had to remain plugged in to wall power. Earl Bakken, who in 1949 had founded Medtronic as a medical device repair service for hospitals, worked with the leading University of Minnesota cardiac surgeon C. Walton Lillehei to develop a battery-powered pacemaker appropriate for the newly developed surgically implantable myocardial wire. Bakken claimed that in 1957 he had a flash of inspiration when he saw a plan for a transistorized, electronic metronome in a back issue of *Popular Electronics* magazine. He quickly created a prototype; within days, the device was being successfully used on Lillehei's patients. The next year, the first fully implantable pacemaker was used. Almost overnight, a market for pacemakers, and the underlying miniaturized electronics, expanded greatly.[21]

The second-generation SCS device was designed by Mortimer in collaboration with Medtronic engineer Norm Hagfors. Together they adapted Medtronic's Barostat stimulator, originally marketed to treat hypertension and angina pectoris through stimulation of the carotid sinus. The stimulator was powered by an external radiofrequency (RF) generator, eliminating the need for transcutaneous leads. Hagfors and Mortimer's device was implanted into a patient with pain from a pelvic carcinoma, who experienced 4 years of improved pain control. In 1968, Medtronic began marketing a version of this device, dubbed the Myelostat. The commercial availability of an SCS device marked an important turning point, at which neuromodulation jumped from the laboratory into clinical practice.[13]

Growth and Competition in Spinal Cord Stimulation

The next phase of development in SCS focused on making lead implantation safer and technically easier as well as making SCS more effective. In 1970, Charles Burton and others developed intradural lead implantation to avoid known complications of subdural implantation, including cerebrospinal fluid (CSF) leak, spinal cord injury, and arachnoiditis.[22]

In 1968, Roger Avery started Avery Labs out of his garage.[23] In 1971, Avery released an SCS device that also used a single-lead design. However, unlike the Medtronic Myelostat, the lead was implanted in the epidural space and the RF receiver was implanted in the anterior abdomen to facilitate easier coupling to the RF generation unit.[24]

Regulation and a Changing Market

In response to a spate of medical device–related recalls, injuries and deaths, the FDA gained regulatory authority for medical devices with passage of the 1976 Medical Device Regulation Act.[25] The FDA was now given the mandate to independently verify that medical devices were safe and effective.[26] Devices already on the market were exempted, but any new devices were subject to FDA review, increasing development costs. In response, a committee was formed that met at two neurosurgical conferences in 1977 to discuss the safety of neuromodulation devices.[13,27] The unanimous opinion of the committee was that SCS was a safe and effective treatment for pain.[28]

With the basic design in place, device companies looked to improve the convenience and efficacy of their SCS devices (Fig. 1.3). New companies entered the market, including Neuromed and Cordis, the latter of which released the first fully implantable SCS device, termed an *implantable pulse generator (IPG)*.[29] The device, based on a mercury battery–powered cardiac pacemaker, required no external power. Medtronic followed suit, releasing their first IPG, the Itrel I, in 1984.[30] The Itrel I could be used with percutaneously inserted leads, a Medtronic development from 1978.[31] A few years earlier, the current technique had been developed—inserting a catheter into the epidural space through a needle placed between adjacent lamina.[32] With time, this development would transform the dominant setting for SCS implantation from the operating room to the procedure suite, opening the door for physicians in nonsurgical specialties.

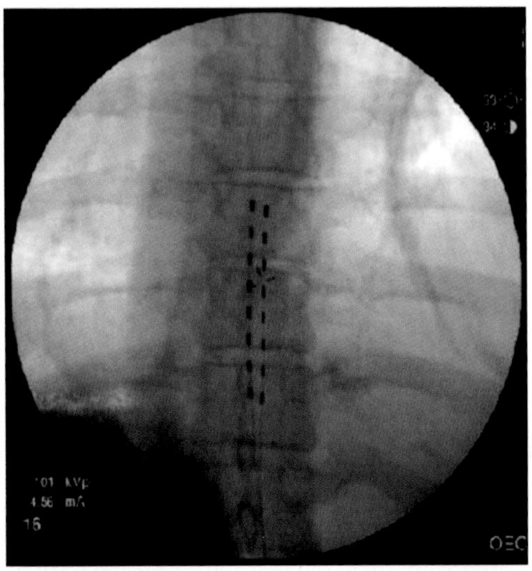

Fig. 1.3 Fluoroscopic image depicting percutaneously inserted spinal cord stimulation leads. (From Benedetti EM. Thoracic spinal cord stimulation is useful for pain treatment after incomplete cervical spinal cord injury. *Rev Col Anest.* 2013;41(2):146-149.)

It was a time of rapid change. In 1981, Avery Labs left the SCS market to focus on its core product, phrenic nerve pacemakers, which became the second type of neuromodulation device to receive FDA approval, in 1986.[13]

In the next phase of development, the remaining SCS device manufacturers focused on increasing flexibility and coverage of the electromagnetic field generated by their devices. Greater coverage could better accommodate minor lead migration and reported changes in sensation with spine flexion and extension. Neuromed released the Octrode, an RF system powering a single lead with eight electrodes, in 1986.[33] Medtronic responded in 1988 with the Xtrel RF system, which used dual electrodes, each with two leads.[34] Neuromed tested an IPG in the early 1990s, but it never came to market. In 1995, Neuromed was acquired by Quest Medical and was renamed Advanced Neuromodulation Systems (ANS).[35]

In this era of SCS, the main development goals remained in conflict. It was understood that the most effective pain relief would be provided by broad electrode coverage and a range of programming settings, increasing energy demands. This ran contrary to the other main goal, which was to make devices fully implantable and nonobtrusive. For these reasons, RF devices continued to be marketed alongside IPG devices for decades. In the late 1990s, a patient may have been asked to consider the choice between a Medtronic Itrel 3, an IPG with a two-by-two electrode lead structure, or the RF-powered ANS Renew system available in 1999, which offered the coverage of two-by-eight electrodes and an array of programming settings.[36]

In 2004, Advanced Bionics, previously known for producing cochlear implants, won FDA approval for the first rechargeable IPG stimulator, the Precision.[37] This device was small and well tolerated by patients, yet featured 16 electrodes and a range of programming settings. Medtronic and ANS, which was purchased by St. Jude in 2005, worked quickly to develop their own rechargeable IPG devices. Throughout the 2000s, rechargeable IPG devices competed against traditional IPG devices, including several larger models with expanded battery capacity.

On May 10, 2005, the FDA published a letter banning physicians from performing magnetic resonance imaging (MRI) on patients with implanted SCS devices. This controversial decision came with little warning, forcing patients, physicians, and the medical device industry to confront new trade-offs. Medtronic won approval in 2008 to allow 1.5T head MR imaging on patients implanted with the Restore Ultra IPG device. In 2013, the FDA allowed full-body MRI with the Restore Sensor SureScan.[38]

Now that issues such as battery capacity, lead coverage, and MRI restrictions had been addressed, attention turned to device programming. St. Jude released the Protégé in 2014, which allowed for software updating after the device had been implanted.[39] This and subsequent devices could be programmed in burst mode or tonic mode. Tonic, or conventional SCS, is paresthesia based, operating at a regular frequency below 1.5 kHz. A typical burst SCS device delivers 5 pulses at 800 Hz. These groupings of pulses are delivered at 40 times per second, which is often able to provide pain relief without producing noticeable paresthesias.[40] The Nevro Senza, released in 2015, operates at 10 kHz, which has been shown to deliver true paresthesia-free pain relief.[41] Three-dimensional (3D) neural targeting, an anatomically guided programming technique, was shown to be superior to traditional SCS programming in the landmark 2017 LUMINA trial.[42] Later, differential target multiplexed (DTM) SCS was developed based on preclinical data suggesting that glial cells played a role modulating ascending neural pathways.[43]

In the mid-2010s, dorsal root ganglion (DRG) stimulators became a popular option in treating painful conditions associated with particular dorsal roots. In these devices, leads are positioned in the lateral epidural space within the spinal foramen (Fig. 1.4). This was thought to decrease changes in sensation associated with changes in body position,[44] which continues to challenge SCS design despite innovations in programming and the addition of accelerometers in some models.[45]

Other uses have been explored for SCS, including to treat spasticity in multiple sclerosis and to improve chronic wound healing in peripheral vascular disease.[46] While these have shown some promise, they are no longer routinely performed in the United States.

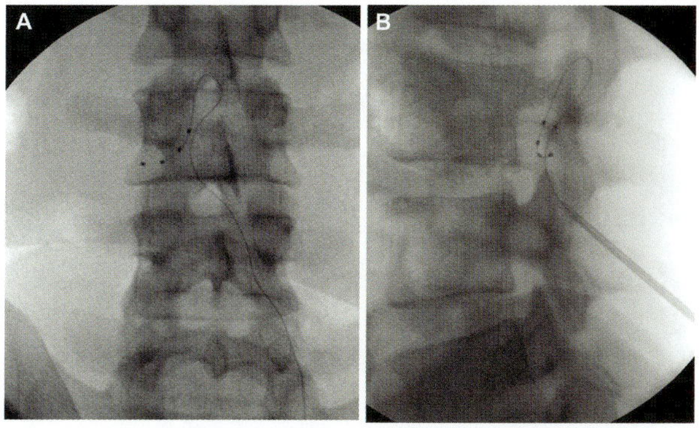

Fig. 1.4 AP and lateral fluoroscopic images of dorsal root ganglion lead placement. *AP*, Anteroposterior. (From Martin SC, Macey AR, Raghu A, et al. Dorsal root ganglion stimulation for the treatment of chronic neuropathic knee pain. *World Neurosurg*. 2020;143:e303-e308.

Deep Brain Stimulation

Deep brain stimulation (DBS) emerged from the same 19th-century experiments that inspired gate theory and SCS. Building on his earlier work stimulating the human cortex intraoperatively, Horsley, alongside Robert Clarke, developed the first stereotactic surgical apparatus.[47] In a landmark 1908 paper, they laid out a system of conventions for describing the 3D position of any point within the stereotactic frame.[48]

The principle was established; a generation later, Ernest Spiegel and Henry Wycis pioneered the first human stereotactic surgery in 1947.[49] This development, combined with work mapping human functional neuroanatomy, such as the landmark 1954 atlas by Wilder Penfield and Herbert Jasper, set the stage for a flood of developments in functional neurosurgery.[50] Penfield led the way in the 1930s, describing a successful ablative technique for epilepsy, known as the *Montreal procedure* (Fig. 1.5).[51] Ablative surgeries were especially useful in treating Parkinson disease (PD) and psychotic disorders, which lacked effective alternative treatments prior to the development of antipsychotics in the 1950s and the development of levodopa in the 1960s.[52] By 1968, approximately 25,000 stereotactic ablation surgeries had been performed worldwide for PD.[53] This allowed for the production of detailed neurophysiological atlases, such as Robert Tasker's definitive atlas of the thalamus.[54] This breadth of collective experience with

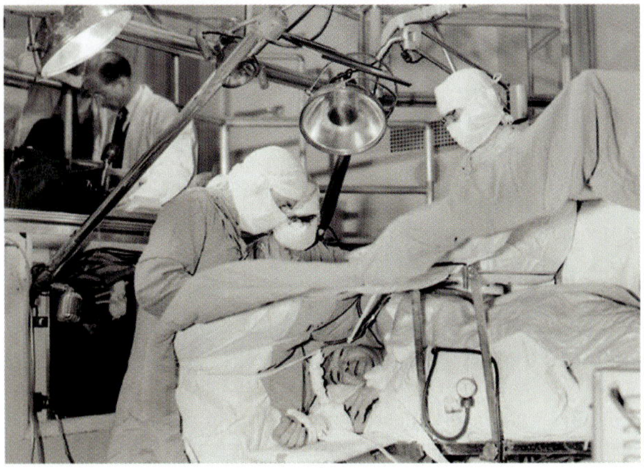

Fig. 1.5 An operating theater at the Montreal Neurological Institute, where the Montreal procedure was developed. (From Ladino LD, Rizvi S, Téllez-Zenteno JF. The Montreal procedure: the legacy of the great Wilder Penfield. *Epilepsy Behav.* 2018;83:151-161.)

neurostimulation in motor disorders also bore out an important heuristic: lower-frequency stimulation tended to exacerbate symptoms, whereas higher-frequency stimulation reduced symptoms.[55]

The finding that electrical stimulation could produce clinically useful effects led some to suggest therapeutic chronic neurostimulation. One of the early uses of chronic stimulation, by Carl Wilhelm Sem-Jacobsen in 1966, was to improve target localization for later ablative surgeries.[56] However, the development of levodopa in 1968 spelled disaster for the growing field of stereotactic neurosurgery. Surgery could no longer be justified but for a few cases of otherwise untreatable PD.[53] Development of effective antipsychotics, as well as a campaign against psychosurgery—led in part by psychiatrist Peter Breggin, who argued that psychosurgery was disproportionately performed on minority patients[57]—led practitioners to abandon stereotactic neurosurgery en masse.

The revival of stereotactic neurosurgery and birth of modern DBS required not only the persistence of stereotactic surgical knowledge in large academic centers but also the advancements in miniaturization led by cardiac pacemaker developers.[55] Neurosurgeon Yoshio Hosobuchi continued to offer stereotactic ablative operations for chronic pain; in 1973, he reported the first use of modern DBS. The operation was deemed successful in three of his four initial patients. Device makers were quick to seize on the opportunity—within a few years Medtronic, Avery Labs, and Cordis marketed DBS devices, all developed from cardiac pacemakers.[58] Throughout the late 1970s and early 1980s, neurosurgeons released case series of patients with treatment-resistant chronic pain, PD, epilepsy, and dystonia that responded well to DBS.[59]

However, DBS ran into the same barrier as SCS: the 1976 Medical Device Regulation Act. All DBS manufacturers opted against pursuing the FDA-mandated device trials; thus, strict limits were placed on the sale of DBS devices. DBS was rescued again from obscurity when it became clear that there was a limit to the effectiveness of levodopa in treating PD, meaning that there was a large population who could potentially benefit from DBS.[55] Clinical trials followed, and in 1997 the FDA approved use of Medtronic's DBS leads and Itrel stimulation system in PD.

Since achieving regulatory approval, over 150,000 patients worldwide have undergone DBS surgery for PD.[60] DBS trials are currently underway in patients who suffer from depression, obsessive-compulsive disorder, schizophrenia, Alzheimer disease, substance abuse, anorexia nervosa, and chronic pain, to name just a few.[61]

Other Neuromodulation Therapies

Several other neuromodulation technologies have come to represent a significant portion of the current 5.8 billion US dollar global neuromodulation market.[62]

INTRATHECAL DRUG DELIVERY

Delivery of drugs into the spinal canal dates back at least to the late 19th century, when neurologist James Corning injected cocaine into the intrathecal space of a patient undergoing surgery.[63] Early experiments were considered successful; other drugs, including morphine, were also delivered in single-dose intrathecal injections in the following decades. In 1935, Mayo Clinic neurosurgeon Grafton Love proposed using a catheter to achieve continuous spinal anesthesia. In 1940, surgeon William Leonard described the use of procaine to achieve spinal anesthesia in over 200 patients. The technique quickly grew in popularity and, in 1945, was further improved by the invention of a directional spinal needle by Edward Tuohy.[64]

The discovery of the opioid receptor in 1971 prompted a series of animal studies confirming the theoretical advantage of decreased adverse effects in intrathecal opioid delivery compared with systemic opioid delivery.[65] It was widely recognized that continuous delivery improved safety and efficacy over single-shot spinal anesthesia. In 1982, the first human implantation of a targeted intrathecal drug delivery system (TIDD) was performed by an M.D. Anderson team led by Milam Leavens. Approval for Medtronic to market a TIDD device delivering preservative-free morphine came in 1991.[66] Since that time, tens of thousands of TIDD devices have been implanted into patients, and multiple opioid and nonopioid drug monotherapies and combination therapies have been recommended in the literature.[67] Of particular interest, a drug based on a marine snail toxin, ziconotide, remains the only FDA-approved nonopioid TIDD agent.[68]

PERIPHERAL NERVE STIMULATION

In the decades after Wall and Sweet demonstrated peripheral nerve stimulation (PNS) in 1967, the use of PNS was largely limited to academic centers and the technique was plagued by morbidity and inconsistent outcomes.[69] A revival of the field occurred with increasing use of clinical ultrasound as well as development of percutaneous implantation techniques.[70] Several device manufacturers now supply PNS devices, and the technique continues to be studied in peripheral neuralgias.[71]

VAGUS NERVE STIMULATION

As early as 1880, James Corning recognized a role for carotid compression in modulating seizure activity. The idea was revived in 1938 by Percival Bailey and Frederic Bremer, who demonstrated that experimental electrical stimulation to feline vagus nerves could directly influence brain activity, as demonstrated by electroencephalogram.[72] These and other contributions formed the basis of Jacob Zabara's argument in a series of 1985 articles arguing that vagus nerve stimulation (VNS) should be explored to treat seizures.[73] The first case report of a vagus nerve stimulator being implanted in a human was published in 1990.[74] In 1997, the FDA approved vagal nerve stimulators for use in epilepsy.[73] As of 2012, over 100,000 VNS devices have been implanted worldwide.[75]

GASTRIC ELECTRICAL STIMULATION

In 1963, Aydin Bilgutay published a case series of patients with postoperative ileus who underwent stimulation by an electrical nasogastric probe.[76] While the initial results were promising, the technique was superseded when Medtronic started marketing an implantable pulse generator under an FDA Humanitarian Device Exemption in 2000. This device, implanted laparoscopically into the greater curvature of the gastric wall, stimulates and entrains gastric electrical activity to promote gastric emptying.[77]

Gastric neuromodulation has also been studied as a treatment for morbid obesity. At the time of this writing, at least three different devices have been studied, though long-term efficacy has yet to be conclusively demonstrated.[78]

SACRAL NERVE STIMULATION

Many neuromodulatory techniques have been proposed to treat various bladder conditions, including a proposal in the early 1970s by Blaine Nashold to treat neurogenic bladder with SCS.[79] These early proposals proved ineffective, in part because CNS stimulation produced sustained activation of the external urinary sphincter alongside the intended activation of the detrusor muscle.[80] The British physiologist Giles Brindley hypothesized that pulsed stimulation of the sacral nerve could exploit the differences between the striated muscle of the external urethral sphincter and the smooth muscle detrusor.[81] Stimulation of the anterior roots of the S2 through S5, termed the *Brindley procedure*, was first employed clinically in 1976. Since then, increasingly sophisticated devices have been successfully used to treat neurogenic bladder. Sacral neuromodulation remains under investigation as a treatment for other urinary disorders.

Conclusion

Any brief review of neuromodulation makes clear that clinical improvement has followed developments in the underlying technologies and advancements in scientific understanding of neurophysiology. Strong levels of funding in neuroscience and materials science portends an exciting future for neuromodulation.[82]

REFERENCES

1. Kellaway P. The part played by electric fish in the early history of bioelectricity and electrotherapy. *Bull Hist Med*. 1946;(20):112-137.
2. Heidland A, Fazeli G, Klassen A, et al. Neuromuscular electrostimulation techniques: historical aspects and current possibilities in treatment of pain and muscle waisting. *Clin Nephrol*. 2013;79(suppl 1):S12-S23.
3. Gensel L. The medical world of Benjamin Franklin. *J R Soc Med*. 2005;98:534-538. doi:10.1258/jrsm.98.12.534.
4. Piccolino M. Animal electricity and the birth of electrophysiology: the legacy of Luigi Galvani. *Brain Res Bull*. 1998;46(5):381-407. doi:10.1016/s0361-9230(98)00026-4.
5. Piccolino M. The bicentennial of the Voltaic battery (1800-2000): the artificial electric organ. *Trends Neurosci*. 2000;23(4):147-151. doi:10.1016/s0166-2236(99)01544-1.
6. Figlio KM. Theories of perception and the physiology of mind in the late eighteenth century. *Hist Sci*. 1975;13(3):177-212. doi:10.1177/007327537501300302.
7. Hagner M. The electrical excitability of the brain: toward the emergence of an experiment. *J Hist Neurosci*. 2012;21(3):237-249. doi:10.1080/0964704X.2011.595634.
8. Bartholow R. Experiments on the functions of the human brain. *Br Med J*. 1874;1(700):727.
9. Horsley V. The cerebellum. *Hospital (London, 1886)*. 1909; 46(1197):410.
10. Electreat Instruction Sheet. *Detroit Historical Society*. c. 1920. Available at: https://detroithistorical.pastperfectonline.com/archive/3B720A84-BCFE-486C-9E8E-394505705129. Accessed June 21, 2022.
11. Ottestad E, Orlovich DS. History of peripheral nerve stimulation—update for the 21st century. *Pain Med*. 2020;21(supp 1):S3-S5. Available at: https://doi.org/10.1093/pm/pnaa165.
12. Shealy CN, Mortimer JT, Reswick JB. Electrical inhibition of pain by stimulation of the dorsal columns: preliminary clinical report. *Anesth Analg*. 1967;46(4):489-491.
13. Gildenberg PL. Chapter 2–neuromodulation: a historical perspective. In: Krames ES, Hunter Peckham P, Rezai AR, eds. *Neuromodulation*. Cambridge, MA: Academic Press; 2009:9-20.
14. Melzack R, Wall PD. On the nature of cutaneous sensory mechanisms. *Brain*. 1962;85:331-356. doi:10.1093/brain/85.2.331.
15. Mendell LM. Constructing and deconstructing the gate theory of pain. *Pain*. 2014;155(2):210-216. doi:10.1016/j.pain.2013.12.010.
16. Szentagothai J. Neuronal and synaptic arrangement in the substantia gelatinosa rolandi. *J Comp Neurol*. 1964;122:219-239. doi:10.1002/cne.901220207.
17. Melzack R, Wall PD. Pain mechanisms: a new theory. *Science*. 1965;150(3699):971-979. doi:10.1126/science.150.3699.971.
18. Wall PD, Sweet WH. Temporary abolition of pain in man. *Science*. 1967;155(3758):108-109. doi:10.1126/science.155.3758.108.
19. North RB, Prager JP. Chapter 45—history of spinal cord stimulation. In: Krames ES, Hunter Peckham P, Rezai AR, eds. *Neuromodulation*. 2nd ed. Cambridge, MA: Academic Press; 2018:587-596.
20. Shealy CN, Mortimer JT, Reswick JB. Electrical inhibition of pain by stimulation of the dorsal columns. Preliminary clinical report. *Anesth Analg (Cleve)*. 1967;46:489-491.
21. Aquilina O. A brief history of cardiac pacing. *Images Paediatr Cardiol*. 2006;8(2):17-81.
22. Shealy CN, Stern R, Schneider C, Burton C, Brownell E, Fox J. Seminar on dorsal column stimulation. Summary of Proceedings. Edited by Dr. Charles Burton. *Surg Neurol*. 1973;1:285-289.
23. Deaths: Avery, Roger E. *New York Times*; November 4, 2001. Available at: https://www.nytimes.com/2001/11/04/classified/paid-notice-deaths-avery-roger-e.html. Accessed June 21, 2022.
24. Ranu E. Chapter 10, electronics. In: *Essential Neuromodulation*. Elsevier; 2011:213–251.
25. Foote SB. Loops and loopholes: hazardous device regulation under the 1976 medical device amendments to the Food, Drug and Cosmetic Act. *Ecol Law Q*. 1978;7:101-135.
26. U.S. Food and Drug Administration. *A History of Medical Device Regulation & Oversight in the United States*. June 24, 2019. Available at: https://www.fda.gov/medical-devices/overview-device-regulation/history-medical-device-regulation-oversight-united-states. Accessed June 21, 2022.
27. Mount LA. Neurosurgery 1977: problems and attainments. *J Neurosurg*. 1977;47(5):647-652. Available at: https://thejns.org/view/journals/j-neurosurg/47/5/article-p647.xml. Accessed April 27, 2021.
28. Gildenberg PL. Neurosurgical statement on neuroaugmentive devices. *Appl Neurophysiol*. 1977;40:69-71.
29. U.S. Food and Drug Administration. *Premarket Approval. Docket number 81M-0136*. April 14, 1981. Available at: https://www.accessdata.fda.gov/scripts/cdrh/cfdocs/cfpma/pma.cfm?id=P800040. Accessed June 21, 2022.
30. U.S. Food and Drug Administration. *Premarket Approval. Docket number 81M-0415*. November 30, 1984. Available at: https://www.accessdata.fda.gov/scripts/cdrh/cfdocs/cfpma/pma.cfm?id=P840001. Accessed June 21, 2022.
31. U.S. Food and Drug Administration. *510(k) Premarket Notification. 510k number K812154*. September 20, 1981. Available at: https://www.accessdata.fda.gov/scripts/cdrh/cfdocs/cfpmn/pmn.cfm?ID=K812154. Accessed June 21, 2022.
32. Hoppenstein R. Percutaneous implantation of chronic spinal cord electrodes for control of intractable pain: preliminary report. *Surg Neurol*. 1975;4(1):195-198.
33. U.S. Food and Drug Administration. *510(k) Premarket Notification. 510k number K860158*. March 7, 1986. Available at: https://fda.report/PMN/K860158. Accessed June 21, 2022.
34. U.S. Food and Drug Administration. *510(k) Premarket Notification. 510k numberK883780*. Available at: https://www.accessdata.fda.gov/scripts/cdrh/cfdocs/cfpmn/pmn.cfm?ID=K883780. Accessed June 21, 2022.
35. Bloomberg. *Advanced Neuromodulation Systems Inc*. Available at: https://www.bloomberg.com/profile/company/ANSI:US#:~:text=Advanced%20Neuromodulation%20Systems%2C%20Inc.,of%20the%20central%20nervous%20system. Accessed June 21, 2022.
36. U.S. Food and Drug Administration. *510(k) Premarket Notification. 510k number K992946*. September 24, 1999. Available at: https://www.accessdata.fda.gov/scripts/cdrh/cfdocs/cfpmn/pmn.cfm?ID=K992946. Accessed June 21, 2022.
37. *PrecisionTM Spinal Cord Stimulator System Clinician Manual*. 2004. Available at: https://www.bostonscientific.com/content/dam/Manuals/us/current-rev-en/91083273-02_Precision_Clinician_Manual_Entrada_2_DFU_en-US_S.pdf. Accessed June 21, 2022.
38. Medical Company Product News. *Medtronic Launches RestoreSensor SureScan MRI Neurostimulation System*. April 14, 2021.

Available at: https://www.zenopa.com/news/801622708/candidate-engagement-policy. Accessed June 21, 2022.

39. *St. Jude's New Upgradeable Protégé Spinal Cord Stimulator Stays Up to Date with New Software Updates*. MedGadget; April 7, 2014. Available at: https://www.medgadget.com/2014/04/st-judes-new-upgradeable-protege-spinal-cord-stimulator-stays-up-to-date-with-new-software-updates.html. Accessed June 21, 2022.
40. De Ridder D, Vanneste S, Plazier M, van der Loo E, Menovsky T. Burst spinal cord stimulation: toward paresthesia-free pain suppression. *Neurosurgery*. 2010;66(5):986-990. doi:10.1227/01.NEU.0000368153.44883.B3.
41. Stauss T, El Majdoub F, Sayed D, et al. A multicenter real-world review of 10 kHz SCS outcomes for treatment of chronic trunk and/or limb pain. *Ann Clin Transl Neurol*. 2019;6:496-507. Available at: https://doi.org/10.1002/acn3.720.
42. Veizi E, Hayek SM, North J, et al. Spinal cord stimulation (SCS) with anatomically guided (3D) neural targeting shows superior chronic axial low back pain relief compared to traditional SCS-LUMINA Study. *Pain Med*. 2017;18(8):1534-1548. doi:10.1093/pm/pnw286.
43. Provenzano DA, Heller JA, Hanes MC. Current perspectives on neurostimulation for the management of chronic low back pain: a narrative review. *J Pain Res*. 2021;14:463-479. doi:10.2147/JPR.S249580.
44. Kramer J, Liem L, Russo M, Smet I, Van Buyten JP, Huygen F. Lack of body positional effects on paresthesias when stimulating the dorsal root ganglion (DRG) in the treatment of chronic pain. *Neuromodulation*. 2015;18(1):50-57; discussion 57. doi:10.1111/ner.12217.
45. Deer TR, Grigsby E, Weiner RL, Wilcosky B, Kramer JM. A prospective study of dorsal root ganglion stimulation for the relief of chronic pain. *Neuromodulation*. 2013;16:67-71. doi:10.1111/ner.12013.
46. Cook AW, Weinstein SP. Chronic dorsal column stimulation in multiple sclerosis. Preliminary report. *N Y State J Med*. 1973;73(24):2868-2872.
47. Compston A. The structure and functions of the cerebellum examined by a new method. By Sir Victor Horsley, FRS, FRCS and R.H. Clarke, MA, MB. Brain 1908:31;45–124. *Brain*. 2007;130(6):1449-1452. Available at: https://doi.org/10.1093/brain/awm115.
48. Horsley V, Clarke RH. The structure and functions of the cerebellum examined by a new method. *Brain*. 1908;31(1):45-124.
49. Spiegel EA, Wycis HT, Marks M, Lee AJ. Stereotaxic apparatus for operations on the human brain. *Science*. 1947;106(2754):349-350. doi:10.1126/science.106.2754.349.
50. Penfield W, Jasper H. *Epilepsy and the Functional Anatomy of the Human Brain*. Boston: Little, Brown; 1954.
51. Penfield W. Epilepsy and surgical therapy. *Arch Neurol Psychiatry*. 1936;36(3):449-484.
52. Mashout GA. Psychosurgery: past, present, and future. *Brain Res Brain Res Rev*. 2005;48(3):409-419.
53. Gildenberg PL. Fifty years of stereotactic and functional neurosurgery. In: Barrow DL, Kondziolka DS, Laws Jr ER, Traynelis VC, eds. *Fifty Years of Neurosurgery*. New York, NY: Lippincott Williams & Wilkins; 2000:295-320.
54. Tasker RR, Organ LW, Hawrylshyn PA. *The Thalamus and Midbrain of Man. A Physiological Atlas Using Electrical Stimulation*. Springfield, IL: CC Thomas; 1982.
55. Gardner J. A history of deep brain stimulation: technological innovation and the role of clinical assessment tools. *Soc Stud Sci*. 2013;43(5):707-728. doi:10.1177/0306312713483678.
56. Sem-Jacobsen CW. Depth-electrographic observations related to Parkinson's disease. Recording and electrical stimulation in the area around the third ventricle. *J Neurosurg*. 1966;24(suppl 1):388-402.
57. Pert C. *The Conscience of Psychiatry: The Reform Work of Peter R. Breggin, MD. Candace Pert*. Ithaca, NY: Lake Edge Press; 2009.
58. Coffey RJ. Deep brain stimulation devices: a brief technical history and review. *Artif Organs*. 2009;33(3):208-220. doi:10.1111/j.1525-1594.2008.00620.x.
59. Cooper IS, Upton AR, Amin I. Reversibility of chronic neurologic deficits. Some effects of electrical stimulation of the thalamus and internal capsule in man. *Appl Neurophysiol*. 1980;43(3-5):244-258. doi:10.1159/000102263.
60. Hariz M. My 25 stimulating years with DBS in Parkinson's disease. *J Parkinsons Dis*. 2017;7(supp 1):S33-S41. doi:10.3233/JPD-179007.
61. Lozano AM, Lipsman N, Bergman H, et al. Deep brain stimulation: current challenges and future directions. *Nat Rev Neurol*. 2019;15(3):148-160. doi:10.1038/s41582-018-0128-2.
62. Markets and Markets. *Neuromodulation Market by Technology—Internal (Deep Brain Stimulation, Vagus Nerve Stimulation), External (Transcranial Magnetic Stimulation), Application (Ischemia, Chronic Pain, Parkinson's, Depression, Tremor, Epilepsy, Migraine) - Global Forecast to 2025*. Available at: https://www.marketsandmarkets.com/Market-Reports/neurostimulation-devices-market-921.html. Accessed June 21, 2022.
63. Rizvi S, Kumar K. History and present state of targeted intrathecal drug delivery. *Curr Pain Headache Rep*. 2015;19(2):474. doi:10.1007/s11916-014-0474-8.
64. Deer TR. History of intrathecal drug delivery. In: Deer TR, ed. Atlas of Implantable Therapies for Pain Management. New York: Springer; 2011:139-141.
65. Yaksh TL, Rudy TA. Analgesia mediated by a direct spinal action of narcotics. *Science*. 1976;192(4246):1357-1358. doi:10.1126/science.1273597.
66. Belverud S, Mogilner A, Schulder M. Intrathecal pumps. *Neurotherapeutics*. 2008;5(1):114-122. doi:10.1016/j.nurt.2007.10.070.
67. Krames E, Peckham PH, Rezai AR. *Neuromodulation*. 1st ed. Cambridge, MA: Academic Press; 2009.
68. Klotz U. Ziconotide—a novel neuron-specific calcium channel blocker for the intrathecal treatment of severe chronic pain—a short review. *Int J Clin Pharmacol Ther*. 2006;44(10):478-483. doi:10.5414/cpp44478.
69. Stanton-Hicks M. Peripheral nerve stimulation for pain, peripheral neuralgia and complex regional pain syndrome. Neuromodulation. In: Krames ES, Hunter Peckham P, Rezai AR, eds. *Neuromodulation*. Cambridge, MA: Academic Press; 2009:397–408.
70. Slavin KV. Peripheral nerve stimulation for neuropathic pain. *Neurotherapeutics*. 2008;5(1):100-106. doi:10.1016/j.nurt.2007.11.005.
71. Nayak R, Banik RK. Current innovations in peripheral nerve stimulation. *Pain Res Treat*. 2018;2018:9091216. doi:10.1155/2018/9091216.
72. Bailey P, Bremer FA. Sensory cortical representation of the vagus nerve. *J Neurophysiol*. 1938;1:405-412.
73. Groves DA, Brown VJ. Vagal nerve stimulation: a review of its applications and potential mechanisms that mediate its clinical effects. *Neurosci Biobehav Rev*. 2005;29(3):493-500.
74. Penry JK, Dean J. Prevention of intractable partial seizures by intermittent vagal stimulation in humans: preliminary results. *Epilepsia*. 1990;31:S40-S43. Available at: https://doi.org/10.1111/j.1528-1157.1990.tb05848.x.

75. Cyberonics Inc. *Cyberonics Announces 100,000th Patient Implant of VNS Therapy*. Cision PR Newswire; December 20, 2012. Available at: https://www.prnewswire.com/news-releases/cyberonics-announces-100000th-patient-implant-of-vns-therapy-184314661.html. Accessed June 22, 2022.
76. Bilgutay AM, Wingrove R, Griffen WO, Bonnabeau Jr RC, Lillehei CW. Gastro-intestinal pacing: a new concept in the treatment of ileus. *Ann Surg*. 1963;158(3):338-348. doi:10.1097/00000658-196315830-00003.
77. Soffer EE. Gastric electrical stimulation for gastroparesis. *J Neurogastroenterol Motil*. 2012;18(2):131-137. doi:10.5056/jnm.2012.18.2.131.
78. Abell TL, Chen J, Emmanuel A, Jolley C, Sarela AI, Törnblom H. Neurostimulation of the gastrointestinal tract: review of recent developments. *Neuromodulation*. 2015;18(3):221-227; discussion 227. doi:10.1111/ner.12260.
79. Nashold Jr BS, Friedman H, Boyarsky S. Electrical activation of micturition by spinal cord stimulation. *J Surgical Res*. 1971;11:144-147.
80. Li LF, Leung GKK, Lui WM. Sacral nerve stimulation for neurogenic bladder. *World Neurosurg*. 2016;90:236-243. Available at: https://doi.org/10.1016/j.wneu.2016.02.108.
81. Brindley GS. Emptying the bladder by stimulating sacral ventral roots. *J Physiol*. 1974;237:15P-16P.
82. New NIH brain initiative awards move toward solving brain disorders. November 23, 2020. National Institutes of Health. https://www.nih.gov/news-events/news-releases/new-nih-brain-initiative-awards-move-toward-solving-brain-disorders. Accessed July 10, 2022.

Chapter 2

Patient Selection

William T. Daprano, Raymon S. Dhall, Kailash Pendem, and Navdeep S. Jassal

Chapter Outline

Introduction

Chronic pain, or pain that persists beyond a normal healing time, has a profound impact on physical and emotional well-being. It results in disability, disruption of ability to work, and is linked to opioid dependence.[1] In the United States, chronic pain is becoming increasingly prevalent. In 2016, 1 in 5 adults had chronic pain per the Centers for Disease Control and Prevention (CDC).[2] Since their development, physicians have been utilizing spinal cord stimulation (SCS) devices to help in the treatment of chronic pain. By delivering electrical stimuli to target locations, traditional SCS devices (40–100 Hz) aim to generate comforting paresthesias via dorsal column stimulation and negate the sensation of pain. More recently, novel waveform devices have become more widely used and demonstrate superiority to traditional tonic SCS devices in the treatment of low back pain. Dorsal root ganglion (DRG) stimulation has also had a widespread impact on a variety of focal pain disorders. Given the rapidly increasing prevalence of chronic pain and the opioid epidemic, SCS and DRG stimulation have emerged as promising therapeutic options to be considered by treating physicians.

Patient Selection

Neuromodulation is an established modality for chronic pain management that should be considered for patients in whom conservative measures have failed. SCS and DRG stimulation are not effective for all patients with all types of pain. Because proper patient selection is an important determinant of successful SCS therapy, potential candidates should be evaluated based on chronic pain etiology and neurostimulation appropriateness. Patients should be screened for comorbidities and contraindications to implantation. Furthermore, a psychological evaluation should be performed to identify patients who will achieve the maximum benefit from an implanted device.[3] This will be further discussed in the following sections.

Indications

The primary indication for SCS is chronic neuropathic pain secondary to altered nerve function or nerve damage. Peripheral neuropathy, complex regional pain syndrome (CRPS), peripheral nerve injury, spinal cord injury, ischemia (peripheral vascular and cardiac disease), postlaminectomy syndrome (PLS) or central neuropathic pain (secondary to stroke) are examples of conditions that may be treated with SCS. SCS can induce functional change based on involved spinal cord segments (not vertebral levels). Due to the targeted nature of SCS, it is important to keep in mind anatomical correlates when considering this therapy. Specific pathologies and potential targets of SCS therapy may be found in Tables 2.1 and 2.2, respectively.

TABLE 2.1 Spinal Cord Stimulation Pathologies[4]

- Abdominal pain
- Angina
- Central neuropathic pain
- Chronic critical limb ischemia
- Complex regional pain syndrome
- Headache/cephalalgia
- Multiple sclerosis
- Peripheral neuropathy
- Postherpetic neuralgia
- Spinal disorders (including postlaminectomy syndrome)

US Food and Drug Administration–Approved Indications

Given the many targets of SCS, there are many conditions and etiologies to which it may be applied. Of these, the US Food and Drug Administration (FDA) has approved SCS primarily for the treatment of chronic intractable pain of the trunk and/or limbs, including unilateral or bilateral pain associated with PLS, CRPS types I and II, intractable low back pain, and leg pain.[5] In this chapter, we will cover the most common and successful FDA-approved SCS applications.

Postlaminectomy Syndrome	PLS, or failed back surgery syndrome, is defined as persistent or recurrent pain, usually in the back or legs, that remains following spinal surgery. There has been a rise in spinal surgeries given the aging population, resulting in an increased prevalence of PLS. Estimates of PLS prevalence within 2 years of back surgery are between 20% to 40%.[6] Given these high rates, it comes as no surprise that PLS is one of the most common indications for SCS therapy in the United States. The data for SCS efficacy in the treatment of PLS is well studied. In 2005, the multicenter, prospective, randomized, controlled PROCESS study compared SCS combined with conventional medical management (CMM) versus CMM alone. Kumar and colleagues found that 37% of SCS + CMM patients versus 2% of CMM-alone patients had 50% or greater pain relief in the legs at 24 months' follow-up.[7] Most recently, in 2019, the multicenter, prospective, randomized, controlled PROMISE study compared SCS to optimal medical management (OMM) in PLS patients. The study found positive outcomes associated with SCS + OMM versus OMM alone in low back pain reduction, leg pain reduction, change in disability status, and quality of life.[8] With recent improvements in technology, these lifestyle improvements for PLS may also be achieved via novel waveforms. Randomized controlled trials (RCTs) with these waveforms will be discussed later in this chapter. PLS is a diagnosis of exclusion. Given the limitations of the physical examination, a PLS diagnosis must be accompanied with imaging studies and possible surgical consultation. These studies can help narrow the differential diagnosis by identifying surgically correctable lesions and may also further warrant SCS therapy by visualizing pathologies such as concomitant arachnoiditis or epidural fibrosis.[9]

Radiculopathy and Plexopathy

Radiculopathy is the radiation of pain due to nerve root or spinal nerve dysfunction or damage. An excellent indication is leg pain associated with radiculopathy due to its great response to SCS therapy. Radiculopathy commonly arises secondary to disc herniation, spondylosis, PLS, or facet joint hypertrophy. It is thus important to rule out other causes of referred pain such as spinal stenosis, facet disease, myofascial pain, sacroiliitis, internal disk disruption, or piriformis syndrome.[10]

Downstream from nerve roots, a plexus of nerves may be found, such as the brachial plexus or the lumbar plexus. When neuropathy affects these plexuses, they become known as plexopathy. With this background knowledge, it is easy to see why SCS therapy that targets upstream of the involved plexus can be effective in treating this pathology. While the physical examination may identify a plexopathy, electromyography and nerve conduction studies are more specific in the confirmatory process of a plexopathy diagnosis.

Complex Regional Pain Syndrome

There are two types of CRPS: type I, formerly referred to as *reflex sympathetic dystrophy*, and type II, formerly referred to as *causalgia*. Differentiating the two types requires the absence (type I) or presence (type II) of a known nerve lesion. CRPS is characterized by the presence of spontaneous, evoked regional pain that is disproportionate in severity in typical courses of pain following similar tissue trauma. Both autonomic and inflammatory symptoms are present in CRPS, such as burning, hyperesthesia, allodynia, trophic skin changes, edema, altered hair growth patterns, skin color or skin temperature changes relative to the unaffected side, reduced strength, tremors, and dystonia.[11] To aid in the diagnosis of CRPS, the Budapest criteria (Table 2.3) have become widely adopted and accepted as the gold standard behind any CRPS diagnosis.

After meeting the Budapest criteria and establishing a CRPS diagnosis, concurrent therapeutic disciplines should be utilized, including medical, rehabilitative, and psychological management, with the clinical picture dictating further interventional therapy. In patients with either type of CRPS, SCS may be considered after exhausting traditional therapies, including medications such as anticonvulsants or tricyclic antidepressants, nonpharmacological therapies such as physical therapy or occupational therapy, and psychological treatment such as cognitive behavioral therapy.[11] Current Neurostimulation Appropriateness Consensus Committee (NACC) recommendations on SCS for CRPS management advise the requirement of 3-month duration of pain or a severe, rapidly progressing clinical picture unresponsive to conservative measures.[12,13] SCS should be trialed in CRPS patients, particularly in those who do not experience an improvement in condition with conservative treatment.[11,14] If the trial is successful, patients may undergo SCS implantation with focus on optimizing function and normalizing their daily activities.

Arachnoiditis	Arachnoiditis is a chronic inflammation and scarring of the meninges of the spinal cord, particularly after surgery or myelogram. The condition is characterized by gradual fibrosis of the arachnoid, an avascular membrane that lies between the arachnoid mater and pia mater. Subsequent to this fibrosis, the vascular supply and cerebrospinal fluid (CSF) supply is interrupted in affected areas.
Epidural Fibrosis	Epidural fibrosis is the scarring and presence of adhesions in the epidural space, especially following spinal surgery. This condition is most associated with PLS given the formation of adhesions as part of the natural healing process. The insidious course of epidural fibrosis normally occurs over 2 to 3 months following spinal surgery and is often seen with a postoperative period of relief followed by persistent leg pain.
Painful Peripheral Neuropathy	There is a plethora of peripheral neuropathy classifications that present with differing patterns of recognition, etiologies, and prognosis. The anatomical involvement varies with both regional and local nerve involvement as well as involvement varying by nerve types (motor, autonomic, sensory). Most recently, high-frequency stimulation was studied in the treatment of painful diabetic neuropathy.[15]
Conditions Associated with Reduced Probability of Success	• Axial spine pain associated with PLS • Incomplete spinal cord injury • Intercostal neuralgia • Phantom pain • Postherpetic neuralgia • Post-thoracotomy pain Patients with conditions associated with an unfavorable prognosis generally make excellent candidates for SCS implantation. The literature on these conditions demonstrates that SCS has a favorable effect on pain reduction. Despite this, these conditions may experience less success with SCS treatment due to poorly understood mechanisms in the current body of medical knowledge. It can never be certain how a patient may respond to neuromodulatory therapy given the variation of nervous system pathologies and the body's responses to such disease processes. However, there have been a plethora of new studies supporting patients with back pain having a long-term favorable response to SCS (as opposed to trunk and limb pain).

TABLE 2.2 Neurostimulation Anatomical Targets[4]

Organ/anatomic Location → SCS Target Segment → Function

- Brain → C2–C3 → Cerebral vasodilation
- Lungs → C2–C3 → Bronchodilation
- Hands/upper extremity → C3–C6 → Peripheral vasodilation
- Heart → T1–T5 → Pain reduction/improved cardiac function
- Gastrointestinal tract → T6–T8 → Pain reduction/improved gastrointestinal function
- Feet/lower extremity → L1–L4 → Peripheral vasodilatation
- Bladder/genitourinary → T11–L2/S2–S4 → Decreased bladder spasticity/increased stretch tolerance

TABLE 2.3 Budapest Criteria

- Continuing pain, which is disproportionate to any inciting event
- Must report at least one symptom in three of the four following categories:
  - Sensory: Reports of hyperalgesia and/or allodynia
  - Vasomotor: Reports of temperature asymmetry and/or skin color changes and/or skin color asymmetry
  - Sudomotor/edema: Reports of edema and/or sweating changes and/or sweating asymmetry
  - Motor/trophic: Reports of decreased range of motion and/or motor dysfunction (weakness, tremor, dystonia) and/or trophic changes (hair, nails, skin)
- Must display at least one sign at time of evaluation in two or more of the following categories:
  - Sensory: Evidence of hyperalgesia (to pinprick) and/or allodynia (to light touch or deep somatic pressure, or joint movement)
  - Vasomotor: Evidence of temperature asymmetry and/or skin color changes and/or asymmetry
  - Sudomotor/edema: Evidence of edema and/or sweating changes and/or sweating asymmetry
  - Motor/trophic: Evidence of decreased range of motion and/or motor dysfunction (weakness, tremor, dystonia) and/or trophic changes (hair, nails, skin)
- There is no other diagnosis that better explains the signs and symptoms

Off-label Applications

Headache

- Neuromodulation therapy is effective for the treatment of headache disorders, including chronic migraines, chronic tension headaches, and trigeminal autonomic cephalgias (TACs). TACs are a group of headache disorders that include cluster headaches, paroxysmal hemicrania, and short-lasting unilateral neuralgiform headache attacks. Headaches may be treated via SCS centrally and peripherally. Deep-brain stimulation (DBS) may be considered in patients with TACs, especially those with cluster headaches or epilepsy. Peripheral stimulation is directed at specific targets, such as the trigeminocervical complex, occipital nerve, auriculotemporal nerve, supraorbital nerve, or auriculotemporal nerve. Preliminary studies of occipital nerve stimulation in particular suggest that it may be efficacious for the treatment of chronic migraine headache.[16]
- Peripheral stimulation is thought to work by activating Aβ fibers that then inhibit the Aδ and C fibers responsible for nociceptive pain while producing paresthesia along the nerve distribution.[4] With this understanding, the downstream benefits of targeted neuromodulation therapy are clear. For example, given the trigeminocervical complex innervation of a large portion of the anterior head, stimulation of this target can be an indicated therapy in patients with chronic migraine or tension headache. There are now devices with nonimplantable internal pulse generators that may prove to make this therapy more favorable than traditional implantation.

Refractory Angina

- In the case of refractory angina (RA), the chest is an appropriate anatomical target for SCS. RA is the presence of chronic angina secondary to coronary insufficiency that is unable to be managed by first-line therapies such as medication, angioplasty, or coronary artery bypass grafting. RA patients should have a disease duration of greater than 3 months with clinical evidence of reversible myocardial ischemia. Significant attention should be given to less invasive alternative RA therapies such as transcutaneous or subcutaneous electrical nerve stimulation. While there are limitations to these modalities, their risk of vascular and infectious complications is lower when compared with SCS placement. Regardless, if these therapies are subtherapeutic or contraindicated in a patient, SCS can be a viable therapy for RA.[17]
- SCS is thought to alleviate RA pain via activation of $\alpha 1$-adrenergic pathways resulting in vasodilation and inhibition of the sympathetic nervous system along the spinal segment target distribution. After nerve terminal depolarization, calcitonin gene-related peptide (CGRP), a substance known for its vasodilatory properties, is released and acts to induce nitric oxide release.[4] It is through the combined effects of these substances that SCS therapy is thought to produce a benefit in microcirculatory perfusion.

Peripheral Vascular Disease

- SCS targeting the upper or lower extremities is used when treating CRPS type 1 and type 2, peripheral neuropathy, and/or peripheral vascular disease. The diagnosis and management of CRPS is complex. In the case of peripheral neuropathy or peripheral vascular disease, SCS is again an excellent therapeutic option when more conservative measures have failed.[16] After appropriate workup, often involving an appropriate physical examination and electromyography or nerve conduction studies, a conservative approach dictated by the clinical picture should be utilized.
- First-line therapies for peripheral vascular disease should include medical management with gabapentinoids or antidepressants and nonpharmacologicals such as foot hygiene, weight loss, or physical therapy. If the patient's pain remains refractory to these therapies, SCS may be utilized to great effect due to its potential activation of second-order spinothalamic neurons and interneurons at these targets as well as the potential vasodilatory benefits of neuromodulatory therapy.[4]

Unsuccessful Applications

SCS application has been trialed and adopted as a treatment modality for many conditions. Of the pathologies trialed for SCS therapy, some have returned unfavorable results. This may be due to an anatomical disruption in the stimulation pathway or nervous system mechanisms beyond the current medical literature's understanding. These pain syndromes include:

- Nerve root avulsion[10,18]
  - Including avulsive plexopathy[18]
- Nonischemic, nociceptive pain[10]
- Paraplegia and quadriplegia[10]
- Spinal cord injury with complete transection[10]
- Partial spinal cord injury that involves dorsal column loss of function[18]
- Central pain of nonspinal origin[18]

Contraindications

Before beginning a trial or permanent implantation of SCS, patients must be evaluated for absolute or relative contraindications. Relative contraindications would warrant the delay or modification of a SCS trial. Contraindications can be found in Table 2.4.

Medical Considerations

Before implementing a treatment plan involving SCS, it is imperative to consider three aspects pertaining to patient safety: neurological injury prevention, infection prevention, and coagulation management. The NACC is a group of experts on neuromodulation. They have released and revised a series of recommendations on the topics mentioned earlier, the most recent revision being in 2017. An update will be provided in 2022.

Foremost, a review of preoperative advanced imaging, magnetic resonance imaging (MRI) or computed tomography (CT) in most cases, is indicated.[21] By reviewing favorable versus unfavorable anatomy on imaging, risks of SCS placement can be mitigated. In addition, review may reveal conditions amenable to conservative management for which SCS would not be indicated. For percutaneous and surgical SCS placements, patient coagulation status should be optimized to prevent neurological injury secondary to spinal hematoma.[21] When managing coagulation medications used as prophylaxis to prevent thrombosis, care should be coordinated with patients and managing medical physicians. Infection prevention for SCS treatments should involve following CDC infection-control measures, treating remote infections preoperatively, and using preoperative antibiotics for neuromodulation trials and implants.[22] Aspirin should be discontinued for 6 days if taken for primary prophylaxis or, if taken for secondary prophylaxis, a shared decision should be made with the prescribing physician.[23] Nonaspirin nonsteroidal antiinflammatory drugs, with an exception given to COX-2 selective inhibitors, should be discontinued for five half-lives of the specific medication to reverse their antiplatelet effect.[23] Further infection control measures can be found in the 2017 article "The Neurostimulation Appropriateness Consensus Committee (NACC) Recommendations for Infection Prevention and Management."[22]

Novel SCS Waveforms

A plethora of new research is being done to compare conventional tonic, high-frequency, and burst devices to optimize therapies for chronic intractable leg and

TABLE 2.4 Spinal Cord Stimulation Therapy Contraindications[12,18–20]

Relative	Absolute
Major psychiatric comorbidity, substance abuse disorder, or cognitive impairment	Patient inability to understand/use/control device
Anticoagulant or antiplatelet therapy	Coagulopathy
Local or systemic infection	Immunosuppression
Pregnancy	Nerve compression best suited for surgical correction
Presence of a pacemaker or defibrillator	
Occupational risk	

back pain. Novel waveform devices now being studied include high-frequency (HF), burst SCS, differential target multiplexed (DTM) stimulation, and multi-waveform capabilities. The underlying theory of HF and burst device preference is that they eliminate paresthesias while still maintaining satisfactory targeted pain control. Comparative studies of conventional versus HF (Table 2.5) and conventional versus burst SCS modalities (Table 2.6) are now available.

Most recently, a prospective, multicenter, randomized clinical trial compared CMM with HF SCS plus CMM for the treatment of refractory painful diabetic neuropathy (PDN). The primary end point of the study was percentage of participants with 50% pain relief or more on the visual analog scale (VAS) without worsening of baseline neurological deficits at 3 months. Of 216 randomized patients, the responder rate of 79% with HF SCS plus CMM was superior to 5% with

TABLE 2.5 Comparative Studies Between Conventional/Tonic and High-Frequency Spinal Cord Stimulation [24]

Study	Study Design	Indication	Outcome Measures	Conclusion
Kapura et al.[32]	RCT	Chronic intractable back and leg pain	Primary outcome >50% reduction in VAS	HF stimulation showed superior analgesia compared with tonic SCS.
Kapura et al.[33]	RCT	Chronic intractable back and leg pain	Primary outcome >50% reduction in VAS	HF stimulation showed superior analgesia compared with tonic SCS.
Ameridelfan et al. [35]	RCT	Chronic intractable back and leg pain	ODI, GAF, CGIC, PSQI, SF-MPQ-2	HF stimulation showed more improved QOL when compared with tonic SCS.
Thomson et al.[34]	RCT	Low back pain ± leg pain more than 90 days	ED-NRS at 3 months	SCS frequencies between 1, 4, 7, and 10 kHz provide equivalent pain relief.

CGIC, Clinical global impression of change; *ED-NRS,* E-Diary Numeric Rating Scale; *HF,* high frequency; *GAF,* global assessment of functioning; *ODI,* Oswestry Disability Index; *PSQI,* Pittsburgh Sleep Quality Index; *QOL,* quality of life; *RCT,* randomized controlled trial; *SCS,* spinal cord stimulation; *SF-MPQ,* Short Form McGill Pain Questionnaire; *VAS,* visual analog scale.

TABLE 2.6 Comparative Studies Between Conventional/Tonic and Burst Spinal Cord Stimulation[24]

Study	Study Design	Indication	Outcome Measures	Conclusion
De Ridder et al.[38]	Retrospective analysis	PLS	NRS, number of responders	Burst stimulation showed superior analgesia compared with tonic SCS.
Deer et al.[37]	RCT	PLS	VAS	Burst stimulation showed superior analgesia compared with tonic SCS.
DeMartini et al.[36]	Multicenter observational study	PLS	1° outcome- reduction of pain in the back and the legs. 2° EG-5D, PCS	Burst stimulation improved leg pain more when compared with tonic SCS.

EQ 5D, European Quality of life scale; *NRS,* Numeric Rating Scale; *PLS,* postlaminectomy syndrome; *RCT,* randomized controlled trial; *PCS,* Pain Catastrophizing Scale; *SCS,* spinal cord stimulation; *VAS,* visual analog scale.

CMM alone. In the same study, neurological examination improvements of 62% with HF SCS plus CMM was superior to 3% with CMM alone at 6 months.[15] Given these results, HF SCS should be considered for patients with painful diabetic neuropathy who fail conservative medical management.

In addition to HF and burst waveforms, a new SCS modality, differential target multiplexed (DTM) stimulation, is of notable mention. DTM SCS uses waveforms that are individually unique from one another and can have different frequencies, pulse rates, and amplitudes. A prospective, multicenter, cohort study comparing traditional SCS to DTM SCS evaluated 134 subjects. Of 94 patients implanted, 46 subjects in each group completed 3-month, 6-month, and 12-month assessments. Responder rates were indicated for low back pain (LBP) with subjects reporting at least 50% pain relief. In the intention-to-treat analysis, the LBP responder rate of 80.1% with DTM SCS was superior to 51.2% with traditional SCS. These results were sustained at 6-month and 12-month assessments.[25] The results of this study are promising given the high percentage of DTM SCS responders with satisfactory pain relief. At this time, further studies are still needed on this novel waveform before it may be considered for implementation into practice.

These studies make it clear that further studies into novel waveforms are warranted owing to the benefits they may be able to provide to patients. With the development of these novel waveforms, there is an expanded scope of application for neurostimulation with proven longevity of outcomes. Future SCS studies may lead to the discovery of new SCS indications and prove to be an invaluable addition in the treatment of patients with chronic pain conditions.

Dorsal Root Ganglion Stimulation Patient Selection

The use of DRG stimulation has proven its worth as an exciting treatment modality. While DRG stimulation can be effective for a variety of pain disorders, including back pain, phantom limb pain, and pelvic pain, it has specifically shown its value as a highly effective treatment for focal pain. Patients with severe neuropathic pain arising from CRPS and causalgia can be extremely difficult to treat with conventional and more conservative methods of management. DRG stimulation has been proven to be a powerful tool to treat focal pain in certain body parts, such as the hip, groin, knee, and foot and ankle.[26-28]

The DRG is located at every vertebral level between the spinal cord and spinal nerve, and houses the somas of the primary sensory neurons. They help transmit sensory signals from the periphery to the central nervous system.[29] Through various studies it is believed that electrical stimulation can modulate these pain signals.[26,27] For example, stimulation at the L3 and/or L4 can be a highly effective form of treatment for chronic knee pain.[28]

The ACCURATE study in 2017 compared SCS with DRG stimulation in patients with CRPS or causalgia in the lower extremities. It was the first RCT that demonstrated the overall superiority of DRG stimulation after 3 months of treatment in terms of pain relief, quality of life, and less postural variation. Pain relief continued at 12 months after treatment.[27] Focal pain can be difficult to treat with SCS. While SCS has shown benefit in patients who have exhausted other options, it is not always the most effective in providing high-level pain relief in patients with CRPS and causalgia. Therapeutic efficacy can fade over time, relief can be incomplete, and it is limited in its ability to target focal regions of pain.

While SCS stimulates the dorsal column and targets large dermatomal areas, stimulation at the relevant DRG will affect the specific dermatome, leading to more precise anatomical targeting. There is significantly less perceived stimulation in nonpainful areas. The DRG is located in a tight space; thus, stimulators are less susceptible to lead migration. There is less variation in cerebrospinal fluid at that location in relation to position and, thus, less postural variation in pain relief.[27-29]

Prior to determining whether a certain patient will benefit from DRG stimulation, a thorough history and physical examination should be performed to ensure successful treatment of CRPS or causalgia in the lower extremities. The proper diagnosis of CRPS should be made based on the Budapest criteria. Peripheral causalgia is diagnosed as nerve damage resulting in chronic pain. This pain of the lower limbs should be intractable for at least 6 months.[27,30] Once a diagnosis is made, patients with CRPS or causalgia should explore other forms of treatment prior to DRG stimulation. These include, but are not limited to, medication therapy from at least two different pharmacological agents from two different classes, sympathetic nerve blocks, and physical therapy. If pain continues to be persistent after 6 months of these other forms of therapy, then the patient should be considered a reasonable candidate for DRG stimulation. If a patient had tried SCS or peripheral nerve stimulation (PNS) with minimal relief for focal pain, DRG stimulation should be considered.[27,28]

Patients must understand and be willing to comply with follow-up. They must be appropriately psychologically screened and demonstrate stable neurological function, as they will have an implantable medical device. Psychiatric comorbidities—such as substance abuse, uncontrolled depression, anxiety, bipolar disorder, schizophrenia, and certain personality disorders—can present challenges for patients with an implanted stimulator. They must be able to sign consent forms and understand risks and benefits of the procedure.[27]

Similar to SCS implantation, DRG stimulation is considered relatively safe but there are certain factors to consider prior to placement. For the procedure itself, anesthesia planning requires a thorough medical history and evaluation. The ACCURATE study looked at subjects between the ages of 22 and 75 years, which should be considered the optimal age range. Subjects were not childbearing, not nursing, and had no plans to become pregnant.[27] The safety profile of a DRG stimulator is unknown on the pregnant patient or developing fetus. The clinician performing the procedure should evaluate the patient's relevant imaging, such as MRI, CT or X-ray findings. These can reveal certain anatomical features related to contraindications to lead placement.[27] While rates of infection or bleeding are rare, they can have devastating consequences. Thus, additional contraindications include coagulation disorders, use of anticoagulation/antiplatelet therapy, or an active systemic infection.[27,31]

When it is determined that the patient is appropriate for DRG stimulation, a trial stimulation is scheduled, with implantation planned 3 to 30 days following a successful trial. The DRG stimulator is an exciting and effective form of treatment providing the opportunity for patients suffering from focal pain from CRPS or causalgia to drastically reduce their pain and improve their overall quality of life. Like any interventional or pharmacological treatment, its success is dependent on accurate patient selection.

REFERENCES

1. Fayaz A, Croft P, Langford RM, Donaldson LJ, Jones GT. Prevalence of chronic pain in the UK: a systematic review and meta-analysis of population studies. *BMJ Open*. 2016;6(6):e010364.
2. Dahlhamer J, Lucas J, Zelaya C, et al. Prevalence of chronic pain and high-impact chronic pain among adults—United States, 2016. *MMWR Morb Mortal Wkly Rep*. 2018;67(36):1001-1006.
3. Campbell CM, Jamison RN, Edwards RR. Psychological screening/phenotyping as predictors for spinal cord stimulation. *Curr Pain Headache Rep*. 2013;17(1):307.
4. Pritzlaff S, Hah JM, Fishman MA, Leong MS. Anatomy of neuromodulatory targets: central nervous system and the periphery. In: Diwan S, Deer TR, eds. *Advanced Procedures for Pain Management: A Step-by-Step Atlas*. Cham: Springer International Publishing; 2018:105-121.
5. Deer T, Masone RJ. Selection of spinal cord stimulation candidates for the treatment of chronic pain. *Pain Med*. 2008;9(suppl 1):S82-S92.
6. Baber Z, Erdek MA. Failed back surgery syndrome: current perspectives. *J Pain Res*. 2016;9:979-987.
7. Kumar K, North R, Taylor R, et al. Spinal cord stimulation vs. conventional medical management: a prospective, randomized, controlled, multicenter study of patients with failed back surgery syndrome (PROCESS Study). *Neuromodulation*. 2005;8(4):213-218.
8. Rigoard P, Basu S, Desai M, et al. Multicolumn spinal cord stimulation for predominant back pain in failed back surgery syndrome patients: a multicenter randomized controlled trial. *Pain*. 2019;160(6):1410-1420.
9. Lee AW, Pilitsis JG. Spinal cord stimulation: indications and outcomes. *Neurosurg Focus*. 2006;21(6):1-6.
10. Kreis PG, Fishman S. *Spinal Cord Stimulation: Percutaneous Implantation Techniques*. Oxford, UK: Oxford University Press; 2009.
11. Bruehl S. Complex regional pain syndrome. *BMJ*. 2015;351:h2730.
12. Deer TR, Mekhail N, Provenzano D, et al. The appropriate use of neurostimulation of the spinal cord and peripheral nervous system for the treatment of chronic pain and ischemic diseases: the Neuromodulation Appropriateness Consensus Committee. *Neuromodulation*. 2014;17(6):515-550; discussion 550.
13. Deer TR, Pope JE, Lamer TJ, et al. The neuromodulation appropriateness consensus committee on best practices for dorsal root ganglion stimulation. *Neuromodulation*. 2019;22(1):1-35.
14. Stanton-Hicks M. Spinal cord stimulation for the management of complex regional pain syndromes. *Neuromodulation*. 1999;2(3):193-201.
15. Petersen EA, Stauss TG, Scowcroft JA, et al. Effect of high-frequency (10-kHz) spinal cord stimulation in patients with painful diabetic neuropathy: a randomized clinical trial. *JAMA Neurol*. 2021;78(6):687-698.
16. Lee S, Abd-Elsayed A. Some non-FDA approved uses for neuromodulation: a review of the evidence. *Pain Pract*. 2016;16(7):935-947.

17. Bagger JP, Jensen BS, Johannsen G. Long-term outcome of spinal cord electrical stimulation in patients with refractory chest pain. *Clin Cardiol.* 1998;21(4):286-288.
18. Atkinson L, Sundaraj SR, Brooker C, et al. Recommendations for patient selection in spinal cord stimulation. *J Clin Neurosci.* 2011;18(10):1295-1302.
19. North R, Shipley J. Practice parameters for the use of spinal cord stimulation in the treatment of chronic neuropathic pain. *Pain Med.* 2007;8(s4):S200-S275.
20. Epstein LJ, Palmieri M. Managing chronic pain with spinal cord stimulation. *Mt Sinai J Med.* 2012;79(1):123-132.
21. Deer TR, Lamer TJ, Pope JE, et al. The Neurostimulation Appropriateness Consensus Committee (NACC) safety guidelines for the reduction of severe neurological injury. *Neuromodulation.* 2017;20(1):15-30.
22. Deer TR, Provenzano DA, Hanes M, et al. The Neurostimulation Appropriateness Consensus Committee (NACC) recommendations for infection prevention and management. *Neuromodulation.* 2017;20(1):31-50.
23. Deer TR, Narouze S, Provenzano DA, et al. The Neurostimulation Appropriateness Consensus Committee (NACC): recommendations on bleeding and coagulation management in neurostimulation devices. *Neuromodulation.* 2017;20(1):51-62.
24. Malinowski MN, Jain S, Jassal N, Deer T. Spinal cord stimulation for the treatment of neuropathic pain: expert opinion and 5-year outlook. *Expert Rev Med Devices.* 2020;17(12):1293-1302.
25. Fishman M, Cordner H, Justiz R, et al. Twelve-month results from multicenter, open-label, randomized controlled clinical trial comparing differential target multiplexed spinal cord stimulation and traditional spinal cord stimulation in subjects with chronic intractable back pain and leg pain. *Pain Pract.* 2021;21(8):912-923.
26. Deer TR, Hunter CW, Mehta P, et al. A systematic literature review of dorsal root ganglion neurostimulation for the treatment of pain. *Pain Med.* 2020;21(8):1581-1589.
27. Deer T, Levy R, Kramer J, et al. Dorsal root ganglion stimulation yielded higher treatment success rate for CRPS and causalgia at 3 and 12 months: randomized comparative trial. *Pain.* 2017;158(4):669-681.
28. Martin SC, Macey AR, Raghu A, et al. Dorsal root ganglion stimulation for the treatment of chronic neuropathic knee pain. *World Neurosurg.* 2020;143:e303-e308.
29. Esposito MF, Malayil R, Hanes M, Deer T. Unique characteristics of the dorsal root ganglion as a target for neuromodulation. *Pain Med.* 2019;20(suppl 1):S23-S30.
30. Harden RN, Bruehl S, Stanton-Hicks M, Wilson PR. Proposed new diagnostic criteria for complex regional pain syndrome. *Pain Med.* 2007;8(4):326-331.
31. Kumar K, Wilson JR, Taylor RS, Gupta S. Complications of spinal cord stimulation, suggestions to improve outcome, and financial impact. *J Neurosurg Spine.* 2006;5(3):191-203.
32. Kapural Leonardo, Yu Cong, Doust Matthew W, et al. Novel 10-kHz high-frequency therapy (HF10 therapy) is superior to traditional low-frequency spinal cord stimulation for the treatment of chronic back and leg pain: the SENZA-RCT Randomized Controlled Trial. *Anesthesiology.* 2015;123(4):851–860. doi:10.1097/ALN.0000000000000774.26218762.
33. Kapural Leonardo, Yu Cong, Doust Matthew W, et al. Comparison of 10-kHz high-frequency and traditional low-frequency spinal cord stimulation for the treatment of chronic back and leg pain: 24-month results from a multicenter, randomized, controlled pivotal trial. *Neurosurgery.* 2016;79(5):667–677. doi:10.1227/NEU.0000000000001418.27584814.
34. Thomson Simon J, Tavakkolizadeh Moein, Love-Jones Sarah, et al. Effects of rate on analgesia in kilohertz frequency spinal cord stimulation: results of the PROCO randomized controlled trial. *Neuromodulation.* 2018;21(1):67–76. doi:10.1111/ner.12746. 29220121.
35. Amirdelfan Kasra, Yu Cong, Doust Matthew W, et al. Long-term quality of life improvement for chronic intractable back and leg pain patients using spinal cord stimulation: 12-month results from the SENZA-RCT. *Qual Life Res.* 2018;27(8):2035–2044. 1573-2649. doi:10.1007/s11136-018-1890-8.29858746.
36. Demartini Laura, Terranova Gaetano, Innamorato Massimo A, et al. Comparison of tonic vs. burst spinal cord stimulation during trial period. *Neuromodulation.* 2019;22(3):327–332. doi:10.1111/ner.12867.30328646.
37. Deer Timothy, Slavin Konstantin V, Amirdelfan Kasra, et al. Success using neuromodulation with BURST (SUNBURST) study: results from a prospective, randomized controlled trial using a novel burst waveform. *Neuromodulation.* 2018;21(1):56–66. doi:10.1111/ner.12698.28961366.
38. De Ridder Dirk, Plazier Mark, Kamerling Niels, Menovsky Tomas, Vanneste Sven Burst spinal cord stimulation for limb and back pain. *World Neurosurg.* 2013;80(5):642–649.e1. 1878-8769. doi:10.1016/j.wneu.2013.01.040.23321375.

Chapter 3

Psychological Evaluation for Neuromodulation

Ashley Katsarakes, Ashley Scherer, Lindsay Kate Wanner, and Michael Alan Fishman

Chapter Outline

Introduction

"Patient-centered care takes into account the biopsychosocial nature of chronic pain."

—Jianguo Cheng, MD, PhD, FIPP[1]

Neuromodulation therapies encompass an array of modalities that interface with the brain and nervous system at a variety of levels, from the deep brain to the peripheral nerve and the spinal cord in between. Recent advances in autonomic neuromodulation have shown promise in the treatment of autoimmune inflammatory conditions such as rheumatoid arthritis, systemic lupus erythematosus, and more.[2,3] The indications for therapies continue to grow as the sophistication of the neural interfaces and programming options evolve.

Neuromodulation has been indicated in the treatment of chronic low back and leg pain stemming from trauma, degeneration, or prior surgical intervention. Most insurance companies require additional imaging and psychometric testing to guarantee approval and monetary coverage. Psychometric testing is primarily a psychological evaluation of the patient's mental status. Typically, these visits involve assessing the patient's past medical and surgical history as well as social history (alcohol and substance use) and family history (medical and psychiatric). In addition, standardized questionnaires to evaluate mood, sleep, anxiety, and depression are utilized as a clear-cut measure of state of mind. Importantly, the psychologist typically discusses the patient's goal in pursuing neuromodulation to ensure that it is realistic in nature. Still, many patients and providers question why this is a necessary step prior to neuromodulation therapies.

Prior studies have shown that there is some correlation between psychological evaluations and outcomes with SCS therapy, though many of these studies have had mixed and inconclusive results. We can attribute these mixed results to the fact that human beings are akin to snowflakes. This is true in that all snowflakes are made up of the same material, but each snowflake has a unique structure. Even patients who present in a very similar way may respond differently to SCS therapy, stemming from anatomical, psychological, and social differences.

Sheldon et al. examined the correlation between family history of psychiatric illness and patient outcomes with SCS. They retrospectively analyzed pre- and post-SCS results of the following assessments: the McGill Pain Questionnaire (MPQ), Oswestry Disability Index (ODI), Beck Depressive Inventory (BDI), Pain Catastrophizing Scale (PCS), and Numeric Rating Scale (NRS). They determined that subjects with psychiatric family history (PFH) experienced less improvement in the aforementioned measures following SCS implementation when compared with subjects without PFH.[4] This means that patients with PFH may take longer to achieve the same improved outcomes if they do at all.

A study from Prabhala et al. created a unique tool for psychometric evaluation. They denoted this the Psychological Evaluation Tool for Spinal Cord Stimulation Candidacy (PETSCSC), which consisted of the NRS, Patient Global Impression of Change (PGIC), PCS, MPQ, ODI, and BDI.[5] They used this tool to evaluate patient improvement over the course prior to and after receiving SCS therapy (Box 3.1). The results of this analysis demonstrated that there was no significant correlation with SCS outcomes, although the total score on the PETSCSC correlated with the PGIC, the affective section of the MPQ, the rumination and helplessness sections of the PCS, and the total PCS score.[5]

Although psychometric testing is commonly required for insurance approval, this should not be the primary reason that it is completed prior to SCS trial and implant. It is well understood in the literature that the "pain experience" is multifaceted. To ensure that patients receive the most comprehensive treatment possible, all aspects of the pain experience need to be considered prior to and after implementing SCS therapy. Neurostimulation Appropriateness Consensus Committee (NACC) and other neuromodulation guidelines do not specifically implicate the importance of psychometric testing as a preoperative measure although psychosocial complications have been shown to play a vital role in influencing the effectiveness of neuromodulation therapies.[6,7]

BOX 3.1 PSYCHOLOGICAL EVALUATION TOOL FOR SPINAL CORD STIMULATION CANDIDACY

EMOTIVE SUBSET		
Aberrant negative thoughts	Yes	No
Aberrant body concerns	Yes	No
Difficulties with autonomous coping	Yes	No
Emotional internalizing disorders	Yes	No
Feelings of demoralization	Yes	No
Less feelings of joy than average	Yes	No
Substance abuse	Yes	No
DEPRESSION SUBSET		
Depression	Yes	No
Depression that would benefit with medication	Yes	No
Depression that would benefit from psychotherapy	Yes	No
OTHER DISORDER SUBSET		
Borderline personality disorder	Yes	No
Personality disorder (other)	Yes	No
Untreated posttraumatic stress disorder	Yes	No
Other untreated psychiatric disorder	Yes	No
THERAPY SUBSET (PATIENT MAY POTENTIALLY BENEFIT FROM):		
Further education about expectations	Yes	No
Medication evaluation with psychiatrist	Yes	No
Psychotherapy	Yes	No
Support group	Yes	No

Adapted from the Psychological Evaluation Tool for Spinal Cord Stimulation Candidacy in Prabhala et al.[5]

The Biopsychosocial Model

SCS is only a part of the complex treatment plan necessary to overcome chronic pain. The biopsychosocial model implicates many factors that contribute to chronic pain, including socioeconomic status, emotions, expectations, genetic factors, attitude, and stress, among others. It is the combination of these diverse factors that encompass the pain experience; see Fig. 3.1 for more factors. SCS is one part of this lifesaving strategy. For the best chance at success, however, the physician should take an individualized and holistic approach.

PROMIS-29 is a questionnaire that is commonly used to assess psychological health in chronic pain patients, although it is relevant across many disease states. Pope et al. retrospectively analyzed PROMIS-29 scores in 19,546 patients across multiple pain management and neurosurgery practices to establish a normative data set. They determined that dysfunction as defined by the PROMIS-29 questionnaire was significantly higher than that of the general population.[8] Fig. 3.2 provides details on scoring the PROMIS-29 questionnaire. Koster-Brouwer et al. analyzed the prevalence of new chronic pain 1 year after intensive care unit (ICU) discharge. They determined that 17.7% of people developed a new chronic pain after

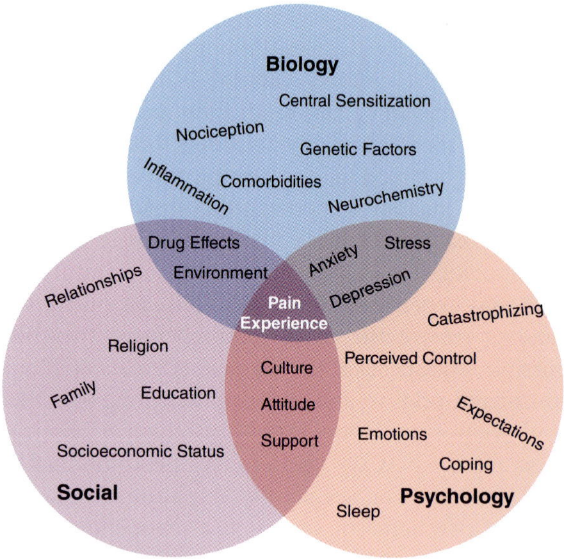

Fig. 3.1 The biopsychosocial model of the pain experience. This diagram shows the biological, social, and psychological factors that affect a patient's experience dealing with chronic pain.

spending time in the ICU, with the average NRS being 4/10. Quality of life was severely impacted by their inability to complete activities of daily living, inability to participate in social activities, and overall decline in mobility.[9] The results of these studies represent the incidence with which we see chronic pain disorders as well as the toll it takes on quality of life in these affected populations.

There is an inherent need for a multimodal approach to pain treatment to ensure that the psychological and social aspects of pain are adequately treated in addition to the physiological symptoms. The US Department of Health and Human Services Pain Task Force recommends a balanced approach that is both individualized to the patient and multidisciplinary in nature. Evidence-based clinical best practices are designed and utilized to optimize patient outcomes. The clinical best practice for chronic pain has evolved to recognize the important relationship between psychological health and the chronic pain experience. Patients with chronic pain are at a much higher risk for psychological distress, maladaptive coping, and physical inactivity related to fear of reinjury.[10] Psychological evaluations commonly refer to "pain impact" as a variable that denotes how much or how often pain interferes with the patient's quality of life.

Approach to the Patient

Approach to the neuromodulation patient is built on providing an understanding of the therapy process, which includes an understanding of the technical procedure risks and pitfalls as well as the appropriate work-up. This includes gently preparing the patient for the psychological evaluation, as an indelicate reference to this prerequisite can be off-putting and erode trust. It is important to share with the patient that a psychological evaluation is required by insurance but is also wise to ensure that we have a complete understanding of the patient's mental health, needs, and expectations for treatment. If a patient is already engaged with a mental health professional (MHP), it is prudent to ask that patient to approach the MHP for a

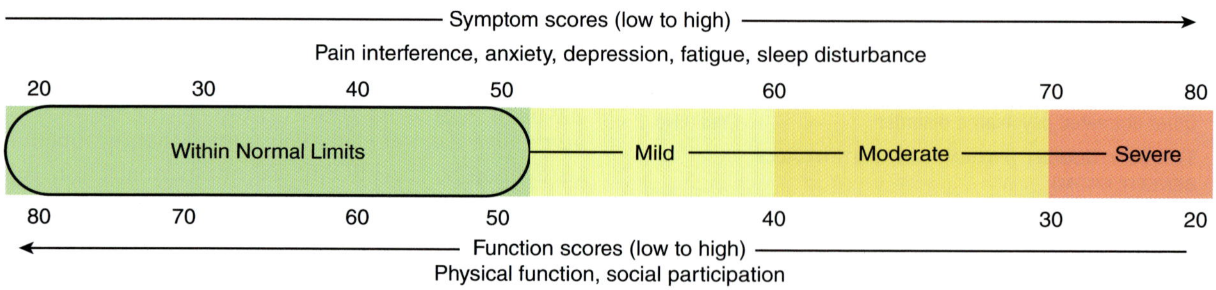

Fig. 3.2 Promis-29 symptom and function score severity. High functional scores and low symptom scores indicate that the results fall within normal limits.

psychological evaluation, as the MHP is already familiar with the patient.

Collaborating with Mental Health Professionals

Collaborating with MHPs is critical to ensure a timely and efficient evaluation of neuromodulation patients that adds to the patient experience. In general, it is ideal to establish a personal relationship with a local MHP or telehealth MHP who understands the general difference between neurostimulation and targeted drug delivery therapies. This is critical to ensuring that the MHP can evaluate the patient's understanding of the procedure. The MHP is also charged with identifying psychogenic barriers to long-term improvement and whether they would be contraindications to these therapies. This includes untreated Axis I or II diagnoses, maladaptive behaviors, poor insight into condition, signs of malingering, somatization, or conversion disorder. Furthermore, during this session it is helpful to establish appropriate objective and subjective expectations in terms of the therapy so that they are documented and can be followed.

Depending on the practice environment, access to in-house MHPs with specialization in chronic pain and chronic medical conditions may be available. If not, define an ad hoc group of MHPs who can be relied on to evaluate patients and help to optimize patients for therapy. Engage these MHPs in learning more about neuromodulation, offer shadowing opportunities to them, and help them understand the reasonable goals and expectations based on the data supporting the therapy being considered.

Evidence Review

There are large numbers of covariates that influence the success and failure of SCS, such as the presence of psychosocial factors or the use of self-management practices. One such psychosocial factor that can play a significant role in determining the effectiveness of a treatment is pain catastrophizing. Catastrophizing is a thought construct consisting of rumination, magnification, and helplessness. It is most commonly measured through the Pain Catastrophizing Scale (PCS).[7] The questionnaire consists of 13 questions rated on a 0 to 4 Likert scale, designed to identify a patient's level of catastrophic thinking related to feelings of chronic pain. Each question is assigned a point value equivalent to the 0 to 4 answer. The total score is a summation of those points, with a higher score indicating greater catastrophizing (see Fig. 3.3 for scoring information). Patients with higher levels of catastrophizing thoughts report a higher pain intensity as determined by the numeric rating scale, poorer pain relief and quality of life, and less satisfaction with the SCS procedure at 6 and 12 months of follow-up as compared with counterparts with lower levels of catastrophizing.[7]

The use of self-management methods, such as meditation or mindfulness practices, has been known to reduce the effects of catastrophizing thoughts, thus improving outcomes for neuromodulation. Conti et al. examined the relationship between trait mindfulness, a predisposition of a person to be mindful, pain catastrophizing, and the psychological distress often observed in chronic pain patients.[11] Patients who exhibited higher levels of trait mindfulness had lower pain catastrophizing, resulting in less depression and

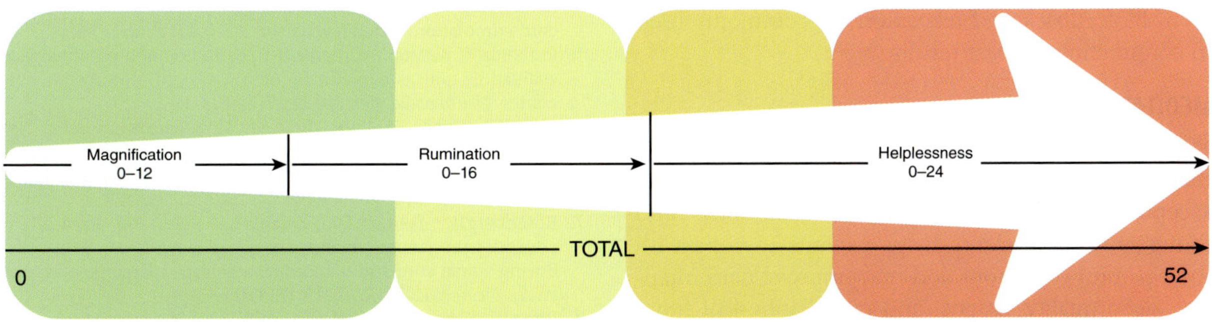

Fig. 3.3 Pain Catastrophizing Scale (PCS) sections: magnification, rumination, and helplessness, totaling from 0 to 52 points.

anxiety.[11] The results of this study, combined with the findings of Rosenberg et al., suggest that patients who exhibit trait mindfulness will have lower pain catastrophizing and, therefore, will have a more successful experience with neuromodulation.[7,11]

The PROMIS-29 questionnaire measures depression, anxiety, and several other biopsychosocial factors. It is commonly utilized by psychiatric professionals in evaluations prior to SCS. High levels of depression and anxiety in chronic pain patients may be indicative of greater catastrophizing thoughts and less trait mindfulness, which could result in neuromodulation treatment failure. The use of psychological evaluations in addition to patient-reported outcome questionnaires such as the PCS and PROMIS-29 is beneficial in attempting to predict patient success with neuromodulation therapy. These evaluations can also be used to suggest additions to the patient's current treatment regime, such as the addition of therapy or mindfulness activities, which can improve the success rate of neuromodulation treatment in chronic pain patients.

Psychological Modalities for Care Optimization

SELF-MANAGEMENT SKILLS

Some patients find benefit in implementing certain mindfulness techniques to help them better manage their psychological state when in painful exacerbations. Monitoring biofeedback allows patients to recognize and understand the physiologic responses associated with increased pain. Improving patient awareness of these biofeedback mechanisms may allow them to apply voluntary control of these biological reactions.[10] Relaxation training alters the patient's attention and helps to distract the patient from the pain. Biofeedback and relaxation are commonly used in conjunction for best results.

MEDITATION

Mindful meditation allows patients to self-regulate their pain experience by developing an awareness and acceptance of present sensations, emotions, and thoughts. This modality helps patients to cope with their painful conditions and may improve pain intensity, sleep quality, fatigue, and overall physical functioning and well-being.[12]

COGNITIVE BEHAVIORAL THERAPY

Cognitive behavioral therapy (CBT) aims to reduce maladaptive behavior and improve functioning.[12] This modality focuses on educating patients about the relationship between thoughts and feelings and painful experiences. Pain coping strategies and restructuring maladaptive thoughts are also included in this type of therapy.

ACCEPTANCE AND COMMITMENT THERAPY

Acceptance and commitment therapy (ACT) is a form of CBT that is focused on accepting thoughts and feelings, living in the present moment, and behaving in a manner that serves chosen values. ACT fosters the awareness and acceptance of pain and directs actions toward fulfilling behavioral functioning.[12] The main goal of ACT is to instill psychological flexibility through the acceptance of psychological and physical experiences.

DIALECTICAL BEHAVIORAL THERAPY

According to Barrett et al., dialectical behavioral therapy (DBT) is a combination of CBT and ACT. This type of therapy may be preferred for some patients as it provides validation and acceptance in addition to changing strategies to help them accept their situation while adding skills to their repertoire which enable them to change their experience.[13]

REFERENCES

1. Cheng J. My take on the biopsychosocial model of patient-centered care. *Pain Med*. 2018;19(11):2101-2103.
2. Chernoff DN. Neuromodulation for rheumatoid arthritis: disrupting the drug treatment paradigm. *Neuromodulation*. 2019;22(3): E255. Available at: https://www.cochranelibrary.com/central/doi/10.1002/central/CN-01937461/full. Accessed June 23, 2022.
3. Levine YA, Chernoff D. 2018 January, First-in-class Bioelectronic Therapy for Rheumatoid Arthritis: Two Year Follow-up [Poster Presentation].
4. Sheldon BL, Khazen O, Feustel PJ, et al. Correlations between family history of psychiatric illnesses and outcomes of spinal cord stimulation. *Neuromodulation*. 2020;23(5):667-672.
5. Prabhala T, Kumar V, Gruenthal E, et al. Use of a psychological evaluation tool as a predictor of spinal cord stimulation outcomes. *Neuromodulation*. 2019;22(2):194-199.
6. Deer TR, Lamer TJ, Pope JE, et al. The Neurostimulation Appropriateness Consensus Committee (NACC) safety guidelines for the reduction of severe neurological injury. *Neuromodulation*. 2017;20(1):15-30.
7. Rosenberg JC, Schultz DM, Duarte LE, Rosen SM, Raza A. Increased pain catastrophizing associated with lower pain relief during spinal cord stimulation: results from a large post-market study. *Neuromodulation*. 2015;18(4):277-284.
8. Pope JE, Fishman M, Chakravarthy K, et al. A retrospective, multicenter, quantitative analysis of patients' baseline pain quality

(PROMIS-29) entering into pain and spine practices in the United States (ALIGN). *Pain Ther*. 2021;10:539-550. Available at: https://doi.org/10.1007/s40122-021-00238-z. Accessed June 23, 2022.
9. Koster-Brouwer ME, Rijsdijk M, van Os WKM, et al. Occurrence and risk factors of chronic pain after critical illness. *Crit Care Med*. 2020;48(5):680-687.
10. US Dept of Health and Human Services Pain Task Force. Draft report on pain management best practices: updates, gaps, inconsistencies, and recommendations. 2018;1-91. Available at: https://www.hhs.gov/ash/advisory-committees/pain/reports/index.html.
11. Conti Y, Vatine JJ, Levy S, Levin Meltz Y, Hamdan S, Elkana O. Pain catastrophizing mediates the association between mindfulness and psychological distress in chronic pain syndrome. *Pain Pract*. 2020;20(7):714-723.
12. Darnall BD, Sturgeon JA, Kao MC, Hah JM, Mackey SC. From catastrophizing to recovery: a pilot study of a single-session treatment for pain catastrophizing. *J Pain Res*. 2014;7:219-226.
13. Barrett D, Brintz CE, Zaski AM, Edlund MJ. Dialectical pain management: feasibility of a hybrid third-wave cognitive behavioral therapy approach for adults receiving opioids for chronic pain. *Pain Med*. 2021;22(5):1080-1094.

Chapter 4

Perioperative Care in Neuromodulatory Systems

Alyson M. Engle

Chapter Outline

Introduction

In 1967, neuromodulation came on the scene as a salvage therapy for chronic refractory neuropathic pain.[1-3] Neuromodulation achieves analgesia through electrical stimulation that affects pain pathways. Neuromodulation devices consist of electrodes on thin flexible wires that supply electrical current to the spinal cord. These electrodes are strategically placed over the area in the spinal cord that is thought to conduct pain signaling. Early progress originally targeted dorsal column electrical stimulation, more commonly referred to as *spinal cord stimulation (SCS)*. Later developments worked to resolve the therapeutic limitations of traditional SCS, in which neurostimulation was advanced to selectively target focal pain generators in the dorsal root ganglion (DRG). Pathological changes occur and are maintained in the DRG. Therefore, selectively targeting the DRG can provide more effective neuromodulation of chronic pain and inflammation.[4] In 2016, neurostimulation devices specific for DRG neuromodulation were approved by the US Food and Drug Administration (FDA).[5] The treatment of intense focal pain of a defined area of the body is approved for DRG neurostimulation therapy.[5]

Both SCS and DRG neurostimulation devices are salvage therapy, utilized when the patient fails conservative therapies. In general, patients with neuropathic pain are the best candidates for neurostimulation therapy. Both SCS and DRG neurostimulation devices are surgically implanted after a successful clinical trial of an external device. These neurostimulation devices consist of electrode leads and an implantable pulse generator. The electrode leads employ electrical field potentials to their targets.[6] Such devices also provide a means for clinicians to deliver personalized drug-free pain therapy for extended periods of time. This chapter's focus is traditional neurostimulation devices.

Anatomical Considerations

SCS lead placement is executed with the goal to place the leads in the dorsal epidural space to effectively stimulate the dorsal column of the spinal cord. Traditional SCS stimulates evoked paresthesias by stimulating the dorsal column over the same region of the patient's pain. The result is pain relief of the area of stimulation. This concept requires the implanting clinician to understand the medial and lateral locations of the nerve fibers to be stimulated.[7] Dorsal columns are organized in a lamellated manner (Fig. 4.1). Caudal to rostral structures are represented in the dorsal columns in a medial to lateral fashion (see Fig. 4.1). For example, the most medial part of the dorsal column contains the sacral and perineal fibers. Lateral to these fibers are the fibers representing S1, then L5, followed sequentially by L4, L3, L2, and L1. Further lateral are fibers representing the low back sensation. This organization follows through to the cervical region.

Neurostimulation devices target structures in the dorsal column. The dorsal column contains white matter composed of diverse pathways that convey sensation. Of primary interest to the interventional pain physician is the transmission of ascending light touch and proprioception, as well as the transmission of pain and temperature, through the spinothalamic tract. There is also evidence of modulation of

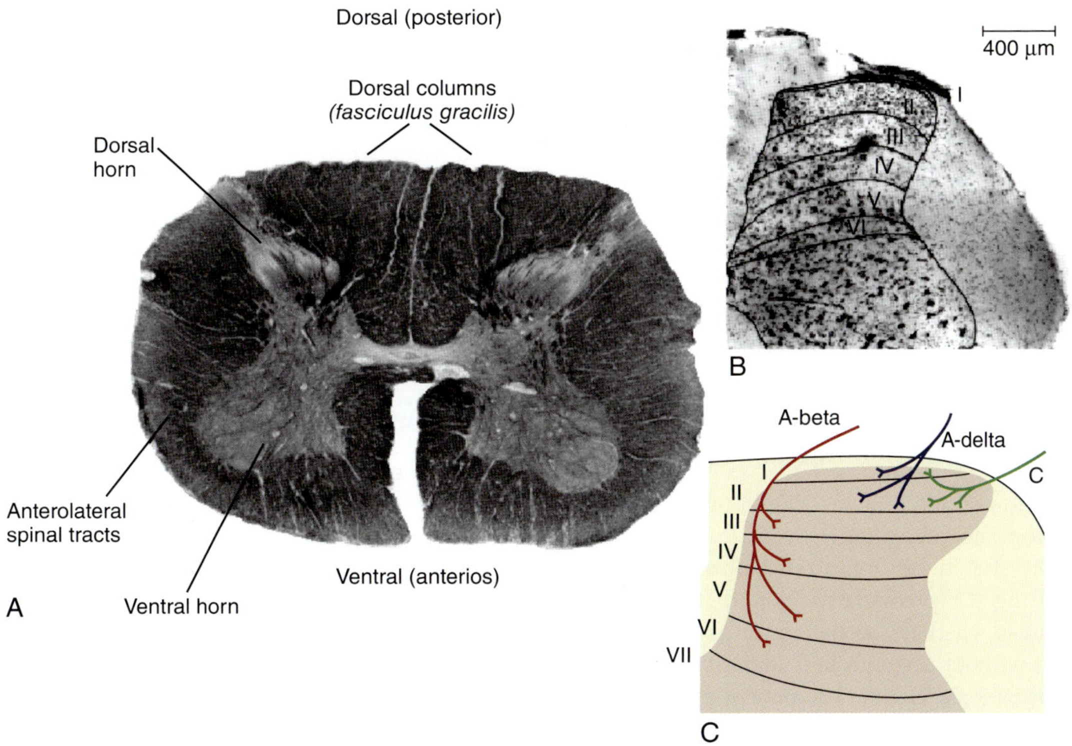

Fig. 4.1 **(A) Histologic sections and schematic diagrams of the spinal dorsal horn. Human lumbar spinal cord is labeled to show the relationship between the major spinal somatosensory structures. The outer heavy lines show the boundary of the spinal gray matter. (B) From rat; the inner heavy lines show the boundaries of Rexed laminae. These boundaries are established by the histological characteristics of each zone and the layers are identified by the numerals at the right of the dorsal horn boundary. (C) Pattern of primary afferent innervation to the nonhuman primate spinal dorsal horn. The large myelinated (Aβ) fibers segregate to the dorsal aspect of an entering rootlet and then course medially in the dorsal horn and terminate in layers III to V. The small myelinated (Aδ) fibers and C fibers, which carry nociceptive information, segregate ventrally in the entering roots, course laterally in the dorsal horn, and then largely terminate in the more superficial layers (I and II) of the dorsal horn.** (From Ringkamp M, Dougherty PM, Raja SN. Anatomy and physiology of the pain signaling process. In: Benzon HT, Raja SN, Liu SS, Fishman SM, Cohen SP, eds. *Essentials of Pain Medicine.* 4th ed. Elsevier; 2018:3-10.e1.)

autonomic tracts, which regulate sympathetic and parasympathetic tone.

Achieving therapeutic pain relief while minimizing the risk of complications requires careful anatomical alignment of the lead(s),[8] as the location of the cathode controls the dispersion of the current. In DRG stimulation, contact leads are placed in proximity to the DRG. The DRG has a lateral positioning in the lumbar spine and more medial positioning in the thoracic spine. Selective neuromodulation of the DRG has several advantages over traditional SCS. DRG stimulation delivers a more precise therapy, with lead positioning closer to the affected location of pathology, reduced contact size, and more specific positioning of leads, which allows for improved pain relief and fewer unwanted side effects.[9-12] This advantage was demonstrated in the ACCURATE study, which showed a higher treatment success rate in patients with CRPS or causalgia in those with DRG stimulation compared to dorsal column SCS.[10] In addition, targeting the L1 and S2 DRGs through neurostimulation has shown promise in chronic pelvic pain.[9] Furthermore, DRG stimulation at the L2 to L3 levels has been shown to effectively relieve low back pain that failed treatment with traditional SCS.[13] Overall, an understanding of the patient's neuroanatomy and related pathophysiology is key to successful outcomes in the use of neurostimulation devices.

Perioperative Considerations

Determination of SCS systems should take place only after appropriate preoperative workup. Medical comorbidities should be optimized before SCS placement. During the preoperative period, the clinician should assess whether the patient is psychologically stable and without uncontrolled addiction to be considered for SCS placement. The patient needs to have psychological clearance by a certified psychologist before SCS. Of note, a history of sexual abuse is a relative contraindication for SCS placement when its indication is for chronic pelvic pain.

Patients should also have baseline laboratory data before proceeding to assess risk factors for complications. For example, coagulation studies and a complete blood count should be done to assess for coagulopathy and blood count problems if applicable. A complete metabolic panel is also helpful to assess for renal dysfunction, electrolyte imbalance, and liver dysfunction that may impact the surgery and selection of postoperative healing. Specifically, patients on anticoagulants need to undergo evaluation with their managing provider as to whether it is safe to with hold the anticoagulant for placement of an epidural lead. Diabetic patients should have their hemoglobin A1C checked and demonstrate acceptable blood sugar control before placement. Immunosuppressed patients need to be optimized in order to decrease infection risk.

Postoperative care includes provider-specific instructions on dressing changes, if desired, and follow-up visits for wound checks and lead pulls. In the case of an SCS trial, the typical time for a trial is 5 to 7 days to follow-up in clinic for removing leads. After implantation of a spinal cord stimulator, the typical follow-up period for wound checks is 7 to 10 days, with variability depending on the clinician's judgment for wound check needs. Sponge baths are allowed, but no soaking in tubs or showers when wires are exposed or with open wounds. Patients are instructed to keep the wounds clean, dry, and intact without manipulation unless specific instructions are given by the provider. During a trial, patients are often instructed not to drive. Patients are often instructed not to engage in heavy lifting or strenuous exercise for the first 6 weeks after implant.

Procedural Description

The patient is brought to the procedure room and positioned prone on the procedure table. Standard sterile technique is carried out with skin preparation, preferably Chloraprep with sufficient dry time. A full-body sterile drape is placed over the thoracic and lumbar spine area. Fluoroscopy is then used to identify the appropriate landmarks for skin and epidural insertion on the anteroposterior (AP) view. An indelible marker is used to mark the needle entry site and relative anatomy to aid in needle positioning. In traditional SCS placement, the epidural space is accessed at midline through the interlaminar space. The length of lead required to extend from the target level to the implant site for the implantable pulse generator (IPG) is determined. Administration of local anesthetic in the subcutaneous space is carried out with approximately 7 mL of lidocaine 1% with 1:100,000 epinephrine.

Fluoroscopy is then used to square off the vertebral body inferior endplate of the target entry site. A 14-gauge Tuohy needle with the bevel facing up is used to enter the skin at one to two levels below the target level of epidural insertion (Fig. 4.2A). The Tuohy needle is advanced at an angle less than 45 degrees under intermittent fluoroscopy until it is engaged in the ligamentum flavum. Confirmation of needle location is checked by visualizing the needle tip depth as it approaches the ventral interlaminar line in the contralateral oblique view and/or the spinolaminar line in the lateral view (Fig. 4.2B). One technique is to touch the lamina with the needle tip and then walk off the lamina until the needle engages in the ligamentum flavum. Once the needle is engaged in the ligamentum flavum, loss of resistance technique is performed to find the epidural space. Needle tip location is confirmed by loss of resistance and on lateral fluoroscopy view. After confirming needle placement in the posterior epidural space, the electrode leads are advanced along the midline until the electrodes reach the level covering the patient's pain. One troubleshooting tip if resistance is encountered is to confirm that the needle is completely in the epidural space and consider removing the needle and reentering with a different angle. Another point of caution is to avoid overmanipulation when in the epidural space to prevent the risk of dural tear or permanent nerve damage. Dorsal lead positioning is confirmed with the lateral view on fluoroscopic imaging (Fig. 4.3). Next, the neurostimulator is tested by connecting the lead wire to the external pulse generator. Stimulation testing is then employed to verify

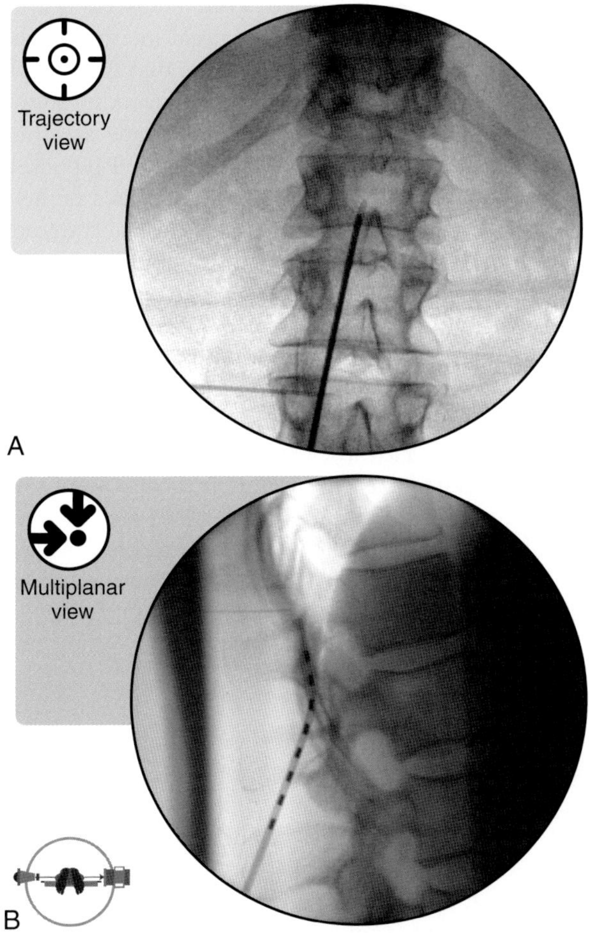

Fig. 4.2 (A) Anteroposterior fluoroscopic view of Tuohy needle trajectory. (B) Lateral fluoroscopic view of Tuohy needle in the dorsal epidural space with initial spinal cord stimulation lead insertion traveling posteriorly in the dorsal epidural space. (From Kim RE, Baez-Cabrera LD, Furman MB. Thoracolumbar spinal cord stimulation. In: Furman MB, ed. *Atlas of Image-Guided Spinal Procedures.* 2nd ed. Elsevier; 2018:325-336.

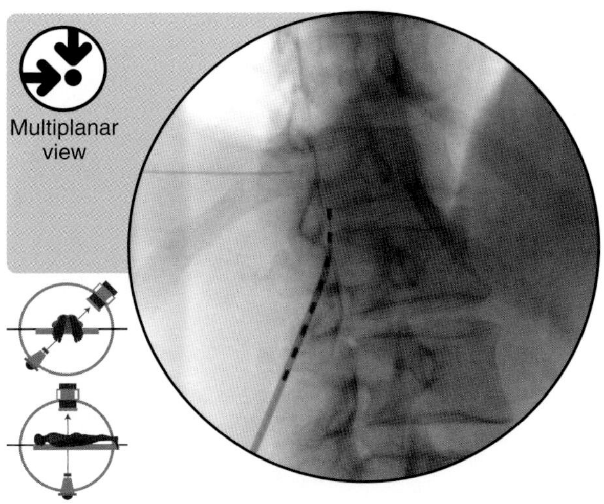

Fig. 4.3 Lateral fluoroscopic view of spinal cord stimulation entering the dorsal epidural space and needle positioned posteriorly to the dorsal epidural space. (From Kim RE, Baez-Cabrera LD, Furman MB. Thoracolumbar spinal cord stimulation. In: Furman MB, ed. *Atlas of Image-Guided Spinal Procedures.* 2nd ed. Elsevier; 2018:325-336.)

electrode leads spread over the area covering the patient's pain.

After appropriate stimulation is ensured and safety views confirm that the leads are dorsal and midline in the epidural space (Figs. 4.4 and 4.5), the guidewire can be removed while holding the leads in place. Next, the needle is carefully removed over the lead under continuous or intermittent AP fluoroscopy view.

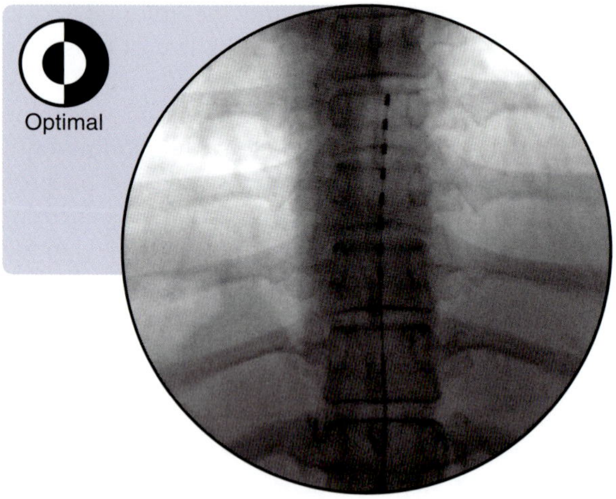

Fig. 4.4 Lateral fluoroscopic view of dorsal column positioning of spinal cord stimulation placement. (From Kim RE, Baez-Cabrera LD, Furman MB. Thoracolumbar spinal cord stimulation. In: Furman MB, ed. *Atlas of Image-Guided Spinal Procedures.* 2nd ed. Elsevier; 2018:325-336.)

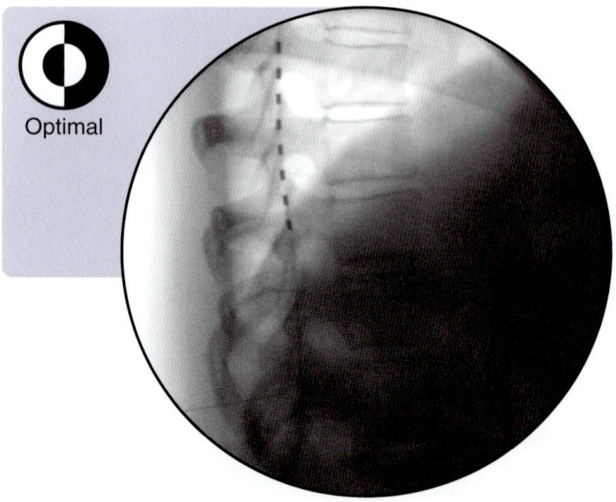

Fig. 4.5 Anteroposterior fluoroscopic view of midline spinal cord stimulation placement. (From Kim RE, Baez-Cabrera LD, Furman MB. Thoracolumbar spinal cord stimulation. In: Furman MB, ed. *Atlas of Image-Guided Spinal Procedures.* 2nd ed. Elsevier; 2018:325-336.)

If implantation is being performed, the next step is creating the IPG pocket. This pocket can be in the paravertebral region, gluteal cleft, or abdominal area, whichever the patient prefers. A skin incision is made over the area where the IPG is to be implanted. The IPG is to be placed below the Scarpa fascia. Blunt dissection is used to make an appropriately sized pocket for the IPG.

After the pocket is created, a tunneling tool is used to the pass the leads from the spinal incision to the IPG pocket. It is important to ensure that the tunneling device remains in the subcutaneous adipose tissue to avoid damaging organs. The leads are then threaded through the tunneler toward the IPG pocket. Next, the tunneler is removed while the leads are held to avoid inadvertently removing the leads. The leads are then attached to the IPG and strain relief loops are tucked behind the IPG. The IPG pocket and the midline incision must then be thoroughly irrigated with normal saline with or without antibiotics. Once irrigation is performed and hemostasis is confirmed, deep basal sutures are placed in both pockets using 3-0 Monocryl. Fascial closure is followed by subcuticular closure of each surgical incision. After skin closure with good skin approximation, the incisions should be cleaned and covered with sterile dressing. The patient is then moved to the recovery room for observation.

Intraoperative Complications

Neurostimulator insertion and implantation is generally safe overall with proper technique and expertise, but the implanter should be aware of the risks of major and minor complications.[14-18] Complications are classified as procedure related, equipment related, and patient specific. Prevention and management of complications should follow best practices and guidelines published by the Centers for Disease Control and Prevention (CDC) and the Neuromodulation Appropriateness Consensus Committee (NACC).

TABLE 4.1 Complications Associated With Neurostimulator Implantation

Procedure complications
- Bleeding
- Cerebrospinal fluid (CSF) leakage
- Postdural puncture headache
- Seroma formation
- Neurological injury
- Wound dehiscence
- Skin erosion
- Seroma
- Neuroma
- Infection
  - Superficial surgical site
  - Deep infection
  - Discitis
  - Epidural abscess
  - Meningitis

Device complications
- Electrode lead malfunction
  - Migration
  - Malposition
  - Dislodgement
  - Kinking
  - Fracture
- Device malfunction
  - Battery failure
  - Implantable pulse generator rotation

Patient-related complications
- Psychiatric comorbidities
- Cancer metastasis
- Smoking
- Uncontrolled diabetes
- Immunosuppression

PROCEDURE COMPLICATIONS

Procedure complications include bleeding, infection, wound dehiscence and neurological injury. Complications specific to neurostimulation insertion and implantation include cerebrospinal fluid (CSF) leakage, postdural puncture headache, IPG malposition, implant pocket seroma, meningitis, epidural abscess, epidural hematoma, spinal cord injury, and death. See Table 4.1 for a list of complications.

Bleeding

An epidural hematoma is a serious complication that requires prompt attention. Bleeding into the epidural space is rare during neurostimulation insertion. Bleeding of the surrounding tissue is more common and can result from a trauma during epidural access, ineffective intraoperative hemostasis, and a coagulopathic state. The implanting provider should be aware of the signs and symptoms of an acute epidural hematoma and be able to appropriately manage the patient if such an event occurred. The clinical presentation of an epidural hematoma is severe back pain, acute leg weakness or spasms, loss of distal extremity reflexes, or acute loss of bowel or bladder control. Any suspicion of an epidural hematoma is a neurosurgical emergency, requiring immediate neurosurgery consultation. Magnetic resonance imaging (MRI), or non-contrast computed tomography (CT) if MRI is unavailable or contraindicated should be obtained.

Identifying risk factors for bleeding complications in the preoperative period is the first step toward reducing complications. For example, coagulopathy concerns should be noted, which may be due to comorbidities, use of anticoagulants, antiplatelet agents, nonsteroidal antiinflammatory medications, and herbal supplements, such as garlic, ginseng, ginkgo, and turmeric. Other factors that increase bleeding risk include quantitative or qualitative platelet abnormalities, abnormalities in clotting factors, vitamin K deficiency, and hepatic synthesis dysfunction. Decision-making for medications that influence clotting function should be discussed with the patient's managing provider along with the 2017 guidelines from the NACC and the American Society of Regional Anesthesia and Pain Medicine (ASRA) for interventional spine and pain procedures in patients on antiplatelet and anticoagulant medications.[16,19]

Neurological Injury

Neurological injury is an uncommon but serious complication, which can result in permanent neurological injury, including paralysis, hypesthesia, and incontinence. The incidence of neurological injuries ranges from 0.6% to 10.5%.[20,21] Neurological injury can result from direct needle trauma, guidewire manipulation, or can be secondary to bleeding or an infection. Bleeding around the neuroaxis can cause diminished spinal cord blood flow that leads to nerve compression and ischemia. The provider should be able to recognize and manage any sign or symptoms of neurological injury during or after neurostimulator placement. Best practice recommendations are to place the leads in an awake and conversant patient. When performed under general anesthesia, the use of intraoperative neurophysiological monitoring (IONM) should be employed.[17] IONM aids in the detection of neurological deficits through early recognition of changes in electromyography (EMG) and somatosensory evoked potentials (SSEPs).

Cerebrospinal Fluid Leak

Dural puncture, intended or unintended, may lead to CSF leak. The reported incidence for this complication ranges from 0.3% to 7%.[17,20,22,23] During needle placement, a large-bore Touhy needle may puncture the dura. Also, during lead insertion, the electrode and guidewire are threaded through this needle. Accidental dural puncture may be encountered during Touhy needle insertion or electrode lead placement. If dural puncture occurs, CSF leak may result in a postdural puncture headache (PDPH). PDPHs present clinically as positional headaches with exacerbation in the upright position and alleviation when supine. Treatment of PDPH starts with conservative therapy (e.g., hydration, abdominal binder, positioning, caffeine, sumatriptan, and theophylline). When conservative therapy fails, the patient and provider may decide to proceed with an epidural blood patch. An epidural blood patch is performed with aseptic technique by taking 15 to 20 cc of autologous blood at the puncture site. Fluoroscopic guidance is used as an aid to avoid infection and damage to the patient or neurostimulator device. Once the blood is injected, it acts to seal off the dural puncture and the symptoms should then resolve quickly. Preventing CSF leaks includes measures taken preoperatively and the use of careful intraoperative technique. For example, one may choose an appropriate path of needle entry, using a shallow angle technique, and utilizing the lateral view during loss of resistance technique.

Seroma Formation

A seroma develops when serosanguinous fluid collection occurs. A seroma is a less serious complication and is usually self-limiting with no clinical consequence. It can last a few days to a couple of months postimplantation. This complication is more common with poor surgical technique, such as inadequate hemostasis and tissue trauma. Management includes patient reassurance and observation. If the fluid collection is excessive, persistent to uncomfortable, then aspiration may be considered. Strict aseptic technique should be followed if aspiration is performed. Conservative treatments include postoperative abdominal binders. However, abdominal binders should be used with caution due to the risk of the potential to cause local tissue ischemia and wound breakdown.

Wound Dehiscence

Wound breakdown and dehiscence are troubling complications that are not uncommon. Such complications occur due to poor suture technique, improper IPG depth, and improper IPG size-to-pocket ratio. Other factors include significant weight loss after implantation, infection, comorbidities such as uncontrolled diabetes, poor nutrition, chronic illness, obesity, high opioid intake, immunosuppression, smoking, and direct compression due to being bed bound or wheelchair dependent. Unresolved seroma or hematoma may also result in wound dehiscence and breakdown. To avoid dehiscence, preoperative evaluation of risk factors should be considered. For example, preexisting scars, ostomy sites, belt preference styles, and barriers to the patient's daily routine, such as wheelchair needs, should be evaluated and discussed. These factors influence surgical site preference because they could lead to excessive pressure over the wound, causing dehiscence or device malposition.

Infection

An infected implanted device is a serious complication with major consequences. The incidence ranges from 0.7% to 10%, with some reports as high as 40%, citing most infections presenting within the first 3 months postimplantation.[24-27] Infection of the surgical site presents with surgical-site pain, induration at the incision or pump site, poor wound healing, erythema, edema, fluctuant pocket, wound exudate, foul smell, skin erosion, and, if systemic, fever and chills. Most superficial infections do not require device explant. However, the provider must rule out deeper infections, including epidural abscess and meningitis. The clinical workup includes a focused history and physical examination followed by laboratory studies, such as white blood cell count, erythrocyte sedimentation rate (ESR), and C-reactive protein. Aspiration of the pocket fluid for cultures may also be performed. Imaging should be obtained if there is concern for an epidural abscess. MRI or CT scan should be ordered along with a neurosurgical evaluation. Deep infections, including epidural abscess and meningitis, require hospital admission, intravenous antibiotics based on culture sensitivities, and immediate explantation.[24] In the serious but rare case of postoperative discitis early detection is key. Management includes antibiotics, analgesics, bed rest and, if needed, neurosurgical exploration with debridement of the disc space granulation tissue.[28] Preventing infection begins in the preoperative setting with evaluation and optimization of risk factors as well as adherence to established guidelines by the CDC and NACC for reducing surgical site infections.[15,29]

GENERAL CONSIDERATIONS

Device-Related Complications

Device-related complications comprise migration, malfunction of device hardware, or battery failure. The annual incidence of complications requiring surgical revision ranges from 5.9% to 49.8%.[12,13,30] The implanting provider should follow the NACC recommendations that focus on risk reduction and mitigation of complications.[14,17]

The most common SCS complication is lead migration, with a reported incidence ranging from 13.2% to 22.6%.[23,31,32] Lead fracture or migration usually occurs due to lack of adequate strain relief loops or lack of electrodes positioned through the ligaments.[24] Catheter migration, fracture, kink, occlusion, or dislodgement may present with increased pain, nerve irritation, CSF leak, or symptoms of spinal cord trauma. Often, the clinical presentation of lead migration is only loss of therapeutic efficacy. Radiography is used to detect lead migration or fractures. Management includes revision, replacement, or device explant. Prevention relies on placing the leads under direct fluoroscopic visualization, anchoring appropriately, creating adequate strain relief loops, and proper lead placement through the ligaments.

Battery failure occurs when the battery reaches the end of its life span, requiring battery replacement. Battery life span depends on the energy use due to programming needs of the patient as well as the number of leads placed. Battery failure happens to a lesser extent than lead failures per reports. The reported incidence is around 1.7%.[23] Management of battery failure begins with having the manufacturer representative assess the device in the office.

Device hardware failure can transpire in the setting of MRI, primarily with 90-cm leads, which are not MRI approved. Many SCS and DRG neurostimulation systems with 50-cm leads are MRI conditional. Management of IPG device failure is IPG replacement.

Patient-Related Complications

Some comorbidities increase the risk of SCS complications. Examples include psychosocial pathologies, such as personality disorders, conversion disorder, and poor coping mechanisms, among others. Other factors involve poor anatomy, prior scar tissue, uncorrected coagulopathy, anticoagulant medications, active infections, active smoking status, insulin-dependent diabetes, and immunosuppression. Minimizing these risk factors begins with optimization in the preoperative period and following the most up-to-date guidelines and best practices provided by the NACC, CDC, and the ASRA.[14,19,29]

Conclusion

SCS is a salvage therapy with several risks and complications. Neuromodulation with SCS is relatively safe with appropriate patient selection, preoperative planning, and when the health care provider follows best practices and updated guidelines from the NACC (2018), CDC (2017), and the ASRA (2018).[14,19,29] See Table 4.2 for more information.

TABLE 4.2 Summary of Infection Management Practices from the Neurostimulation Appropriateness Consensus Committee and the Centers for Disease Control and Prevention (CDC) Guidelines for the Prevention of Surgical Site Infections, 2017[15,29]

Perioperative measures

- Optimize glucose control before device implantation
- Discontinue tobacco use before device implantation
- Decolonize methicillin-susceptible *Staphylococcus aureus* and methicillin-resistant *S. aureus* carriers with mupirocin nasal ointment and chlorohexidine baths
- Antibiotics
  - Use prophylactic antibiotics for both trials and implantation.
  - Dose antibiotics based on weight.
  - Use appropriate timing of prophylactic antimicrobial such that the bactericidal concentration is established in the serum and tissues at incision.
  - Do not routinely use vancomycin.
  - In clean and clean-contaminated procedures, do not administer additional prophylactic antimicrobial agent doses after the surgical incision is closed in the operating room, even in the presence of a drain.
- If hair is removed, use electric clippers immediately before surgery.
- Keep nails short and do not wear artificial nails for both trials and implantation.
- Do not wear hand or arm jewelry for trials or implantation.

Intraoperative measures

- Utilize chlorhexidine gluconate for preoperative skin antiseptic agent.
- Perform preoperative surgical scrub for a minimum of 2–5 minutes with an appropriate antiseptic prior to trials and implantation.
- Limit operating room traffic.
- Maintain positive pressure ventilation and HEPA filters in the operating room for implantation
- Keep the operating room doors closed during the procedure.
- Wear a surgical mask and fully cover hair for both trials and implantation.
- Wear sterile gown and gloves for both trials and implantation.
- Double glove.
- When using an incise drape, use an iodophor-impregnated drape for implantation.
- Handle tissue gently, eradicate dead space, maintain hemostasis, and avoid electrocautery at tissue surface.
- Irrigate with saline through bulb syringe prior to closure of surgical wound.
- Limit operation time.

Postoperative measures

- Use an occlusive sterile dressing following trials and implantation for 24–48 hours postoperatively.
- Do not routinely use topical antimicrobial agents for surgical wounds that are healing by primary intention.
- If a dressing change is required, use hand washing and sterile technique.
- Do not continue antimicrobial agents beyond 24 hours.
- A deep surgical site infection (SSI) of an implanted device is possible up to 1 year postimplantation.
- Educate patient and caregiver on proper incision care, signs of infection, and how and when to communicate with a health care professional.
- When SSI is suspected, prescribe an antibiotic that covers the likely causative organisms.

CDC Evidence Rankings. IA: Strongly recommended for implementation and supported by well-designed experimental, clinical, or epidemiological studies. IB: Strongly recommended for implementation and supported by some experimental, clinical, or epidemiological studies and strong theoretical rationale. II: Suggested for implementation and supported by suggestive clinical or epidemiological studies or theoretical rationale.

REFERENCES

1. Taylor RS. Spinal cord stimulation in complex regional pain syndrome and refractory neuropathic back and leg pain/failed back surgery syndrome: results of a systematic review and meta-analysis. *J Pain Symptom Manage*. 2006;31(suppl 4):S13-S19. doi:10.1016/j.jpainsymman.2005.12.010.
2. Shealy CN, Mortimer JT, Reswick JB. Electrical inhibition of pain by stimulation of the dorsal columns: preliminary clinical report. *Anesth Analg*. 1967;46:489-491.
3. Slavin KV. Spinal stimulation for pain: future applications. *Neurotherapeutics*. 2014;11(3):535-542. doi:10.1007/s13311-014-0273-2.

4. Bevan S, Yeats J. Protons activate a cation conductance in a sub-population of rat dorsal root ganglion neurones. *J Physiol.* 1991;433:145-161. Available at: https://dx.doi.org/10.1113%2Fjphysiol.1991.sp018419.
5. International Neuromodulation Society 12th World Congress Neuromodulation: medicine evolving through technology. Montreal, Canada. *Neuromodulation.* 2015;18:e107-e399. doi:10.1111/ner.12333.
6. Vuka I, Marciuš T, Došenović S, et al. Neuromodulation with electrical field stimulation of dorsal root ganglion in various pain syndromes: a systematic review with focus on participant selection. *J Pain Res.* 2019;12:803-830. doi:10.2147/JPR.S168814.
7. Levy RM. Anatomic considerations for spinal cord stimulation. *Neuromodulation.* 2014;17(suppl 1):2-11. doi:10.1111/ner.12175.
8. Falowski S, Celii A, Sharan A. Spinal cord stimulation: an update. *Neurotherapeutics.* 2008;5(1):86-99. doi:10.1016/j.nurt.2007.10.066.
9. Hunter CW, Yang A. Dorsal root ganglion stimulation for chronic pelvic pain: a case series and technical report on a novel lead configuration. *Neuromodulation.* 2019;22(1):87-95. doi:10.1111/ner.12801.
10. Deer TR, Levy RM, Kramer J, et al. Dorsal root ganglion stimulation yielded higher treatment success rate for complex regional pain syndrome and causalgia at 3 and 12 months: a randomized comparative trial. *Pain.* 2017;158(4):669-681. doi:10.1097/j.pain.0000000000000814.
11. Liem L, Russo M, Huygen FJPM, et al. A multicenter, prospective trial to assess the safety and performance of the spinal modulation dorsal root ganglion neurostimulator system in the treatment of chronic pain. *Neuromodulation.* 2013;16(5):471-482. doi:10.1111/ner.12072.
12. Liem L, Russo M, Huygen FJPM, et al. One-year outcomes of spinal cord stimulation of the dorsal root ganglion in the treatment of chronic neuropathic pain. *Neuromodulation.* 2015;18(1):41-49. doi:10.1111/ner.12228.
13. Huygen F, Liem L, Cusack W, Kramer J. Stimulation of the L2–L3 dorsal root ganglia induces effective pain relief in the low back. *Pain Pract.* 2018;18(2):205-213. doi:10.1111/papr.12591.
14. Deer TR, Pope JE, Lamer TJ, et al. The Neuromodulation Appropriateness Consensus Committee on best practices for dorsal root ganglion stimulation. *Neuromodulation.* 2019;22(1):1-35. doi:10.1111/ner.12845.
15. Deer TR, Provenzano DA, Hanes M, et al. The Neurostimulation Appropriateness Consensus Committee (NACC) recommendations for infection prevention and management. *Neuromodulation.* 2017;20(1):31-50. doi:10.1111/ner.12565.
16. Deer TR, Narouze S, Provenzano DA, et al. The Neurostimulation Appropriateness Consensus Committee (NACC): recommendations on bleeding and coagulation management in neurostimulation devices. *Neuromodulation.* 2017;20(1):51-62. doi:10.1111/ner.12542.
17. Deer TR, Lamer TJ, Pope JE, et al. The Neurostimulation Appropriateness Consensus Committee (NACC) safety guidelines for the reduction of severe neurological injury. *Neuromodulation.* 2017;20(1):15-30. doi:10.1111/ner.12564.
18. Van Buyten JP. Neurostimulation for chronic neuropathic back pain in failed back surgery syndrome. *J Pain Symptom Manage.* 2006;31(suppl 4):S25-S29. doi:10.1016/j.jpainsymman.2005.12.012.
19. Narouze S, Benzon HT, Provenzano D, et al. Interventional Spine and Pain Procedures in Patients on Antiplatelet and Anticoagulant Medications (Second Edition): Guidelines from the American Society of Regional Anesthesia and Pain Medicine, the European Society of Regional Anaesthesia and Pain Therapy, the American Academy of Pain Medicine, the International Neuromodulation Society, the North American Neuromodulation Society, and the World Institute of Pain. *Reg Anesth Pain Med.* 2018;43(3):225-262. doi:10.1097/AAP.0000000000000700.
20. Deer T, Pope J, Hunter C, et al. Safety analysis of dorsal root ganglion stimulation in the treatment of chronic pain. *Neuromodulation.* 2020;23(2):239-244. doi:10.1111/ner.12941.
21. Deer TR, Levy RM, Kramer J, et al. Dorsal root ganglion stimulation yielded higher treatment success rate for complex regional pain syndrome and causalgia at 3 and 12 months: a randomized comparative trial. *Pain.* 2017;158(4):669-681.
22. Hussain A, Erdek M. Interventional pain management for failed back surgery syndrome. *Pain Pract.* 2014;14(1):64-78. doi:10.1111/papr.12035.
23. Cameron T. Safety and efficacy of spinal cord stimulation for the treatment of chronic pain: a 20-year literature review. *J Neurosurg Spine.* 2004;100(3):254-267. doi:10.3171/spi.2004.100.3.0254.
24. Malinowski MN, Bremer N, Kim CH, Deer TR. *Intrathecal Drug Delivery: Indications, Risks, and Complications.* (Khelemsky Y., Malhotra A. GK, ed.). Springer; 2019. doi:10.1007/978-3-030-18005-8_22.
25. Flückiger B, Knecht H, Grossmann S, Felleiter P. Device-related complications of long-term intrathecal drug therapy via implanted pumps. *Spinal Cord.* 2008;46(9):639-643. doi:10.1038/sc.2008.24.
26. Kumar K, Taylor RS, Jacques L, et al. Spinal cord stimulation versus conventional medical management for neuropathic pain: a multicentre randomised controlled trial in patients with failed back surgery syndrome. *Pain.* 2007;132(1-2):179-188. doi:10.1016/j.pain.2007.07.028.
27. Eldabe S, Buchser E, Duarte RV. Complications of spinal cord stimulation and peripheral nerve stimulation techniques: a review of the literature. *Pain Med.* 2016;17:325-336. doi:10.1093/pm/pnv025.
28. Luzzati R, Giacomazzi D, Danzi MC, Tacconi L, Concia E, Vento S. Diagnosis, management and outcome of clinically-suspected spinal infection. *J Infect.* 2009;58(4):259-265.
29. Berriós-Torres SI, Umscheid CA, Bratzler DW, et al. Centers for Disease Control and Prevention Guideline for the prevention of surgical site infection, 2017. *JAMA Surg.* 2017;152(8):784-791. doi:10.1001/jamasurg.2017.0904.
30. Sivanesan E, Bicket MC, Cohen SP. Retrospective analysis of complications associated with dorsal root ganglion stimulation for pain relief in the FDA MAUDE database. *Reg Anesth Pain Med.* 2019;44(1):100-106. doi:10.1136/rapm-2018-000007.
31. Kumar K, Hunter G, Demeria D. Spinal cord stimulation in treatment of chronic benign pain: challenges in treatment planning and present status, a 22-year experience. *Neurosurgery.* 2006;58(3):481-496. doi:10.1227/01.NEU.0000192162.99567.96.
32. Mekhail NA, Mathews M, Nageeb F, Guirguis M, Mekhail MN, Cheng J. Retrospective review of 707 cases of spinal cord stimulation: indications and complications. *Pain Pract.* 2011;11(2):148-153. doi:10.1111/j.1533-2500.2010.00407.x.

Chapter 5

Surgical Instruments

Nomen Azeem and Andrew J. Duarte

Chapter Outline

Introduction

As with any surgical procedure, access to the appropriate surgical instrumentation is imperative for a safe and successful outcome. Neuromodulation has been utilized effectively in chronic pain patients for well over 6 decades. Spinal cord stimulation (SCS) and dorsal root ganglion (DRG) stimulation are advanced procedures for patients who suffer from failed back surgery syndrome, radiculopathy/plexopathy, complex regional pain syndrome, or other peripheral neuropathic conditions.[1] Both procedures utilize wire leads applied to the target structure and an implantable unit to provide neurostimulation. Surgical instruments and equipment required to successfully perform this advanced procedure include those that permit the surgeon to incise, retract structures, maintain hemostasis, suction, perform tunneling, irrigate incisions, and close the resected layers of tissue. The surgical kit provided by the device manufacturer contains the implantable unit and all associated equipment. This is a fluoroscopy-guided or computed tomography (CT)–guided procedure. Fluoroscopy is a type of medical imaging that shows a continuous X-ray image on a monitor. During a fluoroscopy-guided procedure, an X-ray beam is passed through the body and transmitted to a monitor to visualize bone and joint anatomy. A CT scan combines a series of X-ray images taken from different angles that are combined to produce a more detailed image than a fluoroscopic image. Both imaging modalities require the surgeon and operating room staff to wear lead aprons with thyroid guards for protection from radiation exposure.

Anatomical Considerations

Both SCS and DRG implant procedures are preceded by trials to confirm successful neuromodulation. Although in recent years multiple mechanisms of action have been found, SCS and DRG stimulation utilize the fundamental principles of neuromodulation including the Gate Control Theory by Melzack and Wall.[2] In order to provide patients with relief from their chronic pain, it is essential to understand the different anatomical considerations between the two procedures.[3]

Regarding SCS, the primary target is the dorsal column, achieved by placing the leads into the epidural space. Recall that the borders of the epidural space include the ligamentum flavum posteriorly, the pedicles and intervertebral foramina laterally, and the dura anteriorly. The layers pierced en route to the epidural space are as follows, starting most superficial: skin, subcutaneous tissue (adipose and connective tissues, fascial layers), paraspinous muscles, supraspinous ligament, interspinous ligament, and the ligamentum flavum. Placement of the leads into the epidural space is contingent on the desired region of stimulation: C1 to C4 for the neck, C5 to C6 for upper extremities, T6 to T9 for the low back, and T10 to T11 for lower extremity, among others.

Regarding DRG stimulation, the target is the DRG itself, which is a structure located just distal to the posterior (dorsal) spinal nerve roots between each spinal level. There is variability at spinal segments as to whether the DRG is at the intraforaminal, extraforaminal, or intraspinal location.[4] The DRG itself is a collection of primary sensory neuronal cell bodies with axons that project bidirectionally to the spinal cord as well as peripheral nociceptors, mechanoreceptors, and proprioceptors. Afferent signals are transmitted from the periphery through the DRG to the spinal cord synapse in Rexed laminae, which are then routed to the ascending fibers that project into the thalamus and other supraspinal regions of the central nervous system (CNS). DRG stimulation aims to interrupt these neurons. The DRG stimulator pads are placed in the epidural space over the DRG.

Step-by-Step Description of the Procedure

PATIENT POSITIONING AND PREPARATION

Prior to starting the procedure, it is prudent to review the basic steps of the procedure with the patient along with risks, benefits, and alternatives. A preoperative review of medical problems, medications, allergies, marking of the anatomical location(s), and a quick examination should be performed to ensure that there are no contraindications to the procedure. The patient is then brought into the operating room, where they must be positioned prone on the table for the duration of the procedure. The proper position for SCS or DRG stimulator implantation must minimize lordosis of the cervical or lumbar spine to maximally expose the desired interlaminar spaces and to minimize any pressure points on the patient's body. This positioning can be accomplished with a Wilson frame. Wilson frame–induced kyphosis significantly increased flexion at L4 to L5 and L5 to S1 by 47% and 21%, respectively. In addition, it was found that the surgical technique of inducing kyphosis with the Wilson frame prior to incision significantly optimized exposure.[5] If a Wilson frame is not accessible, then a bump (i.e., a gel bump or rolled up towels) underneath the chest or abdomen may be utilized.

Once positioned, the patient's skin is sterilized with an appropriate antiseptic agent such as iodophors and/or chlorhexidine gluconate. The first use of an antiseptic skin agent in surgery is credited to the English surgeon Joseph Lister (1827–1912). Prior to the mid-19th century, limb amputation was associated with an alarming 50% postoperative mortality from sepsis. Lister began treating wounds with carbolic acid (phenol) in an effort to prevent tissue decay and the resultant infectious complications. Consequently, the incidence of surgical sepsis fell dramatically, catalyzing the adoption of modern antiseptic techniques, including instrument sterilization, the use of surgical scrubs and rubber gloves, and sterile patient preparation.[6,7] A recent study assessed the efficacy of chlorhexidine gluconate versus povidone iodine prior to sterilization, after preparation, and after wound closure for posterior spine surgeries among 190 patients. This study found that after skin sterilization, skin culture positivity rates improved from 83% pre-sterilization to 3.1% in the chlorhexidine group and 5.1% in the povidone iodine group post-sterilization. The significant reduction in skin flora persisted to the time of wound closure, with culture positivity rates of 5.1% in the chlorhexidine group and 14.1% in the povidone iodine group.[8] It is also prudent to establish a sterile field with the use of towels and/or drapes to safeguard against cutaneous microorganism contamination.

NONSURGICAL INSTRUMENTS

In addition to surgical tools, it is worth detailing the pertinent instruments that are utilized in planning, administration of local anesthetic, hemostasis, and advancement of the stimulator leads. Under fluoroscopy with a radiopaque instrument/pointer such as forceps or ring forceps as a surface indicator, the target interlaminar levels are viewed and optimized with angulation of the fluoroscope. The skin is then marked with a sterile marking pen. Local anesthetic (with or without epinephrine) is injected via syringe (10 cc) with a skin needle (25-gauge, 1 ½ inch) topically at the skin and along the anticipated trajectory to the target spinal level. A spinal needle (22-gauge, 3 ½ inch) is often utilized to provide local anesthetic along the intended trajectory of the Tuohy needle (Fig. 5.1). Sterile surgical sponges are often utilized to absorb fluids and may be used to hold pressure for hemostasis. Normal saline (with or without antibiotic) should be available to irrigate the surgical wound prior to closure. Suction tubing with a tip should be supplied to remove excessive fluid from the incision and sterile field (Fig. 5.2). Last, sterile dressing (wound-closure strips, gauze, occlusive dressing) should be available to provide the surgical incision physical barrier from environmental elements and may absorb any residual postsurgical fluid.

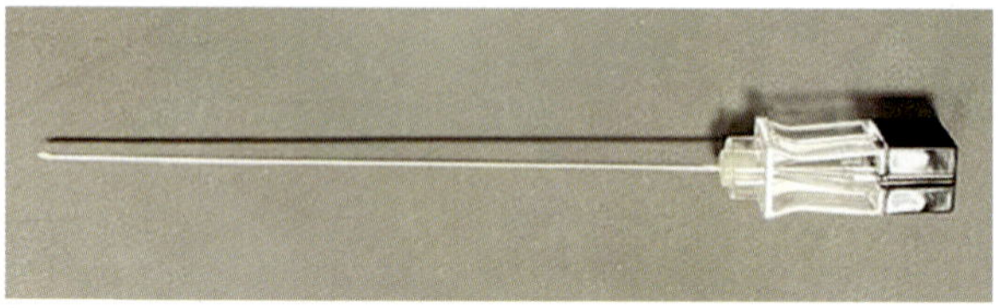

Fig. 5.1 Spinal needle.

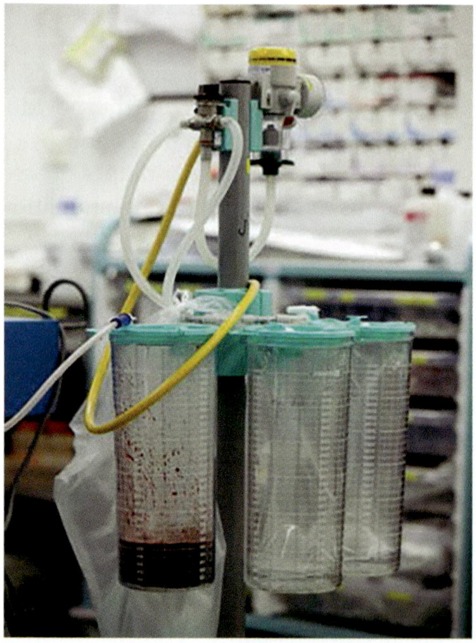

Fig. 5.2 Surgical suction.

DEVICE MANUFACTURER KIT

SCS device kits vary by vendor but contain common elements (Fig. 5.3). In addition to the implantable pulse generator (IPG), there is a device registration form and patient identification card for patients to keep on their person. There is also a device manual with information on the product. These kits typically contain a Tuohy needle (14 gauge), 1 or 2 wire leads with both a curved and straight stylet, lead anchors, tunneling tools, and an IPG. DRG device kits vary only in that they provide two introducer sheaths for the DRG lead, one with a larger curved tip and one with a lesser curved tip. Refer to the device manufacturer for the exact contents of the kit for each device (Fig. 5.4).

For SCS, the Tuohy needle is introduced and advanced under fluoroscopy at a 30- to 45-degree angle medially and cephalad until contact is made with the targeted lamina. The needle is guided to the medial edge of the lamina where the stylet is then removed and a loss-of-resistance (LOR) syringe (Fig. 5.5) is attached. The needle engages with the ligamentum flavum until LOR demonstrates entry into the epidural space. The LOR syringe is removed and the

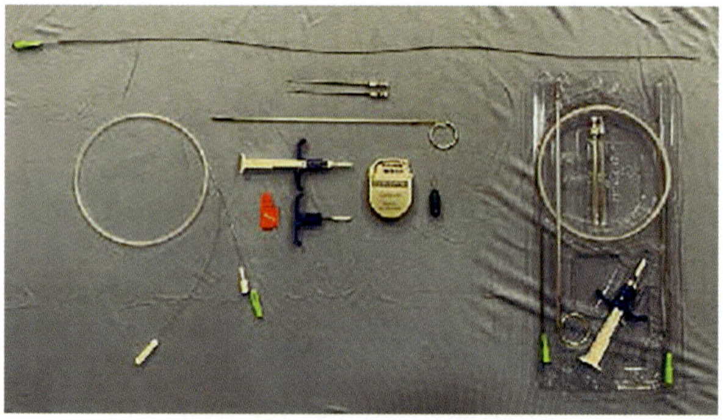

Fig. 5.3 Spinal cord stimulation kit.

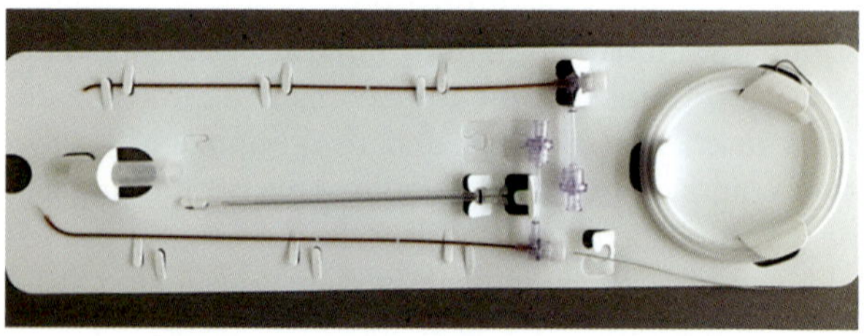

Fig. 5.4 Dorsal root ganglion stimulation kit.

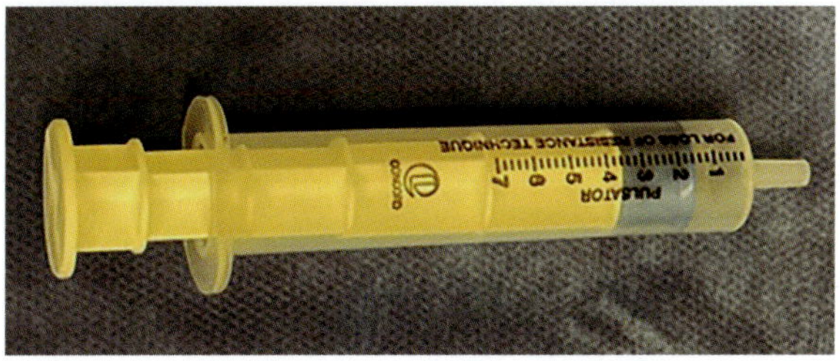

Fig. 5.5 Loss-of-resistance syringe.

percutaneous leads are advanced through the Tuohy needle into the epidural space. These leads are maneuvered to the desired target level; it is prudent to confirm lead placement with lateral fluoroscopic images to ensure that the leads are placed in the posterior aspect of the epidural space. If more than one lead is being placed, the subsequent lead is introduced in a similar manner as above on the contralateral side or on the ipsilateral side above or below the newly placed lead.

DRG stimulator lead placement requires a basic approach of advancing a needle under fluoroscopy similar to SCS. With DRG stimulation, the angle of entry is typically less steep than for SCS to permit lead steering. An important difference is the target: the needle's bevel is aimed toward the contralateral pedicle at the desired level. The use of a curved sheath increases maneuverability; physicians skilled in this procedure can place leads ipsilateral to needle placement should patient anatomy warrant it. As the curved sheath is directed toward the foramen and the sheath containing the lead advanced into the intraforaminal space, the sheath is retracted, allowing 3 to 4 cm of lead slack to form an S-shaped tension release loop around the DRG. This tension release loop reduces the risk of lead migration.[9] Once the leads are placed, the sheath, stylet, and needle are removed. Anchoring of the leads to the subcutaneous tissue is possible but varies by surgeon's preference.

SURGICAL INSTRUMENTS

The pertinent surgical instruments that should be supplied by the facility (Fig. 5.6) for SCS/DRG stimulator implantation should allow for incising/dissecting, hemostasis, handling of instruments provided by the vendor, and surgical wound closure (Table 5.1).

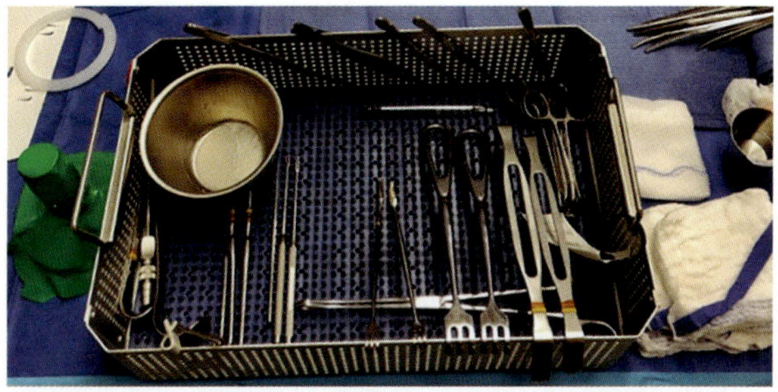

Fig. 5.6 Surgical tray (includes forceps, needle holders, handheld retractors, and bowl for irrigation fluid).

TABLE 5.1 Surgical Instruments Required For SCS/DRG Implantation, Provided By Facility

Surgical Instrument	Use	Types
Scalpel	Incision of superficial tissue	• 10 blade: Larger skin incision • 11 blade: Stab incision • 15 blade: Finer skin incision
Electrosurgery	Dissection of deeper tissue/coagulation	• Bipolar • Monopolar
Sponge clamps	Pointer	

Forceps	Holds skin edges, needles	• Adson
		  ◦ With or without teeth
		  ◦ Most commonly used
		• DeBakey
		  ◦ Longer, more delicate
		  ◦ No teeth

Needle holder	Holds suture needle	• Large • Small

Continued

TABLE 5.1 Surgical Instruments Required For SCS/DRG Implantation, Provided By Facility—cont'd

Surgical Instrument	Use	Types
Surgical retractor	Separate edges of incised surgical incision Holds back layers of incised tissue	• Handheld (Senn, Army-Navy) • Self-retaining (Weitlaner, Gelpi) • Varying sizes
Suction	Removes excess fluids from field	• Plugged into OR
Suture	Incision closure	• Absorbable • Nonabsorbable
Suture scissors	Cuts suture	• Mayo • Straight = "suture scissors" used to cut suture

There are typically two incisions utilized for SCS/DRG stimulator implantation: the IPG pocket incision and lead placement/lead anchor incision. The timing of skin incision for lead placement varies by implanter choice to make the incision prior to needle and lead placement versus after needle and lead placement. The skin is marked and anesthetized. The incision is made with a scalpel (Fig. 5.7). Then, a combination of electrosurgery with a cautery pen (Figs. 5.8 and 5.9) and blunt dissection is utilized for both the IPG pocket and lead placement. Forceps (Fig. 5.10) are utilized to hold skin edges during dissection. Retractors, both handheld and self-retaining (Figs. 5.6 and 5.11) are utilized for sustained skin and superficial tissue retraction during dissection and after for visualization.

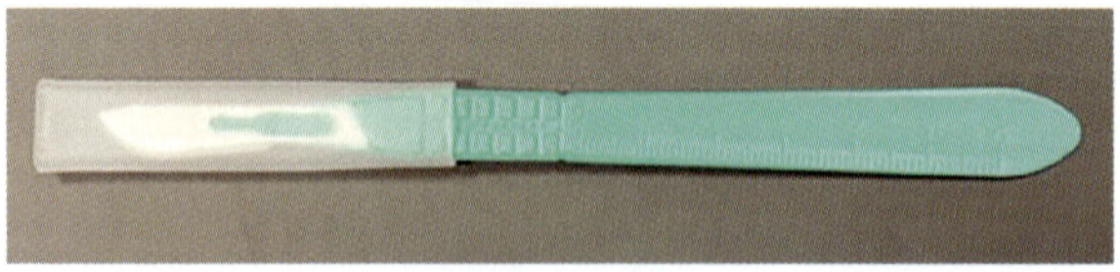

Fig. 5.7 Scalpel.

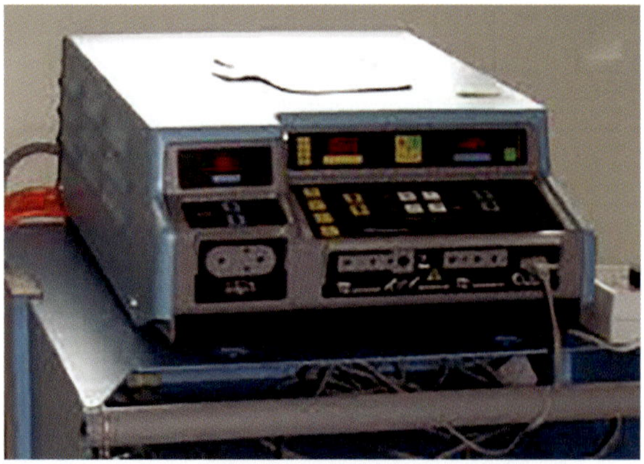

Fig. 5.8 Electrosurgery.

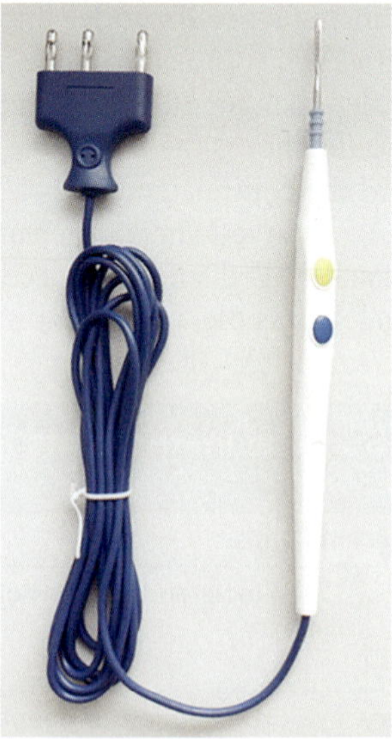

Fig. 5.9 Cautery Pen.

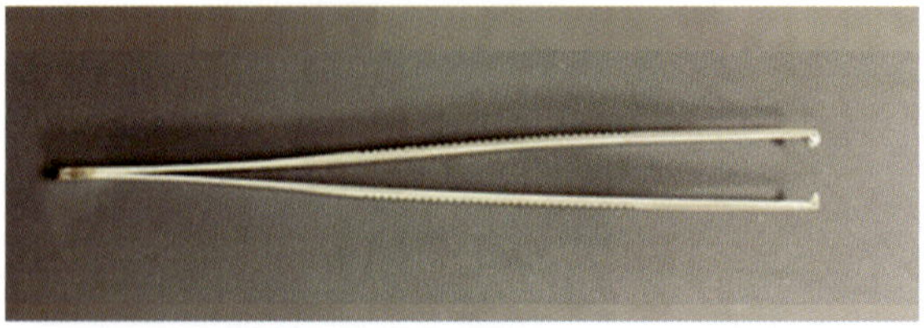

Fig. 5.10 Forceps (colloquially known as "pick ups").

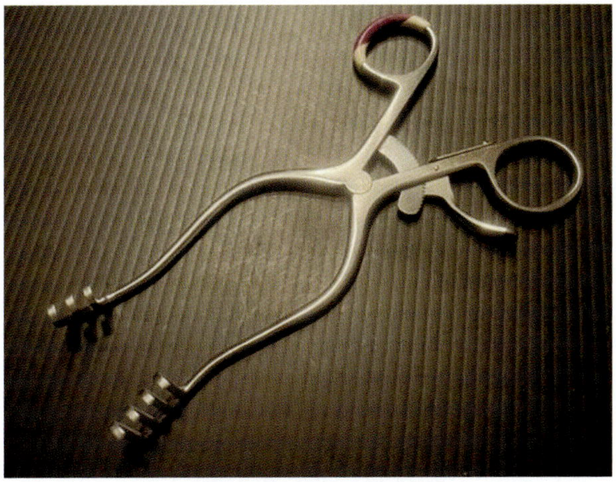

Fig. 5.11 Weitlaner retractor.

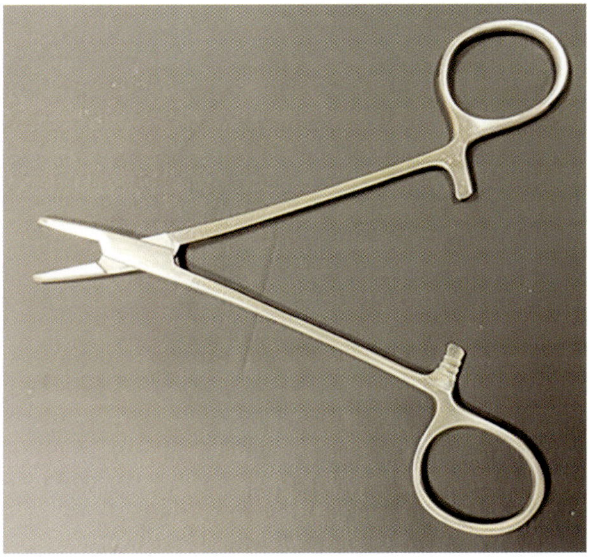

Fig. 5.12 Needle holder.

Once the leads are positioned properly, with confirmation on fluoroscopic imaging, they are anchored. Anchoring of wire leads is achieved with an anchor included in the manufacturer's kit, a nonabsorbing nylon or silk suture to anchor the leads into the connective tissue. Typically, forceps, needle holder, and suture scissors are needed for this step (Figs. 5.10, 5.12–5.14). It is prudent to gently tug on the leads to ensure proper anchoring. Blunt dissection

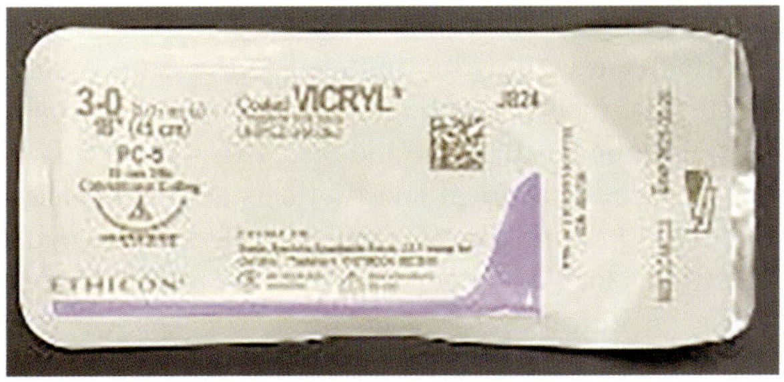

Fig. 5.13 Suture.

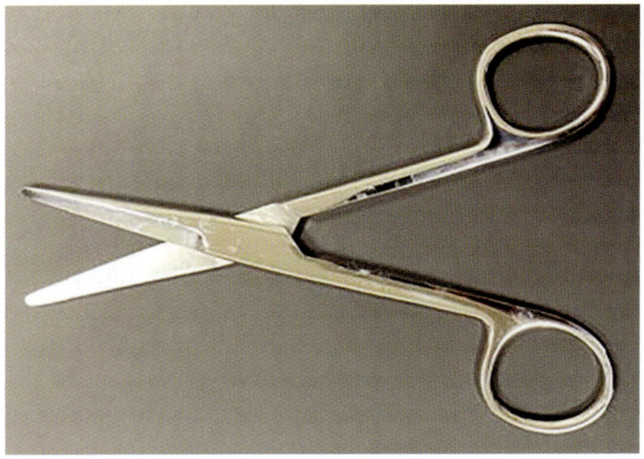

Fig. 5.14 Suture scissors.

at the lead placement incision allows the physician to place tension strain relief loops, which minimize migration.

The IPG pocket dissection is typically located in the superior gluteal region or the low back. Again, using a sterile skin marker, the skin is marked and subsequently anesthetized with a local anesthetic as detailed earlier. Using a scalpel, the skin and superficial fascial layers are incised. A combination of electrosurgery and blunt dissection is then used to extend the pocket along fascial planes. The size of the pocket is dictated by the IPG. The pocket should be deep and large enough to enclose the IPG without tension on the overlying tissue. The IPG is typically placed about 1 to 2 cm beneath the skin surface as this permits recharging for rechargeable IPGs while mitigating the risk for surface tissue erosion. For units with nonrechargeable batteries, the IPG can be placed 2 to 4 cm beneath the skin.

With the leads secured and IPG implanted, the lead wires must now be tunneled to the unit. A sterile surgical marker can be used to demarcate the path between the lead wires and the IPG. The path is anesthetized with local anesthetic as detailed earlier. Utilizing the tunneling device (provided in the manufacturer's kit), advance along the planned trajectory while making sure not to drive the device into deeper structures. Once the device has bridged the discrete surgical areas, the tunneling device is removed, leaving the sheath in the tract. The electrode(s) are tunneled through the sheath and advanced into the IPG pocket, where they are connected to the device.

With the leads, lead wires, and IPG in place and connected, it is advisable to irrigate the pockets with saline with or without antibiotics using forceps to lift skin edges and a syringe to administer irrigation. Splash can be mitigated by placing a towel around the surgical site while suction is applied. The IPG pocket is closed by first suturing deep fascial layers followed by dermal layers. The skin can be approximated with suture or staples. Similarly, the tissue surrounding the leads is closed and skin approximated with suture or staples. Occlusive dressings are applied to the two surgical incisions.

Intraoperative Complications

There are several intraoperative complications that the physician should be aware of and anticipate to avoid harm to the patient. As with any surgical procedure, there is the possibility for hemodynamic instability. A thorough review of the patient's medical history, including recent changes in the patient's medications, can mitigate this risk. Additionally, the participation of an experienced practitioner of perioperative care, such as an anesthesiologist, can provide support for any unanticipated complications pertaining to patient physiology. A possible cause of hemodynamic instability is an anaphylactic reaction to a medication or agent; thus, a thorough preoperative review of allergies is standard of care.

There are several risks to be aware of during permanent lead placement. While injecting local anesthetic, it is important to be cognizant of local anatomy and avoid vasculature as intra-arterial injection of local anesthetics can yield toxicity. This has serious implications across several organ systems, with arrhythmias being the most worrisome. Aspirating before injecting is a common practice to avoid this potentially fatal adverse event. Another potential complication is dural puncture, or worse, subarachnoid administration of an agent (such as a local anesthetic). Dural puncture constitutes any interruption of the dura, which can have postprocedure sequelae, including postdural puncture headache or epidural fibrosis as well as increased risk for direct spinal cord or nerve root injury or infection, such as an epidural abscess. Placement of leads in the thoracic spine carries the risk of pleural puncture and pneumothorax. As with any fluoroscopically guided intervention, multiplanar imaging should be used to ascertain the location of the needle tip to avoid a perforated viscus.

Finally, there are risks related to IPG implantation, most notably dehiscence of the pocket or surgical site. Adequate depth of implantation and pocket size will prevent this complication.

General Considerations

Postoperative evaluation of the patient within 1 to 2 weeks is recommended to assess surgical site healing. The patient is regularly in contact with a device representative, who will answer questions and troubleshoot. Postoperative activity should be minimized to mitigate lead migration. Theoretically, scarring occurs in the weeks after the procedure to secure the leads further. A general rule is avoiding exercise or other vigorous activity for at least 4 to 6 weeks.

As with any procedure, success is often a function of the candidacy for the procedure. Be sure to select the appropriate patients and ensure that they are willing to work with the physician and the entire interdisciplinary team to promote success of the modality. SCS and DRG stimulation technologies have come a long way in both the software (stimulator protocols, remote controls, and more) and hardware (battery technologies, IPG size, leads, and so forth). Thus, they are an integral tool for the treatment of chronic pain.

REFERENCES

1. Diwan S, Deer TR. *Advanced Procedures for Pain Management: A Step-by-Step Atlas*. Cham, Switzerland: Springer; 2018.
2. Melzack R, Wall PD. Pain mechanisms: a new theory. *Science*. 1965;150(3699):971-979.
3. Vallejo R, Gupta A, Cedeño D, et al. Clinical effectiveness and mechanism of action of spinal cord stimulation for treating chronic low back and lower extremity pain: a systematic review. *Curr Pain Headache Rep*. 2020;24(11):70.
4. Moon HS, Kim YD, Song BH, Cha YD, Song JH, Lee MH. Position of dorsal root ganglia in the lumbosacral region in patients with radiculopathy. *Korean J Anesthesiol*. 2010;59(6):398-402.
5. Cardoso MJ, Rosner MK. Does the Wilson frame assist with optimizing surgical exposure for minimally invasive lumbar fusions? *Neurosurg Focus*. 2010;28(5):E20-E21.
6. Hemani ML, Lepor H. Skin preparation for the prevention of surgical site infection: which agent is best? *Rev Urol*. 2009;11(4): 190-195.
7. Newsom B. Surgical wound infections–a historical review. *Int J Infect Control*. 2008;4(1).
8. Yoshii T, Hirai T, Yamada T, et al. A prospective comparative study in skin antiseptic solutions for posterior spine surgeries: chlorhexidine-gluconate ethanol versus povidone-iodine. *Clin Spine Surg*. 2018;31(7):E353-E356.
9. Verrills P. Dorsal root ganglion stimulation for pain control. In: Krames ES, Peckham PH, Rezai A, eds. *Neuromodulation: Comprehensive Textbook of Principles, Technologies, and Therapies*. London: Elsevier; 2018:683-692.

Chapter 6

General Review of Wound Closure in Neuromodulation Cases

Wendell Bradley Lake

Chapter Outline

Introduction

Wound closure is an important step of any surgical procedure. However, this step takes on special significance in neuromodulation procedures due to the risk of device erosion and infection. In fact, infection is one of the most common complications in neuromodulation. In one large review of the literature, the rate of infection for placement of spinal cord stimulation (SCS) devices is 3% to 10%.[1] In the case of intrathecal medication delivery, some series cite an infection rate of 13%.[2] While patient selection, equipment preparation, and postoperative care all play a role in wound healing and infection rate, closure technique is often the area in which surgeons can have the greatest impact in reducing infection and complication rate. Wound closure in the case of neuromodulatory devices is also important because the same incision may have to be opened multiple times over the patient's lifetime for replacement. As such, preserving an appropriate vascular supply and incision geometry is key.

Closure in the case of neuromodulation devices can be broken down into two areas: anchoring the device and skin closure. As previously mentioned, careful attention to skin closure is important to mitigate the risk of infection. However, device anchoring is also key as device migration is a significant source of complication as well. Reviews of SCS have shown that lead migration may be 13% to 20%.[1,3] Additionally, implantable pulse generators (IPGs) can flip in some cases, which can result in lead fracture or patient discomfort. From the standpoint of intrathecal drug delivery, pump flipping can be a significant problem in some patients.[4]

What follows is a discussion of neuromodulation-related wound closure, including deep tissue and skin closure as well as device anchoring. Where appropriate, figures are provided to clarify important concepts.

Anatomical Considerations

Proper closure in the setting of neuromodulation devices requires an understanding of proper device positioning and anatomical tissue layers. The particulars of device positioning on the patient's body and the position of the device relative to the incision are described here. Tissue layers relevant to closure are also described in detail.

One of the first decisions a practitioner faces when implanting a neuromodulation device is where to position the implant. The traditional point of view has been to position the device away from the incision as much as possible to minimize

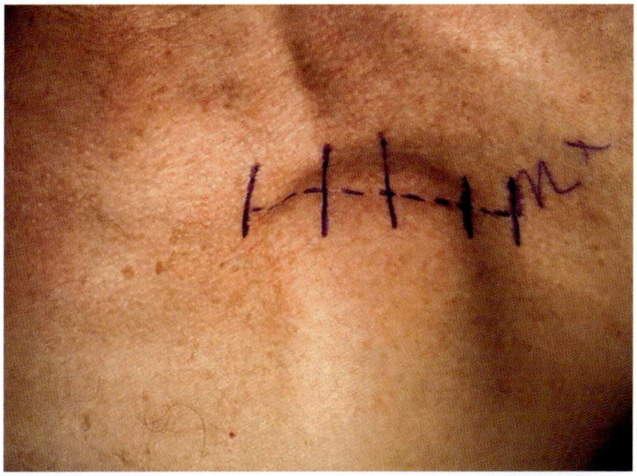

Fig. 6.1 A typical device location, with the smooth portion of the device under the incision if the device cannot be placed completely away from the incision. The feet are toward the bottom of the photograph and the head is toward the top.

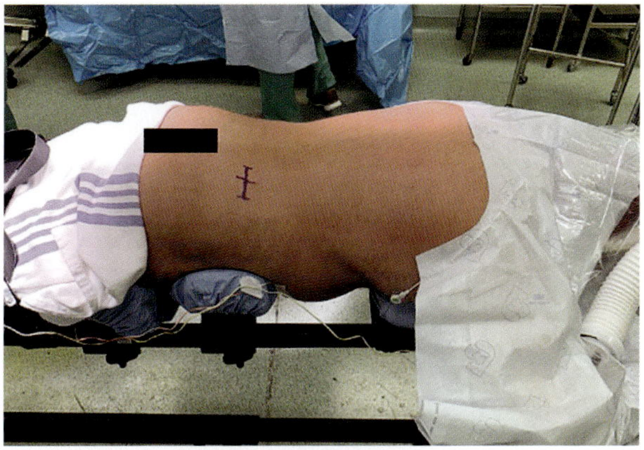

Fig. 6.2 A typical spinal cord stimulation implantable pulse generator location. The incision site avoids painful areas—the waist band and bony prominences.

the risk of erosion through the incision. In some cases, if the device is large (e.g., adjustable pumps for intrathecal drug delivery), some portion of the device will reside under the incision. In this case, the device should be positioned with a flat or smooth surface under the incision (Fig. 6.1). Placing the corner or edge of the device under the incision can increase pressure on the incision and complicate future closure during device replacements.

A second key factor is choosing the position of the device on the patient. For example, in the case of intrathecal pumps and SCS, every effort should be made to ask patients about their habits and preferences. Avoid placing the device under a waistband, for example. Avoid placing the device in an area where it conflicts with the arms of a routinely used wheelchair or other commonly used assistive device. Of course, areas of pain and bony prominences should be avoided—for example, a typical SCS IPG location is above the iliac crest and away from the waist band (Fig. 6.2).[5]

In the closure of a wound, the surgeon must consider the anatomical layers of tissue. In general, each layer that the surgeon encounters during opening must be closed. The layers of the skin include the epidermis, dermis, and subcutaneous tissue. These layers are illustrated in Fig. 6.3.[6] Wound closure for a

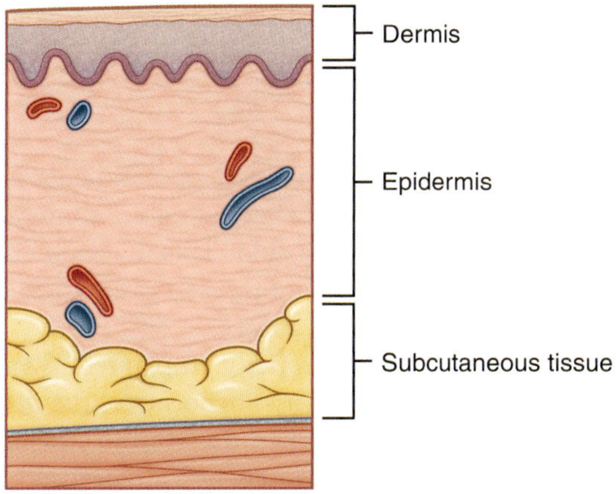

Fig. 6.3 Layers of the skin. (From Wikipedia Commons)

neuromodulation procedure begins with first anchoring the device firmly to a strong tissue layer. In the case of SCS procedures, the leads and IPG should be anchored firmly to the lumbodorsal fascia. In the case of pumps for intrathecal drug delivery, the catheter is anchored to the lumbodorsal fascia and the pump is anchored to the external oblique or the rectus fascia.

Description of the Procedure

Once an appropriate device location has been chosen, the surgeon begins the implantation. With regard to the closure, a key point is the creation of the incision.

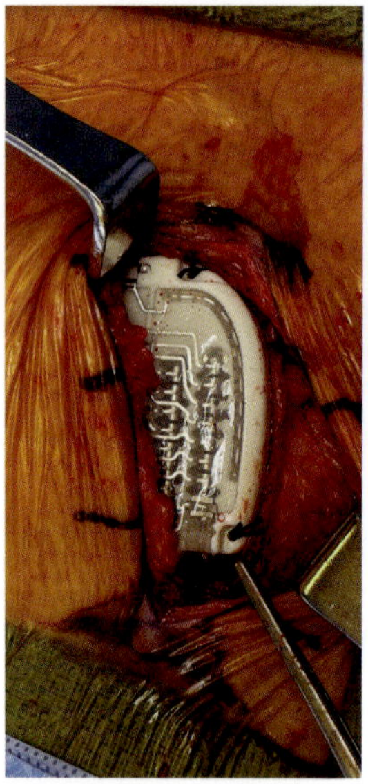

Fig. 6.4 A properly anchored implantable pulse generator. Note the silk sutures. The patient's feet would be toward the left side of the photograph and the head toward the right.

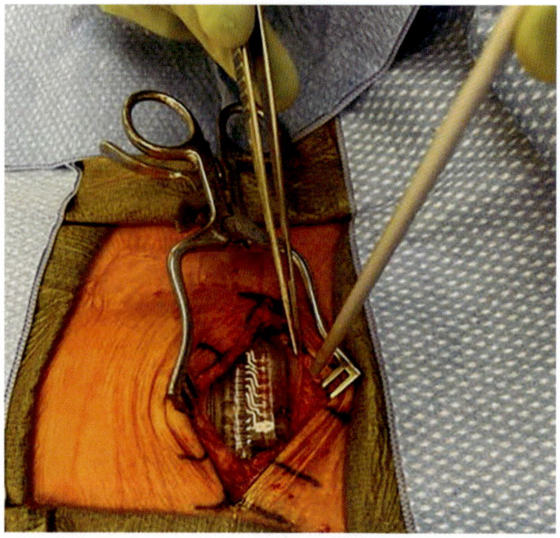

Fig. 6.5 A capsular layer is often encountered at closure of a pocket during implantable pulse generator replacement. In the photograph, the forceps are elevating this pseudocapsular layer.

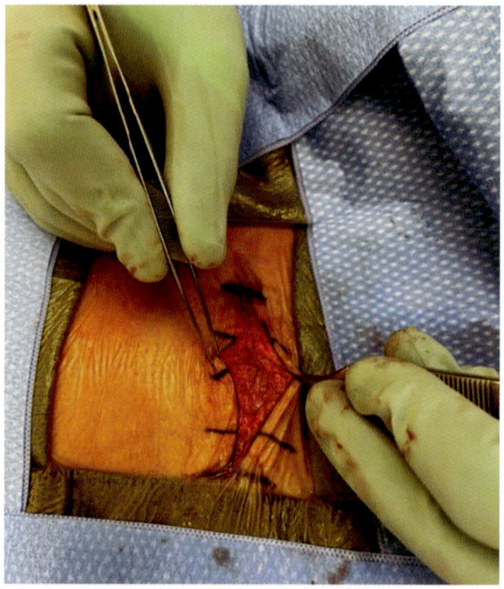

Fig. 6.6 The deep layer closure over implantable pulse generator is shown. Note that the device has complete tissue coverage.

The incision should be oriented perpendicularly to the layers of the skin and, where possible, should follow the Langer lines of the skin. This makes incision layers easier to realign. The first step of incision closure is actually incision creation.

Once the device is properly implanted, wound closure begins in earnest with anchoring of the device in place. As mentioned earlier, this step is crucial, as many complications are caused by catheter/lead migration or by dislodgment of the IPG or pump.[4,7,8] Best practice is to anchor the IPG and leads/catheter with a permanent stitch, such as 2-0 silk. Fig. 6.4 shows a properly anchored IPG.

With the device anchored in place, the process of closing the deep layers of the wound can begin. The deep layers of the wound are closed with 3-0 or 2-0 vicryl suture depending on the size of the individual and the quality of the tissue. Fig. 6.5 shows a capsular layer that may be found during the closure of a pocket with a previously implanted IPG. Fig. 6.6 demonstrates a wound in which its deep layers have been properly closed with vicryl suture.

Next, the deep dermal layers are closed with vicryl suture (Fig. 6.7). The final closure with a subcuticular 4-0 monocryl suture and skin adhesive is shown in Fig. 6.8. Opinions vary on the appropriate method for skin closure in implant cases. A meta-analysis found no evidence that subcuticular sutures reduce the risk of surgical site infection and many patients may prefer avoiding the need to remove sutures.[9]

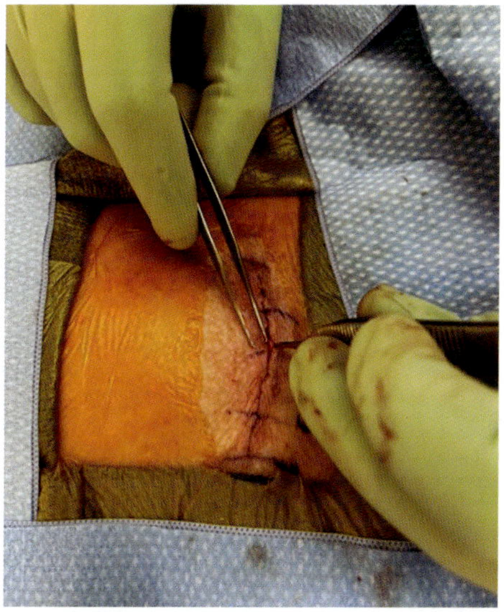

Fig. 6.7 Deep dermal coverage is complete in this photograph, adding another layer of tissue coverage.

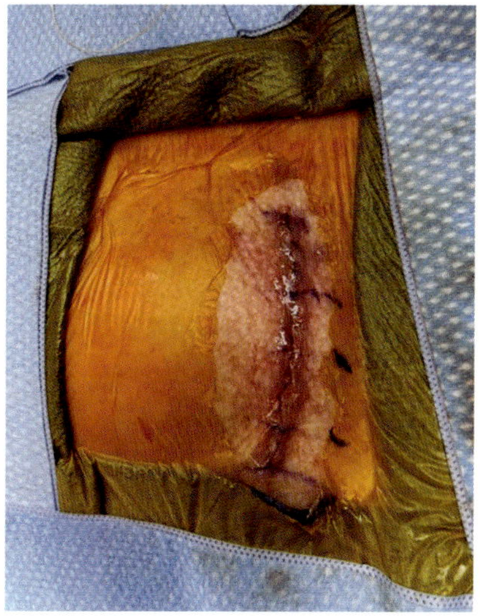

Fig. 6.8 Final wound closure. In this case, closure is accomplished with a subcuticular stitch and skin adhesive. Note the tension-free nature of the closure and the close approximation of the skin edges.

TABLE 6.1 Uses, Pros and Cons for Various Suture Types Commonly Used in Neuromodulation Surgeries

Suture Type	Location, Use	Pros	Cons
Nylon	Skin closure, anchoring device to fascia	Unbraided, strong	Must be removed, can be obscured in dark hair
Prolene	Skin, anchoring device to fascia	Unbraided, strong, blue color makes removal easier	Must be removed, memory makes suture handling more difficult
Monocryl	Skin	Undyed, absorbs, low inflammation	Persists in tissue for a long period
Vicryl	Deep layers or skin	Can be dyed or undyed, absorbs	Braided, may cause inflammation
PDS (polydioxanone)	Deep layers	Unbraided, less inflammation	Requires more knots
Tycron	Anchoring device to fascia	Strong, few knots needed	Braided, dyed
Silk	Anchoring device to fascia	Strong, few knots needed	Braided

Table 6.1 provides a list of commonly employed suture types along with relative pros and cons.

Intraoperative Complications

As mentioned earlier, many complications are likely influenced by wound closure, such as surgical site infection and device erosion. Wound closure and care is one of the key means by which surgeons can influence surgical outcome, along with patient selection. Relatively few intraoperative complications are specific to wound closure. Rarely, when an IPG or pump is being placed in a small patient, obtaining satisfactory tissue coverage for a tension-free closure may be difficult. In these cases, it may be beneficial to use cautery to undermine the skin flaps or expand the pocket in the case of a device replacement in an effort to create a tension-free closure environment conducive to healing. If extensive skin flap undermining or pocket expansion is performed, then a surgical drain could be considered.

General Considerations and Conclusions

Wound healing is the primary goal of wound closure. The approach to closure of a wound is one method by which a surgeon can control the healing of the wound. Another is by patient selection. Several patient factors can negatively affect wound healing and surgical closure. Some common factors are diabetes, obesity, nicotine use, incontinence, nutritional status, and immunosuppression. Surgeons should seek to modify these factors as much as possible to encourage wound healing. However, we do not have as much control over patient factors.[10]

In conclusion, surgical complications, including surgical site infection, are strongly influenced by patient factors and wound closure technique. There is no specific closure method that is appropriate for every neuromodulation patient or device. However, adherence to some general principles to improve closure outcomes is logical. These principles include appropriate device anchoring, good device tissue coverage by closing multiple layers, and ensuring a tension-free closure. If these technical pearls are observed, we can improve outcomes for our patients.

REFERENCES

1. Eldabe S, Buchser E, Duarte RV. Complications of spinal cord stimulation and peripheral nerve stimulation techniques: a review of the literature. *Pain Med.* 2016;17:325-336.
2. Necking E, Levi R, Ertzgaard P. Complications of intrathecal drug delivery therapy (ITDD): a retrospective study of 231 implantations between 1999 and 2014. *Clin Neurol Neurosurg.* 2021;205:106630.
3. Cameron T. Safety and efficacy of spinal cord stimulation for the treatment of chronic pain: a 20-year literature review. *J Neurosurg.* 2004;100(3 Suppl Spine):S254-S267.
4. Abraham M, Gold J, Dweck J, et al. Classifying device-related complications associated with intrathecal baclofen pumps: a MAUDE Study. *World Neurosurg.* 2020;139:e652-e657.
5. Westrup AM, Conner AK. Percutaneous thoracic spinal cord stimulator placement. *Cureus.* 2021;13(3):e13916.
6. Montagna W. Comparative anatomy and physiology of the skin. *Arch Dermatol.* 1967;96:357-363.
7. Sitzman BT, Provenzano DA. Best practices in spinal cord stimulation. *Spine.* 2017;42(suppl 14):S67-S71.
8. Levy R, Henderson J, Slavin K, et al. Incidence and avoidance of neurologic complications with paddle type spinal cord stimulation leads. *Neuromodulation.* 2011;14(5):412-422; discussion 422.
9. Goto S, Sakamoto T, Ganeko R, et al. Subcuticular sutures for skin closure in non-obstetric surgery. *Cochrane Database Syst Rev.* 2020;4(4):CD012124.
10. Bazurro S, Ball L, Pelosi P. Perioperative management of obese patient. *Curr Opin Crit Care.* 2018;24:560-567.

Chapter 7

Waveform Parameters: Electrical Field Interaction on Neuronal Milieu

Gustaf Van Acker, Mark N. Malinowski, and Chong Kim

Chapter Outline

Introduction

At 6:00 PM on March 24, 1967, neurosurgeon C. Norman Shealy, MD, James B. Reswick, PhD, and doctoral candidate J. Thomas Mortimer began applying electrical stimulation to the spinal cord of a patient with malignant pleural and liver cancer pain using a device designed by Mortimer.[1] Stimulation was applied through a single vitallium cathode electrode implanted approximating the dorsal columns, with the electrode sutured to the dura following T2 to T3 laminectomy. The anode electrode was placed intramuscularly nearby. Waveform stimulation parameters were set to a pulse width of 400 msec, frequency of 10 to 50 Hz, and amplitude of 0.36 to 0.52 mA. The patient experienced paresthesia in his chest and abdomen, corresponding to the location of his pain, and reported immediate relief. The patient's relief continued for the duration of the 1-hour session. The next day, stimulation was applied for approximately 10 hours with good relief, occasionally requiring parameter modification. Unfortunately, the patient died the next day due to complications from endocarditis with cerebral embolism. However, this case study would provide the first in vivo human evidence for the potential efficacy of spinal cord stimulation for the abolishment of pain.

The group applied stimulation parameters similar to what they, as well as Wall and Sweet, had applied to peripheral nerves for temporary abolition of pain,[2] which were based on the hypothetical mechanism of action by Melzack and Wall's recently postulated gate control theory. This theory suggested that, because large Aβ fibers are depolarized at a lower threshold than small Aβ and C fibers by an externally applied electrical field, stimulation can selectively activate large fibers, closing the gate and interrupting peripheral pain transmission to the brain at the dorsal horn.[3]

Electrical stimulation of biological tissue utilizes modulation of several key design elements that provide a set amount of electrical charge over time. These elements, or parameters, include but are not limited to stimulus pulse amplitude, pulse duration, pulse frequency, phase, interpulse, and interphase interval (Fig. 7.1A).[4] The combination of these parameters ultimately provides how much electricity, or total charge, is delivered to the central nervous system. *Total charge* can be thought of as the dose of electrical

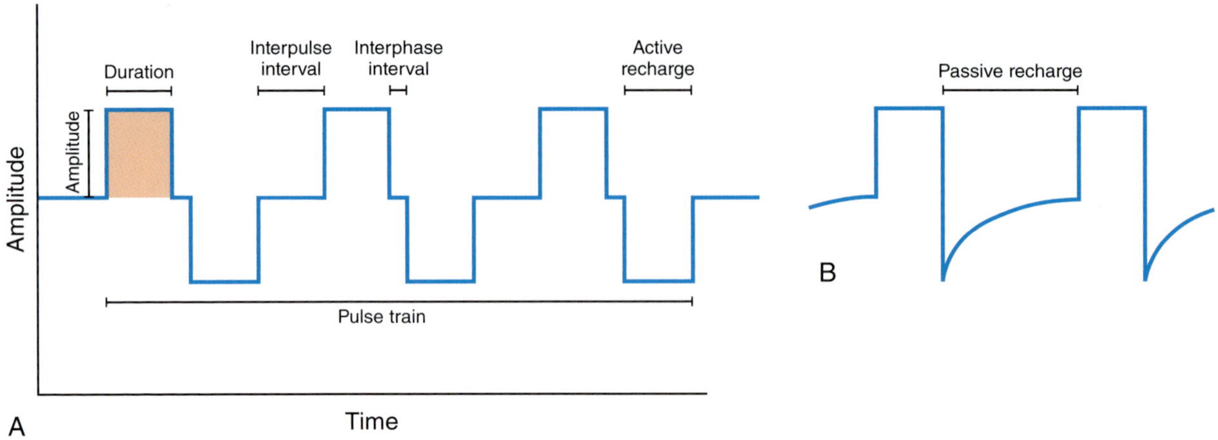

Fig. 7.1 Illustration of waveform components. (A) Pulse train shown, with amplitude on y-axis and time on x-axis. Pulse charge is a product of amplitude and pulse phase duration. Cathodic and anodic pulses are both active, the interpulse interval is the period between two full stimulation cycles, and the interphase interval is the period between phases. Frequency is the number of stimulation cycles per second. (B) Cathodic pulse followed by passive recharge, no interphase interval.

stimulation. Manipulating these parameters can have significant influence on the way that stimulation interacts with the neuronal elements within the electrical field. The neural system being targeted is also important to consider. Whether intracortical, epidural, peripheral, or transcutaneous, the stimulation goals may differ. For example, with spinal cord stimulation, certain parameters can have directly activating effects on large fibers, resulting in perceived paresthesia by the individual receiving the stimulation, whereas other parameters can provide a subthreshold, paresthesia-free interaction. In contrast, the goal of peripheral nerve stimulation may be to directly inhibit nerve conduction. In this chapter, we will discuss waveform parameters as they relate to spinal cord stimulation.

Basic Overview

PULSE

A basic stimulus pulse has four epochs: cathodic phase, interphase interval, anodic phase, and interpulse interval (see Fig. 7.1A). The pulse charge is equal to the product of the cathodic stimulus intensity and its duration. *Total charge* is defined as the product of stimulus intensity, duration, and frequency within a 1-second period. The stimulus intensity can be measured either by current or voltage, and per Ohm's Law $V = IR$, stimulus can be either voltage or current controlled. Current-controlled stimulation requires voltage to adjust with alterations in impedance.

Pulse duration is limited practically by the frequency of the stimulation and recovery method, whether active or passive. Charge balancing allows for recharge so that irreversible biochemical reactions are limited. This requires reversing polarity of the stimulation from anodic to cathodic repetitively. Active charge balance typically uses the same amplitude and duration in polarity opposite to the initial pulse phase in order to provide a net zero charge. However, as pulse charge is equal to the product of pulse intensity and duration, either parameter can be altered and compensated for by the other to obtain the same charge. Charge balancing can also be accomplished through passive recovery (see Fig. 7.1B). This typically takes longer than active recharge and should be taken into account when determining maximum frequency allowed.

A series of consecutive stimulus pulses, typically identified within a 1-second period, is the stimulus train. Stimulus pulses are often delivered at regular repeated intervals; the total number of pulses within a 1-second period is the frequency, measured in hertz. The frequency of pulses is limited by the duration of the pulses and interpulse interval. As the pulse duration increases, the allowable frequency decreases, particularly taking into account active or passive recharge.

Strength–Duration Curve

Activation of axonal fibers requires the charge to meet or exceed the minimum threshold for activation (Fig. 7.2). As charge is the product of amplitude and pulse duration, as amplitude decreases, greater pulse width is needed to achieve the charge necessary for activation.[5] Different nerve types have different diameters and amount of myelination; therefore, they have different strength–duration curves.[6] Activation threshold in the strength–duration curve is dependent on achieving a minimum activation threshold along the curve. *Rheobase* is defined as the minimum intensity, with indefinite pulse duration, required for fiber activation. The *chronaxie* is defined as the minimum pulse duration at an intensity twice the rheobase required for fiber activation. Recently, a group proposed adding patient paresthesia coverage as a variable to the classic strength–duration curve, which allows for optimal programming of the spinal cord stimulation device.[7]

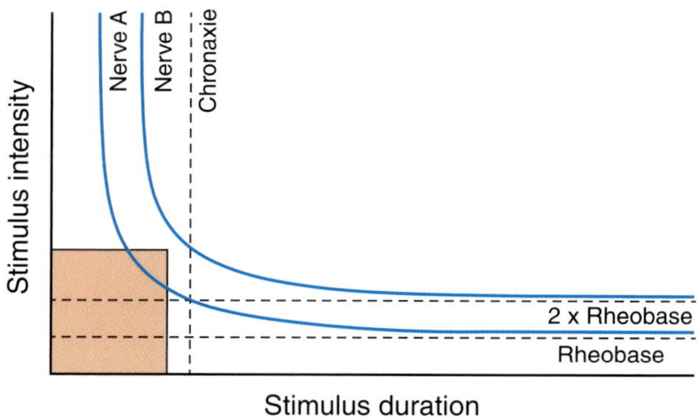

Fig. 7.2 **Strength–duration curve. Parameters required for nerve fiber activation are the product of stimulus intensity and duration exceeding a minimum activation threshold. *Rheobase* is defined as the minimum stimulus intensity required for fiber activation at infinite pulse duration. *Chronaxie* is the stimulus intensity at twice the rheobase. Nerves A and B have different physical properties, and therefore different strength–duration curves. The *red box* is a stimulus pulse with a product of stimulus intensity and duration that exceeds the strength–duration curve of Nerve A, but not Nerve B.**

Paresthesia Versus Nonparesthesia-Based Stimulation

Stimulation delivered to the spinal cord can provide pain relief via either paresthesia or paresthesia-free methods (Table 7.1). Paresthesia-based stimulation provides stimulus pulses to the dorsal column of the spinal cord that exceed the chronaxie, thereby activating nearby axonal fibers. To accomplish this method, surgical implantation of SCS leads over the dorsal columns is performed with the patient awake. Patient perception of paresthesia is mapped corresponding to the painful area, typically the legs or back. Stimulus pulses are delivered with regular interpulse intervals, at a frequency in the 20- to 200-Hz range.

Nonparesthesia stimulation provides subthreshold stimulation to the dorsal columns of the spinal cord. The SCS leads are surgically implanted using anatomical landmarks, typically placing one lead tip at the superior endplate of T8 and the second lead tip at the superior endplate of T9.

TABLE 7.1 Spinal Cord Stimulation Waveform Parameters of Traditional, 10kHz, and BurstDR

	Traditional Tonic	10 kHz	BurstDR
Amplitude (mA)	3.6–8.5	1.6–3.8	0.6
Cathodic phase duration (ms)	~0.2–0.6	0.030–0.040	1
Recharge phase duration (ms)	25	0.030–0.040	1
Interburst phase duration (ms)	—	—	15
Interphase interval (ms)	—	0.010	0
Interpulse interval (ms)	25	0.010	1
Interburst frequency (Hz)	—	—	40
Intraburst frequency (Hz)	~40–80	10,000	500
Intrapulse recharge phase	Passive	Active	Passive
Interburst recharge phase	—	—	Passive
Intraburst polarity	Bipolar	Bipolar	Monopolar
Interburst polarity	—	—	Bipolar
Paresthesia	Present	Absent	Absent

Traditional Paresthesia-Based Stimulation

SCS originally used to treat failed back surgery syndrome utilized paresthesia-inducing pulses covering the topography of pain with subjectively comfortable sensation, often described as tingling, buzzing, pressure, and so on.[8] Providing paresthesia overlying pain in the legs is more readily accomplished than that of the back; therefore, traditional stimulation has typically been employed to provide pain relief for radicular leg pain. The first randomized, multicenter controlled study comparing traditional stimulation to conservative medical management for failed back surgery syndrome with neuropathic leg pain, known as the PROCESS study, utilized a mean of 350 μs pulse width, 49 Hz, and regular interpulse intervals at 3.7V.[9] These general parameters continue to be used for paresthesia-based stimulation, with stimulus pulses usually applied at regular interpulse intervals at a frequency in the 20- to 200-Hz range, with pulse width around 200 to 400 μs (Fig. 7.3A). The product of the pulse width and amplitude exceeds the chronaxie of

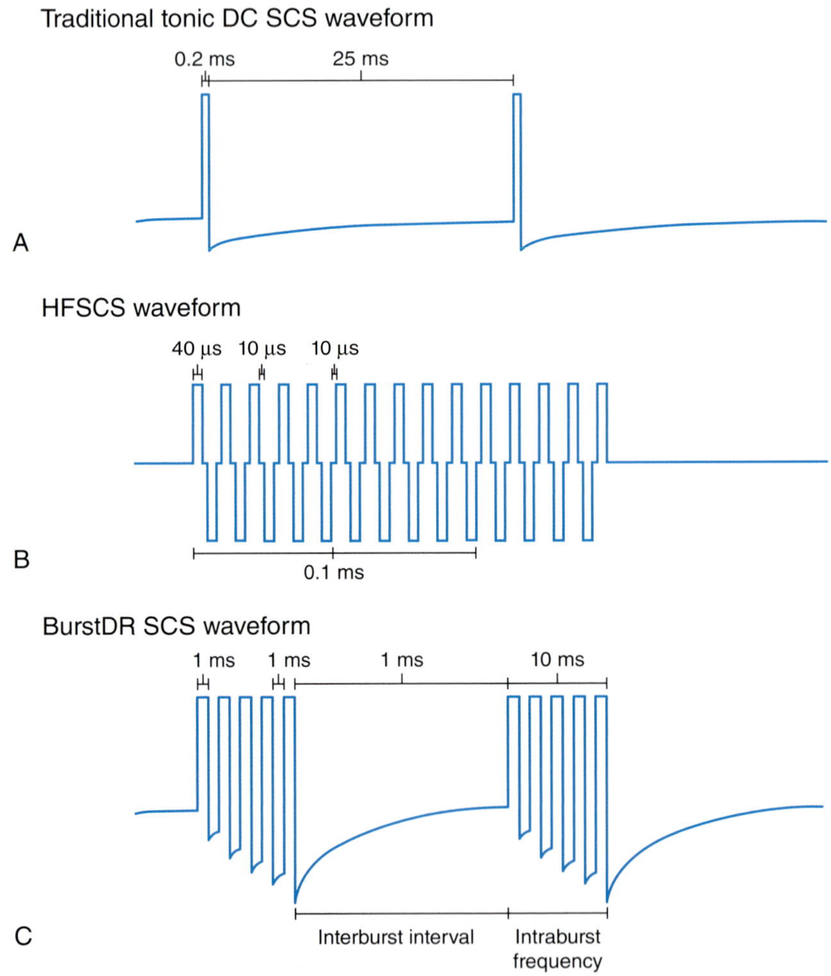

Fig. 7.3 Illustration of spinal cord stimulation (SCS) waveforms. (A) Traditional tonic dorsal column (DC) SCS waveform. Cathodic pulse duration shown at 0.2 ms, with passive recharge phase and interpulse interval at 25 ms; frequency at 40 Hz. (B) High-frequency (HF) SCF waveform. Cathodic and anodic pulse widths shown at 40 μs, each interphase and interpulse interval at 10 μs, and frequency at 10,000 Hz. Recharge phase is active. (C) BurstDR SCS waveform shown with train of 5 monophasic 1-ms pulses with 1-ms intraburst intervals and 15-ms interburst interval with passive recharge. Intraburst frequency of 500 Hz, and interburst frequency of 40 Hz.

fibers within the dorsal column of the spinal cord, which results in perceptive paresthesia. Results from later studies using different stimulation parameters, such as high-frequency stimulation, regularly use the results from the PROCESS study as a comparative measure. Paresthesia-based stimulation has not been shown to be effective for axial low back pain.[10] The proposed mechanism of action of paresthesia-based stimulation is increasing activity of wide dynamic range neurons in the dorsal horn of the spinal cord, releasing excitatory neurotransmitters with decreased release of inhibitory neurotransmitters.[11,12]

High Frequency

High-frequency spinal cord stimulation, or HFSCS, is generally defined as stimulation with a frequency of $\geq$ 1000 Hz.[13] The pulses delivered typically have uniform pulse trains, with regular and equal pulse duration, amplitude and interpulse interval (see Fig. 7.3B). At higher frequencies, including 10,000 Hz that Nevro pioneered in the SCS field and coined *HF10*, charge balancing must be supplied actively as opposed to passively (see Fig. 7.2A). This is because the interpulse interval, or time between pulses, is too short to allow for complete passive recharge.[14] This charge-balanced active recharge pulse train must also use pulse durations less than traditional stimulation due to time constraints. For 10,000 Hz SCS, the pulse duration is usually 30 to 40 μs, compared with 400 μs in traditional stimulation.[14] Interpulse and interphase intervals at 10,000 Hz and 40 μs pulse width are each 10 μs.

Although HFSCS is delivered at a pulse intensity too low to directly depolarize spinal cord axons,[15-17] the total charge of the stimulation train is larger than that of traditional stimulation by an order of magnitude.[18] This may be a key component in HFSCS mechanism of action. As HFSCS is paresthesia free—as opposed to traditional SCS, which utilizes paresthesia overlapping the painful area—the mechanism of action most likely differs. Additionally, unlike kilohertz-frequency alternating current (KHFAC; 10k Hz) stimulation of peripheral nerves, which effectively shuts down nerve fibers through direct nerve depolarization,[19] HFSCS likely acts through a mechanism of action different than direct nerve depolarization.

Modelling studies have shown that this stimulation method is unlikely to directly activate or block dorsal column fibers or dorsal root ganglia.[15] KHFAC stimulation is hypothesized to have distinct sub- and suprathreshold effects that are unique to this frequency range. Neuronal responses to stimuli at this frequency have varied effects, including facilitation, desynchronization, nonmonotonic activation, spike-rate adaptation, conduction block, and synaptic fatigue.[20] One hypothesis for the action of paresthesia-free stimulation is that the low-intensity electrical field may act on axonal branch points and inhibit propagation, such as those of Aβ axons branching off to the dorsal horn circuitry. Aβ ectopic firing has been hypothesized to play a role in central pain perpetuity; its inhibition may attenuate pain propagation.[4] An alternative hypothesis is that high-frequency stimulation of the dorsal spinal cord, with concomitant high total charge, results in heating of the spinal cord. An in vitro modelling study by Zannou et al.[21] suggests that stimulation of the dorsal spinal cord with 10 kHz, 3.5 mA, and a 40- to 10- to 40- to 10-μs biphasic pulse pattern (see Fig. 7.3B) resulted in a temperature increase of 0.18 to 1.72° C.[21] This heating is hypothesized to reduce nuclear factor kappa B (NF-κB)–dependent satellite glial cell activation, thereby reducing inflammatory response.[21] Of note, glial cell overactivity results in increased inflammatory mediators that are hypothesized to be significantly involved in chronic central pain. Modulation of this system may play an important role in pain regulation.[22] However, thermal effects of KHFAC stimulation in vivo remains to be validated.[20]

Other high-frequency parameters have been investigated. For example, Al-Kaisy et al.[23] performed a prospective, randomized, sham-controlled, double-blind crossover of patients with failed back surgery syndrome. The subjects were randomized to 5882 Hz, 3030 Hz, 1200 Hz, and sham. This study demonstrated that 5882 Hz had the greatest reduction in pain score, while 3030 Hz and 1200 Hz had a statistically equal significant decrease in pain scores compared with sham.[23]

As the total charge of an HFSCS stimulation train is a magnitude larger than traditional stimulation,[18] safety of this stimulation has necessarily been carefully evaluated. Neural damage has been well established to be related to charge density.[24] Exceeding the electrochemical water window of irreversible reactions at the electrode surface-neural interface can result in pH changes, redox reactions, and toxic products.[25] The water window is defined as the voltage range at which neither oxidation nor reduction of protons occurs.[26] By these standards, and through subsequent clinical evaluation (SENZA RCT), 10-kHz SCS has been deemed safe.[18,27]

Burst Stimulation

SCS utilizing a burst pattern, rather than tonic, was first proposed for limb and back pain by De Ridder et al.[28] Patients receiving the burst pattern had better results than those receiving the tonic pattern. This pattern, known as BurstDR, utilizes five 1-ms monophasic pulses, with 1-ms interpulse intervals, applied with 1 passive recharge interburst period of 15 ms (see Fig. 7.3C). These 500-Hz bursts are applied at 40 Hz. The reasoning behind this pattern is to simulate a more natural neuronal burst-firing pattern as compared with tonic-firing patterns. Burst stimulation increases synaptic connectivity in short- and long-term anatomical pathways, acting upon short- and long-term plasticity of the thalamic-anterior cingulate pathway.[11] Stimulation through this pathway is hypothesized to interfere with the oscillatory thalamic-cingulate network responsible for pain attention, memory, and anxiety.[29,30] Burst stimulation has been shown to increase dorsal anterior cingulate cortex activation, as imaged through encephalography.[28] Due to low absolute stimulus intensity, burst stimulation tends to be paresthesia free. Burst parameters are lower than traditional tonic parameters and comparatively do not act on wide dynamic range and low-threshold neurons within the gracile nucleus of the dorsal columns, which is involved in tactile sensory information.[31]

Closed Loop

A surgically implanted epidural electrode moves in space relative to the spinal cord with changes in position. Therefore, electrical stimulation arriving at the cord changes strength relative to position. This is the case with SCS devices that use open-loop preset tonic or burst stimulation parameters. To account for this, closed-loop stimulation utilizes recorded evoked compound action potentials (ECAPs) as a measure of relative electrode proximity to the spinal cord. This information is then used to increase or decrease the stimulus output amplitude.[32] The goal is to maintain a relatively constant stimulus amplitude within a therapeutic window arriving at the spinal cord. This closed-loop system has been shown to be effective for both axial back and radicular pain.[33]

Differential Targeted Multiplexed

Development and maintenance of chronic neuropathic pain and nociceptive pain is hypothesized to involve aberrant neuroglial activity. Microglia are known to be involved in the development and maintenance of neuropathic pain states.[34-36] Electrical stimulation of the dorsal column of the spinal cord acts on both neurons and glial cells, and glial cells outnumber neurons 12:1.[37] The electrical resting potential of glial cells are different than that of neurons and are depolarized at different frequencies and amplitudes. Differential targeted multiplexed programming (DTM) utilizes multiple differing waveforms to act on neuronal tissue, including pain fibers and, more importantly, glial cells within the dorsal horn of the spinal cord.[38] Following an inciting event, a phenotypic change occurs that results in a change in the glial cell milieu within the spinal cord. Over time, if glial cell overactivity persists, chronic, centralized pain can develop due to glial cell production of proinflammatory mediators and changes in proteomics, resulting in a chronically inflamed state. This inflamed state is hypothesized to perpetuate central pain state. Vallejo et al., using a scientific model previously described,[39] developed DTM by varying stimulation parameter components delivered to an electrode epidurally implanted over the dorsal columns of rats using a neuropathic pain model.[40] Stimulation was then applied for 72 hours continuously followed by dorsal column tissue sample proteomic analysis. The proteomics of the dorsal column of the rat spinal cord postinjury followed SCS was then compared to a preinjured state. Stimulation using DTM attempts to rebalance the aberrant neuroglial interactions from pain state back to a baseline state using these animal model optimal stimulation parameters. Specific parameter components—such as charge phase, charge balancing, and interphase interval—were optimized to provide the closest return from pain state to pre-pain state. While DTM is not necessarily one signal, or waveform, it currently combines two bipoles for each of four different signals, with frequencies ranging from 50 to 1200 Hz.[39] However, as more effective stimulation parameters are discovered, DTM is likely to continue to be modified in the clinic for optimal pain relief.

Conclusion

Applying electrical stimulation to the spinal cord for pain relief has been utilized for greater than 50 years. For 40 of those years, application was largely premised on the gate control theory of Melzack and Wall. More recently, investigations have yielded more precise mechanisms of cord stimulation. Hypothesis-driven waveform parameter creation, basic science data collection, and industry-driven motivation have prompted advances that have improved the effectiveness of interaction between stimulus and neuronal response. As we improve our understanding of this stimulus parameter and neuronal response interplay, waveform modification will continue to evolve.

REFERENCES

1. Shealy CN, Mortimer JT, Reswick JB. Electrical inhibition of pain by stimulation of the dorsal columns: preliminary clinical report. *Anesth Analg*. 1967;46(4):489-491.
2. Wall PD, Sweet WH. Temporary abolition of pain in man. *Science*. 1967;155(3758):108-109.
3. Melzack R, Wall PD. Pain mechanisms: a new theory. *Science*. 1965;150(3699):971-979.
4. Miller JP, Eldabe S, Buchser E, Johanek LM, Guan Y, Linderoth B. Parameters of spinal cord stimulation and their role in electrical charge delivery: a review. *Neuromodulation*. 2016;19(4):373-384.
5. Crozier WJ. Strength-duration curves and the theory of electrical excitation. *Proc Natl Acad Sci U S A*. 1937;23(2):71-78.
6. Tanaka S, Gomez-Tames J, Wasaka T, Inui K, Ueno S, Hirata A. Electrical characterisation of adelta-fibres based on human in vivo electrostimulation threshold. *Front Neurosci*. 2020;14:588056.
7. Abejon D, Rueda P, del Saz J, Arango S, Monzon E, Gilsanz F. Is the introduction of another variable to the strength-duration curve necessary in neurostimulation? *Neuromodulation*. 2015;18(3):182-190; discussion 190.
8. Burton CV. Safety and clinical efficacy. *Neurosurgery*. 1977;1:214-215.
9. Kumar K, Taylor RS, Jacques L, et al. Spinal cord stimulation versus conventional medical management for neuropathic pain: a multicentre randomised controlled trial in patients with failed back surgery syndrome. *Pain*. 2007;132(1-2):179-188.
10. Kreiner DS, Matz P, Bono CM, et al. Guideline summary review: an evidence-based clinical guideline for the diagnosis and treatment of low back pain. *Spine J*. 2020;20(7):998-1024.
11. Chakravarthy K, Fishman MA, Zuidema X, Hunter CW, Levy R. Mechanism of action in burst spinal cord stimulation: review and recent advances. *Pain Med*. 2019;20(suppl 1):S13-S22.
12. Foreman RD, Linderoth B. Neural mechanisms of spinal cord stimulation. *Int Rev Neurobiol*. 2012;107:87-119.
13. Bicket MC, Dunn RY, Ahmed SU. High-frequency spinal cord stimulation for chronic pain: pre-clinical overview and systematic review of controlled trials. *Pain Med*. 2016;17(12):2326-2336.
14. Russo M, Van Buyten JP. 10-kHz High-frequency SCS therapy: a clinical summary. *Pain Med*. 2015;16(5):934-942.
15. Lempka SF, McIntyre CC, Kilgore KL, Machado AG. Computational analysis of kilohertz frequency spinal cord stimulation for chronic pain management. *Anesthesiology*. 2015;122(6):1362-1376.
16. Tang R, Martinez M, Goodman-Keiser M, Farber JP, Qin C, Foreman RD. Comparison of burst and tonic spinal cord stimulation on spinal neural processing in an animal model. *Neuromodulation*. 2014;17(2):143-151.
17. Song Z, Viisanen H, Meyerson BA, Pertovaara A, Linderoth B. Efficacy of kilohertz-frequency and conventional spinal cord stimulation in rat models of different pain conditions. *Neuromodulation*. 2014;17(3):226-234; discussion 234-235.
18. Kapural L, Yu C, Doust MW, et al. Novel 10-kHz high-frequency therapy (HF10 therapy) is superior to traditional low-frequency spinal cord stimulation for the treatment of chronic back and leg pain: the SENZA-RCT randomized controlled trial. *Anesthesiology*. 2015;123(4):851-860.
19. Kilgore KL, Bhadra N. Reversible nerve conduction block using kilohertz frequency alternating current. *Neuromodulation*. 2014;17(3):242-254; discussion 254-255.
20. Neudorfer C, Chow CT, Boutet A, et al. Kilohertz-frequency stimulation of the nervous system: a review of underlying mechanisms. *Brain Stimul*. 2021;14(3):513-530.
21. Zannou AL, Khadka N, Truong DQ, et al. Temperature increases by kilohertz frequency spinal cord stimulation. *Brain Stimul*. 2019;12(1):62-72.
22. Vallejo R, Bradley K, Kapural L. Spinal cord stimulation in chronic pain: mode of action. *Spine (Phila Pa 1976)*. 2017;42(suppl 14):S53-S60.
23. Al-Kaisy A, Palmisani S, Pang D, et al. Prospective, randomized, shamcontrol, double blind, crossover trial of subthreshold spinal cord stimulation at various kilohertz frequencies in subjects suffering from failed back surgery syndrome (SCS frequency study). *Neuromodulation*. 2018;21(5):457-465.
24. McCreery DB, Agnew WF, Yuen TG, Bullara LA. Relationship between stimulus amplitude, stimulus frequency and neural damage during electrical stimulation of sciatic nerve of cat. *Med Biol Eng Comput*. 1995;33(3 Spec No):426-429.
25. Merrill DR, Bikson M, Jefferys JG. Electrical stimulation of excitable tissue: design of efficacious and safe protocols. *J Neurosci Methods*. 2005;141(2):171-198.
26. Vrabec T, Bhadra N, Van Acker G, Bhadra N, Kilgore K. Continuous direct current nerve block using multi contact high capacitance electrodes. *IEEE Trans Neural Syst Rehabil Eng*. 2017;25(6):517-529.
27. Kapural L, Al-Kaisey A. Ten kilohertz (10 kHz) high-frequency spinal cord stimulation. In: Krames ES, Peckham PH, Rezai AR, eds. *Neuromodulation: Comprehensive Textbook of Principles, Technologies, and Therapies*. UK: Vol 2. Elsevier; 2018:693-699.

28. De Ridder D, Plazier M, Kamerling N, Menovsky T, Vanneste S. Burst spinal cord stimulation for limb and back pain. *World Neurosurg*. 2013;80(5):642-649.e1.
29. Shyu BC, Vogt BA. Short-term synaptic plasticity in the nociceptive thalamic-anterior cingulate pathway. *Mol Pain*. 2009;5:51.
30. De Ridder D, Vanneste S. Burst and tonic spinal cord stimulation: different and common brain mechanisms. *Neuromodulation*. 2016;19(1):47-59.
31. Gong WY, Johanek LM, Sluka KA. A comparison of the effects of burst and tonic spinal cord stimulation on hyperalgesia and physical activity in an animal model of neuropathic pain. *Anesth Analg*. 2016;122(4):1178-1185.
32. Mekhail N, Levy RM, Deer TR, et al. Long-term safety and efficacy of closed-loop spinal cord stimulation to treat chronic back and leg pain (Evoke): a double-blind, randomised, controlled trial. *Lancet Neurol*. 2020;19(2):123-134.
33. Russo M, Brooker C, Cousins MJ, et al. Sustained long-term outcomes with closed-loop spinal cord stimulation: 12-month results of the prospective, multicenter, open-label Avalon study. *Neurosurgery*. 2020;87(4):E485-E495.
34. Vallejo R, Tilley DM, Vogel L, Benyamin R. The role of glia and the immune system in the development and maintenance of neuropathic pain. *Pain Pract*. 2010;10(3):167-184.
35. Ji RR, Berta T, Nedergaard M. Glia and pain: is chronic pain a gliopathy? *Pain*. 2013;154(suppl 1):S10-S28.
36. Grace PM, Wang X, Strand KA, et al. DREADDed microglia in pain: implications for spinal inflammatory signaling in male rats. *Exp Neurol*. 2018;304:125-131.
37. Ruiz-Sauri A, Orduña-Valls JM, Blasco-Serra A, et al. Glia to neuron ratio in the posterior aspect of the human spinal cord at thoracic segments relevant to spinal cord stimulation. *J Anat*. 2019;235(5):997-1006.
38. Vallejo R, Kelley CA, Gupta A, Smith WJ, Vallejo A, Cedeno DL. Modulation of neuroglial interactions using differential target multiplexed spinal cord stimulation in an animal model of neuropathic pain. *Mol Pain*. 2020;16:1744806920918057.
39. Vallejo R. DTM "Differential Targeted Multiplexed" Spinal Cord Stimulation: What Is It, and How Does it Work? Neurovations Virtual Webinar, September 10, 2021. Accessed https://neurovations.com/event/differential-target-multiplexed-dtm-spinal-cord-stimulation-scs-what-isit-and-how-does-it-work/
40. Tilley DM, Lietz CB, Cedeno DL, Kelley CA, Li L, Vallejo R. Proteomic modulation in the dorsal spinal cord following spinal cord stimulation therapy in an in vivo neuropathic pain model. *Neuromodulation*. 2021;24(1):22-32.

Chapter 8

Percutaneous Spinal Cord Stimulator Trial

Neel Mehta, Rohit Aiyer, and Alaa Abd-Elsayed

Chapter Outline

Introduction

Neuromodulation is based on the principle of electrically stimulating the dorsal column in the spinal cord to mask and intercept pain signals that are transmitted to the brain.[1] This concept of spinal cord stimulation (SCS) technology is based on the gate control theory of pain proposed by Melzack and Wall in 1965.[2] In essence, the "gate" in the dorsal horn of the spinal cord regulates signal transduction from the spinal cord to the brain that is indicated in pain perception. Aß fibers (nonnociceptive stimuli) and C fibers (nociceptive stimuli) synapse with the projection neurons of the spinothalamic tract on the dorsal horn of the spinal cord.[3] The gate control theory therefore suggests that stimulating both Aß fibers and C fibers closes the gate, which results in blocking and masking pain transmission signals to the brain.[3] This led to the first dorsal column stimulator in 1967 for treatment of chronic pain.[4] Over the decades, there have been many developments and advances in SCS. Traditional, conventional/tonic stimulation was the only treatment, with low frequency (40–100 Hz), high amplitude (3.6–8.5 mA), and pulse widths ranging between 300 and 600 μs.[3] In recent years, there has been the introduction of high-frequency (10 khz) stimulation with a pulse width at 30 μs and amplitude ranging between 1 and 5 mA. There has also been the development of burst SCS, which is a series of five 1000-μs pulses delivered at 500 Hz followed by a repolarization pulse. This is then repeated at 40 Hz.[3]

The spinal cord stimulator consists of leads placed in epidural space along the dorsal column, which is then connected to an implantable pulse generator (IPG).[5] The IPG contains a battery and processor that is surgically placed in either the gluteal, abdominal, or flank anatomical areas of the patient.[5] The IPG is either rechargeable or nonchargeable depending on the device company.

Anatomical Considerations

Spinal cord anatomy knowledge is critical to understand the principles of SCS in pain relief. Stimulation of rostral lateral fibers is utilized for axial back pain, whereas caudal medial fibers are stimulated for radicular pain.[6] It should be noted that as an electrical field moves laterally, the risk of stimulating anatomical regions such as the dorsal or ventral roots is increased, which can cause muscle contractions or painful sensation.[6] For patients with failed back surgical syndrome, the target area is usually T8 to T9, the lower thoracic spine. For patients with post-cervical surgery pain, the target area is around C4 to C5, the mid-cervical spine.[6]

The dorsal columns are in a lamellated arrangement.[7] The fibers are layered from medial to lateral within the dorsal columns. The initial caudal fibers that create the dorsal columns represent the sacral and perineal regions, which comprise the medial aspect of the dorsal columns. These are then layered on from medial to lateral to represent S11, and then from L5 to L1.[7] This continues from the lumbar to the cervical region. Consequently, knowledge of anatomy is essential to ensure the success of SCS in treating a patient's chronic pain condition.

Step-by-Step Description of the Procedure

1. Place the patient in a prone position with adequate support under the abdomen (pillows often best) to remove any lordotic curve (Fig. 8.1).
2. Place appropriate draping and sterile antiseptic solution, such as 2% chlorhexidine gluconate/70% isopropyl alcohol, on the patient to ensure the proper sterile environment and reduce the risk of bloodstream and surgical site infections. Prepare the patient with sterile drapes in the usual sterile fashion (Figs. 8.2 and 8.3).
3. Fluoroscopy is then utilized for image-guided assistance. Levels of the spine can be confirmed with fluoroscopy in the anteroposterior (AP) position (Fig. 8.4).

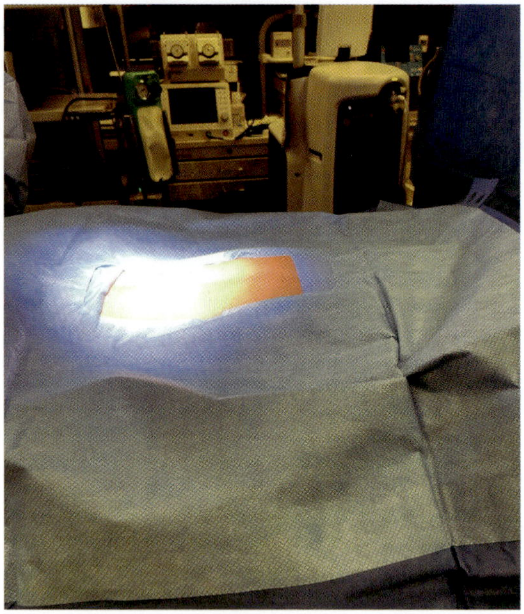

Fig. 8.2 Place appropriate draping and sterile antiseptic solution, such as 2% chlorhexidine gluconate/70% isopropyl alcohol, on the patient to ensure the proper sterile environment and reduce the risk of bloodstream and surgical site infections.

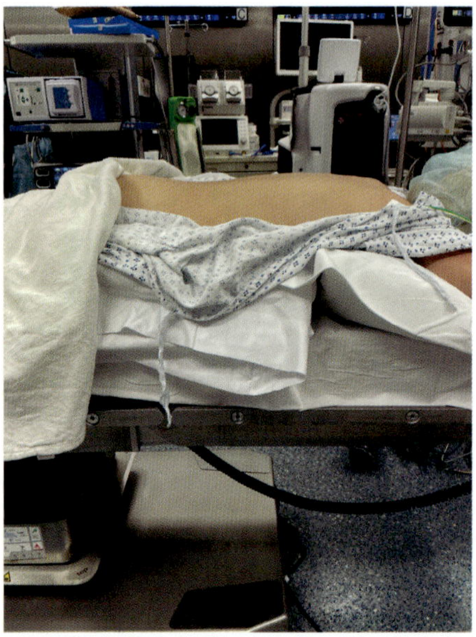

Fig. 8.1 Place the patient in a prone position with adequate support under the abdomen (pillows often best) to remove any lordotic curve.

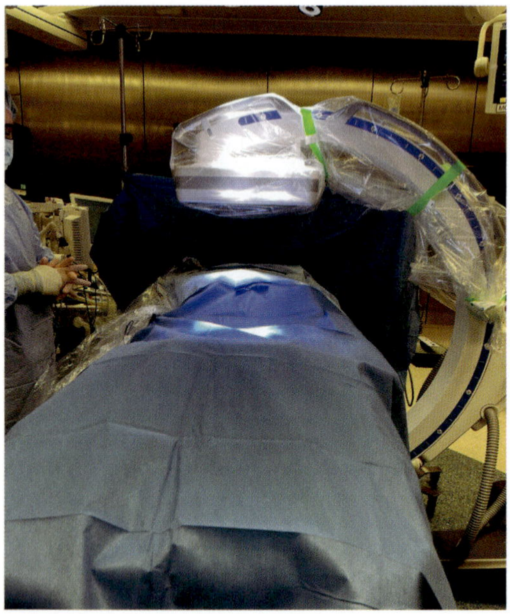

Fig. 8.3 Prepare the patient with sterile drapes in the usual sterile fashion.

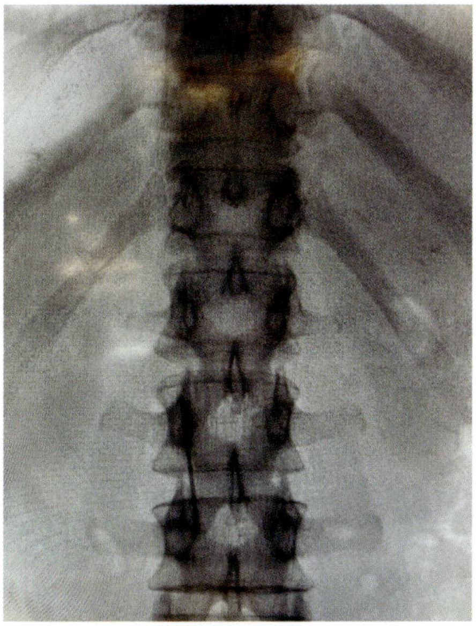

Fig. 8.4 Fluoroscopy is then utilized for image-guided assistance. Levels of the spine can be confirmed with fluoroscopy in the anteroposterior position.

4. Antibiotic prophylaxis can be utilized as per hospital or clinic protocol, such as weight-based intravenous cefazolin.
5. Identify the level appropriate for 14-gauge Touhy needle entry point. The skin entry level of the needle is usually one level below epidural space access. For example, if the epidural access target is T12/L1, the skin entry would be L2. Fig. 8.5 shows a skin needle on the site of the left L2 pedicle.
6. Local anesthetic can be administered at that area to anesthetize the skin and subcutaneous tissues (Fig. 8.5).
7. The Tuohy needle is aligned either just over or slightly medial to the pedicle at the level of skin entry (Fig. 8.6).
8. The Tuohy needle is then inserted at an angle of 30 to 45 degrees, with the bevel facing downward (Fig. 8.7).
9. The Tuohy needle is then directed medially toward the spinous process of the vertebra level above (Fig. 8.8).
10. Once the needle is above the lamina (of the vertebra level above), the needle angle is steepened to make contact with the lamina.

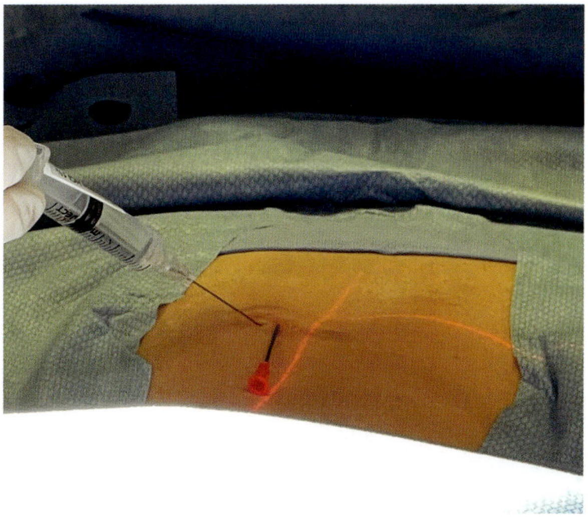

Fig. 8.5 Local anesthetic can be administered at that area to anesthetize the skin and subcutaneous tissues.

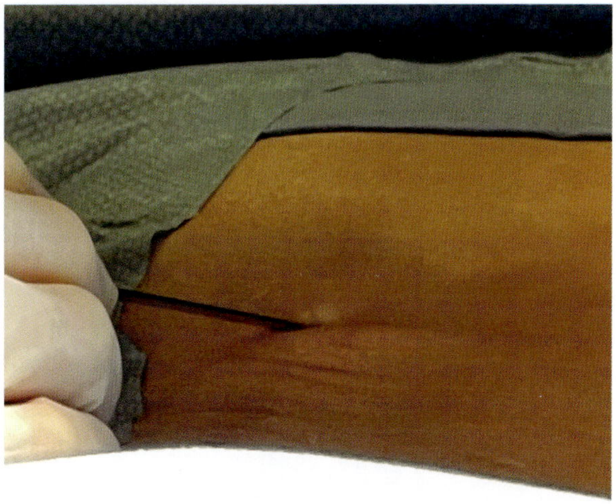

Fig. 8.6 The Tuohy needle is aligned either just over or slightly medial to the pedicle at the level of skin entry.

11. The bevel of the needle is then rotated to face upward.
12. The needle is then slowly moved cephalad "walking along" the lamina.
13. When the needle "walks off" the lamina, it is in close proximity to accessing the epidural space (very close to the ligamentum flavum).
14. This is an appropriate time to consider placing a second needle for an additional lead in

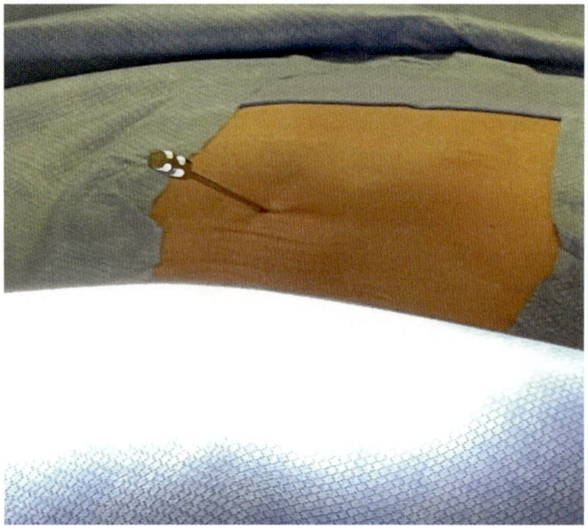

Fig. 8.7 The Tuohy needle is then inserted at an angle of 30 to 45 degrees, with the bevel facing downward.

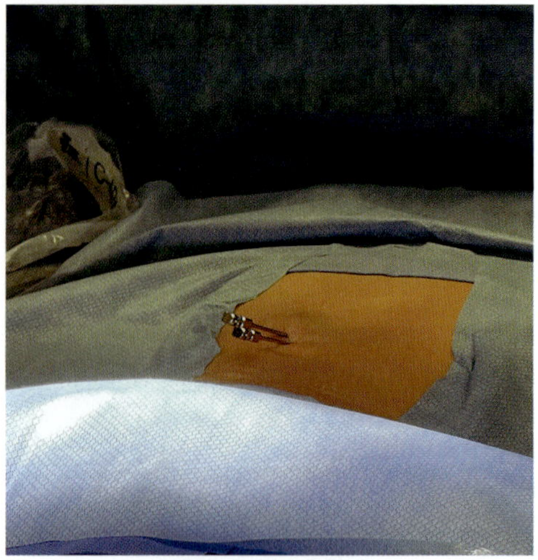

Fig. 8.9 This is an appropriate time to consider placing a second needle for an additional lead in a similar fashion as the first needle.

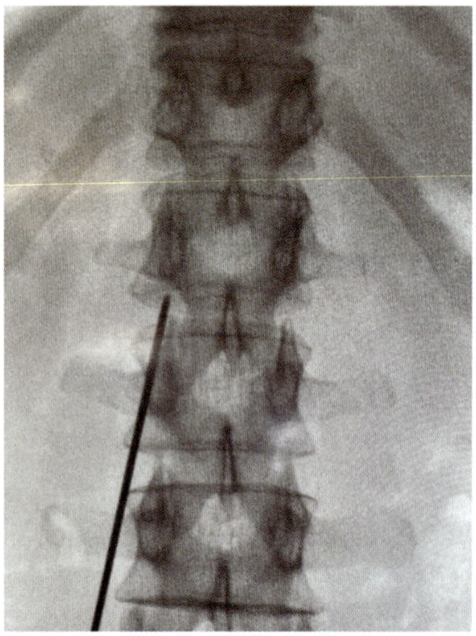

Fig. 8.8 The Tuohy needle is then directed medially toward the spinous process of the vertebra level above.

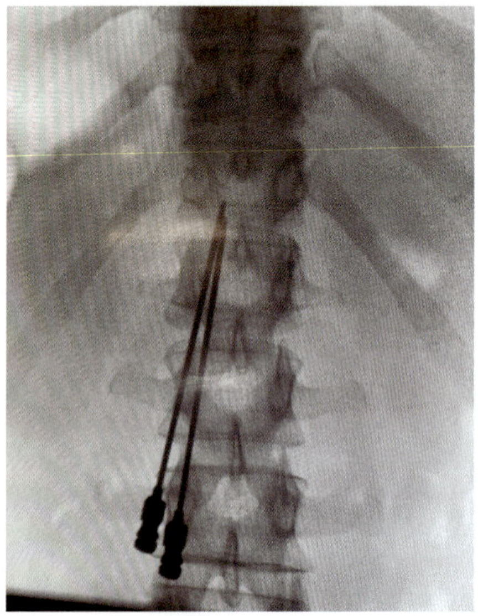

Fig. 8.10 Anteroposterior fluoroscopic view of second needle placement. Note use of the same side and same level approach. This can utilize the same anesthetized track and minimize postoperative pain.

a similar fashion as just described (Figs. 8.9–8.11).

15. Remove the needle stylet from the Touhy needle. Use either a glass or plastic syringe for loss-of-resistance technique.
16. Lateral fluoroscopic images should be used for confirmation of loss of resistance, which is acquired by using either an intermittent or continuous technique or by the guidewire technique (Fig. 8.12).
17. Insert the spinal cord stimulator trial lead into the Touhy needle (Fig. 8.13)
18. After the lead is inserted, visualize it under fluoroscopy in the lateral view. This will help

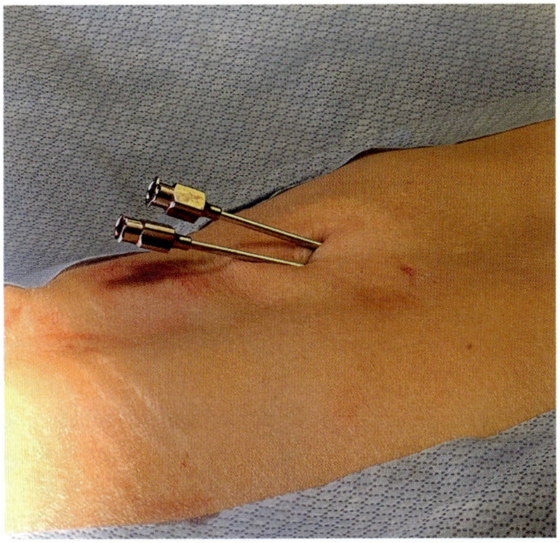

Fig. 8.11 View of two-needle placement, same level, same side. Note the same 30- to 45-degree approach.

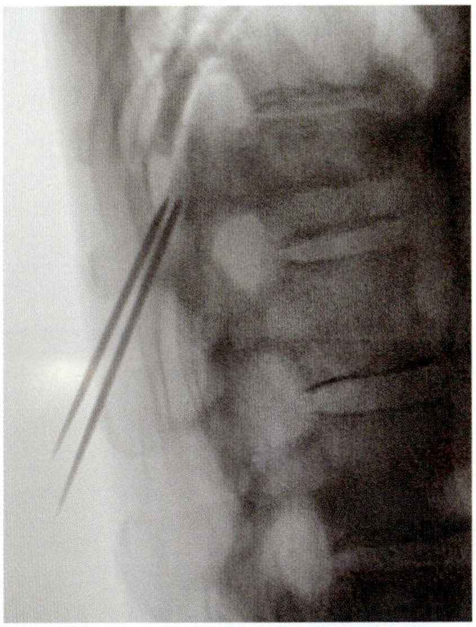

Fig. 8.12 Lateral fluoroscopic view of two-needle placement, same spinal level.

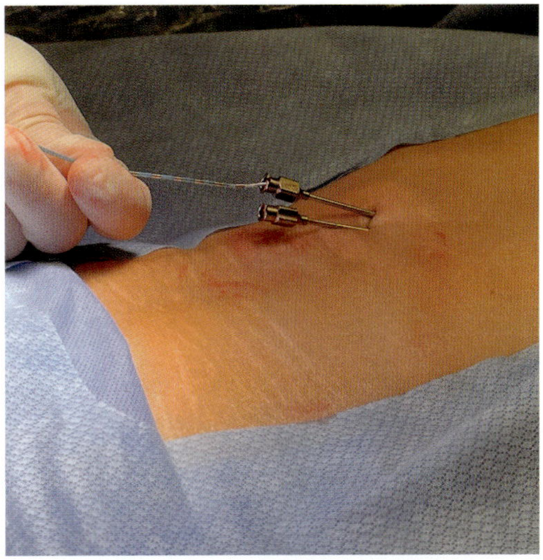

Fig. 8.13 Insert the spinal cord stimulator trial lead into the Touhy needle.

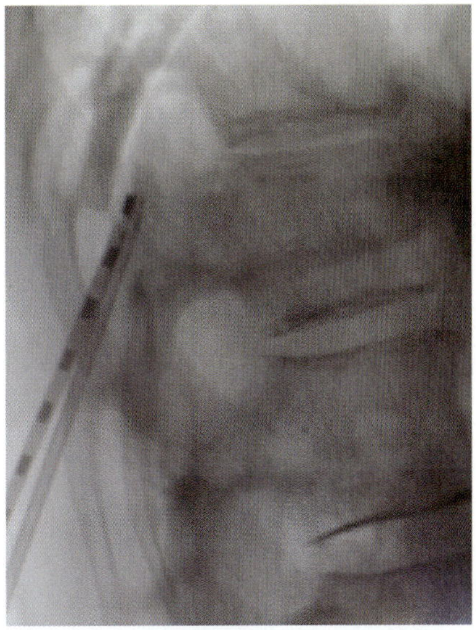

Fig. 8.14 Lateral fluoroscopic images are useful for confirmation of loss-of-resistance entry into the epidural space.

confirm that the lead is located in the posterior epidural space and is not travelling anteriorly (Figs. 8.14 and 8.15).

19. Return the C-arm to AP view. Using a two-hand technique, use your dominant hand to control the lead by holding the stylet with your thumb and index finger (Fig. 8.16).
20. Use your nondominant hand to advance the lead through the epidural space.
21. While advancing the lead with your nondominant hand, control or "steer" the direction of the lead with fine movements, rotations, and adjustments of the stylet with your dominant hand's thumb and index finger (see Fig. 8.16).

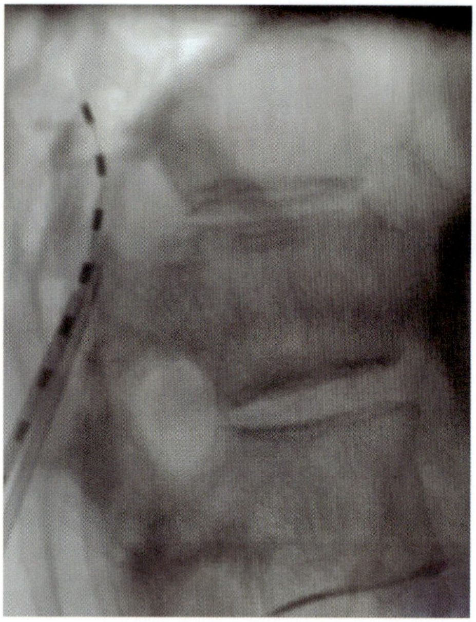

Fig. 8.15 Here, the lead is seen in the lateral view to confirm that the lead is located in the posterior epidural space and not travelling anteriorly.

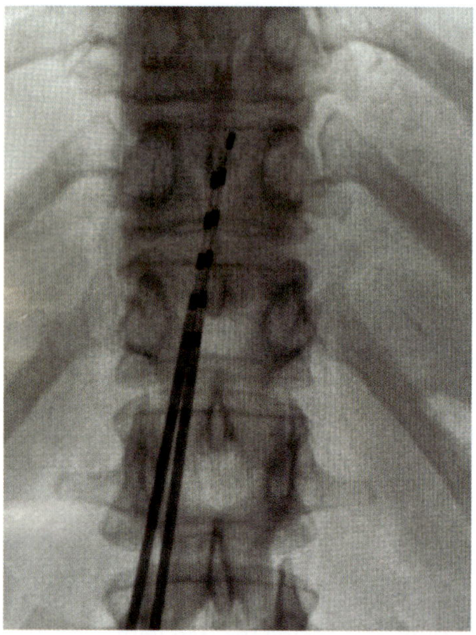

Fig. 8.16 Here, the fingers are performing a two-hand technique. Use the dominant hand to control the lead by holding the stylet with your thumb and index finger. Control or "steer" the direction of the lead with fine movements, rotations, and adjustments of the stylet with your dominant hand's thumb and index finger.

22. While advancing the lead, continuous live fluoroscopy should be used.
23. While advancing the lead, there may be areas of resistance due to possible stenosis or scar tissue. Adjustments of the stylet will be required to maneuver around these areas of resistance.
24. Drive the lead to the target level vertebrae, utilizing fluoroscopy to confirm accuracy and posterior epidural space positioning. Use AP and lateral views (Figs. 8.16 and 8.17).
25. Once at target level, testing can begin to check that maximal and optimal pain relief is obtained for the patient. This is done with the assistance of a SCS device representative. It should be noted that, depending on the patient and SCS device, a second lead may have to be placed in the midline. Therefore, these steps may need to be repeated (Figs. 8.18 and 8.19).
26. Once programming is completed, disconnect the stylet from the lead.
27. Hold the lead tightly proximally to the needle hub. Then, retract the needle from the epidural space while holding the lead in place (Fig. 8.20).
28. After removing the needle, the lead should be exposed.

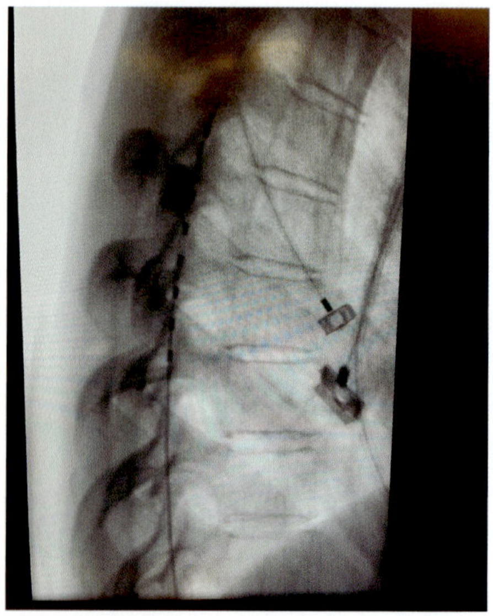

Fig. 8.17 Visualize the midline starting point in an anteroposterior view to help aid a final midline approach.

29. Connect the cable to the leads (see Fig. 8.18).
30. Programming can be confirmed again to ensure that proper coverage of pain relief is maintained for the patient (see Fig. 8.19).

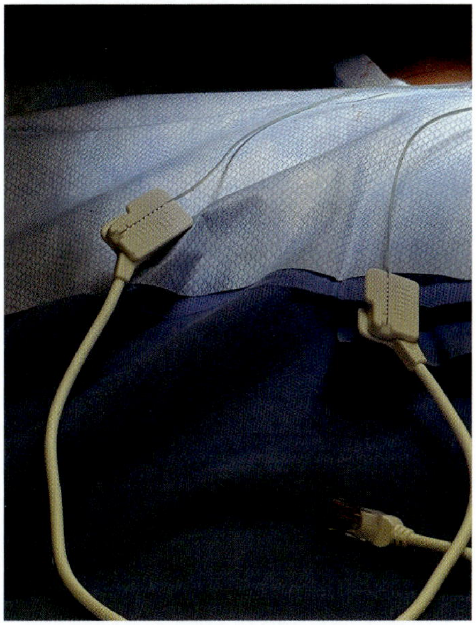

Fig. 8.18 Connect the leads to the temporary lead extensions for programming.

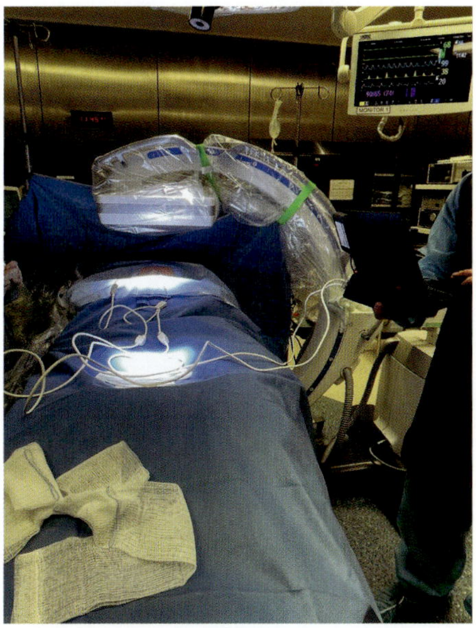

Fig. 8.19 Programming of the system can now begin, with lead impedance check and possible paresthesia mapping.

31. The lead can then be secured with steri-stripes (medical tape) and specialized medicated bandages as seen here, or with simple skin sutures (Figs. 8.21 and 8.22).

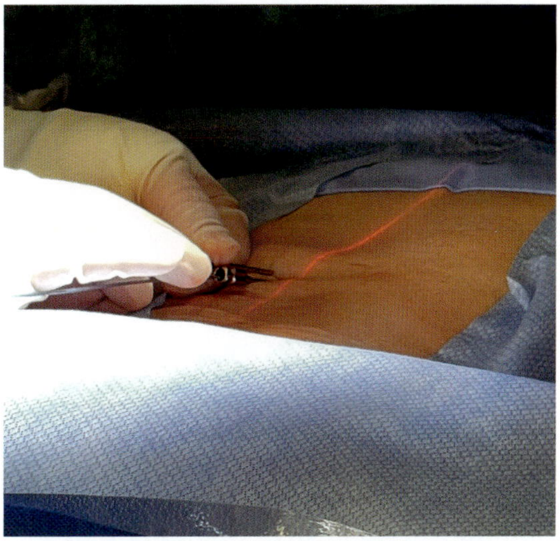

Fig. 8.20 Use the anteroposterior and lateral views to confirm the final lead targets.

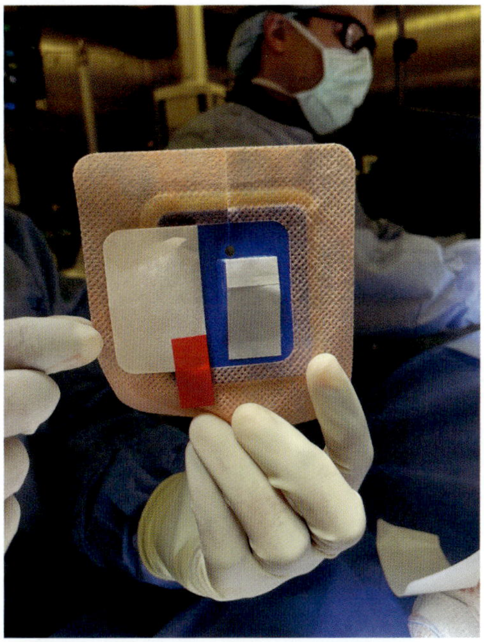

Fig. 8.21 Final dressing to secure leads such as one that holds epidural catheters. Skin sutures can also be used.

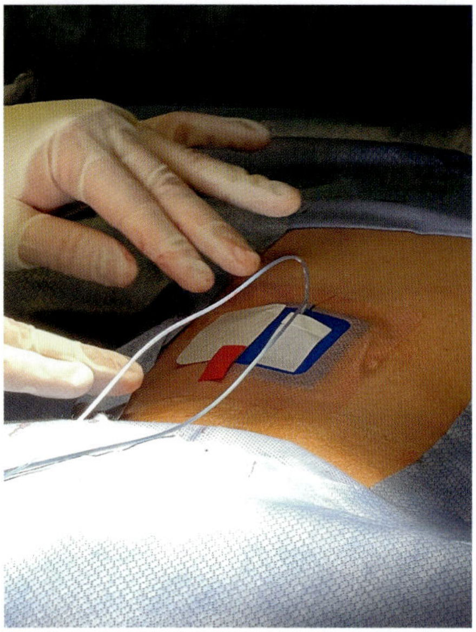

Fig. 8.22 Secure placement of the leads at the site of skin entry.

Handling Intraoperative Complications

Complications can either be device related or biological. Device-related complications include lead breakage, intermittent stimulation, hardware malfunction, battery failure, loose connection, and lead migration.[8] Biological complications include seroma, epidural hemorrhage, infection, cerebrospinal fluid leakage, and pain at implant site.[8] Literature indicates that complications such as epidural abscesses or hematomas are relatively uncommon (> 0.3%).[3] A large retrospective study of over 2700 SCS implants found an overall infection rate of 2.45%.[9]

REFERENCES

1. Deer TR, Mekhail N, Provenzano D, et al. The appropriate use of neurostimulation of the spinal cord and peripheral nervous system for the treatment of chronic pain and ischemic diseases: the Neuromodulation Appropriateness Consensus Committee. *Neuromodulation*. 2014;17:515-550.
2. Melzack R, Wall PD. Pain mechanisms: a new theory. *Science*. 1965;150:971-979.
3. Deer TR, Jain S, Hunter C, Chakravarthy K. Neurostimulation for intractable chronic pain. *Brain Sci*. 2019;9(2):23.
4. Shealy CN, Mortimer JT, Reswick JB. Electrical inhibition of pain by stimulation of the dorsal columns: preliminary clinical report. *Anesth Analg*. 1967;46:489-491.
5. Hong A, Varshney V, Hare GMT, Mazer D. Spinal cord stimulation: a nonopioid alternative for chronic pain management. *CMAJ*. 2020;192(42):E1264-E1267.
6. Moore DM, McCrory C. Spinal cord stimulation. *BJA Educ*. 2016;16(8):258-263.
7. Levy RM. Anatomic considerations for spinal cord stimulation. *Neuromodulation*. 2014;17(11):2–11.
8. Cameron T. Safety and efficacy of spinal cord stimulation for the treatment of chronic pain: a 20-year literature review. *J Neurosurg*. 2004;100(3 Suppl Spine):S254-S267.
9. Hoelzer BC, Bendel MA, Deer TR, et al. Spinal cord stimulator implant infection rates and risk factors: a multicenter retrospective study. *Neuromodulation*. 2017;20(6):558-562.

Chapter 9

Spinal Cord Stimulation Implant (Percutaneous Leads)

Alaa Abd-Elsayed, David Abejón González, and Cristina Abad Salom

Chapter Outline

Introduction

The use of spinal cord stimulation (SCS) first began over 50 years ago, and there has been a notable increase in its use during the last decade. There has been a rise in SCS use for the treatment of chronic back pain refractory to standard treatment; this use has yielded positive results.[1,2]

Different types of programming have been developed for SCS. The waveform[3-7] itself has not changed; however, there has been considerable improvement in the efficacy of the therapy. Studies have demonstrated its superiority compared with conventional treatment methods[8] and compared with reoperation.[9] Recent studies have also proved a significant decrease in opioid intake,[10,11] which is vital in the current opioid epidemic,[12] as well as an important increase in quality of life and cost-effectiveness compared with other treatments.[13]

As discussed, SCS has some notable advantages for treating chronic pain. In this chapter, the essential criteria for SCS indication, the surgical procedure for placement, and postprocedure follow-up are explained. Throughout the chapter, all aspects of SCS therapy that providers need to be aware of are presented.

Patient Preparation and Preoperative Conditioning

The key to success in SCS therapy is following a simple algorithm. To adequately perform this treatment, providers need to take into account five fundamental pillars: correct diagnosis, appropriate selection criteria, perfect surgical technique, selection of the most adequate SCS system for each specific patient's needs, and the patient–doctor relationship (Table 9.1).

The diagnosis (Table 9.2) needs to be appropriate for this type of technique to be completed. For example, in a neuropathic pain case, the patient needs to fulfill the inclusion criteria for the SCS therapy, including achievement of a positive test phase and, during this test phase, selection of the most appropriate system for each patient. Most importantly, a doctor–patient relationship must be developed.

TABLE 9.1 Basic Algorithm for Successful Spinal Cord Stimulation
Correct diagnosis
Patient selection
Test phase
Adequate system selection
Patient–doctor relationship

TABLE 9.2 Indications for Spinal Cord Stimulation[14]
Failed back surgery syndrome
Refractory angina pectoris
Neuropathic pain secondary to peripheral nerve lesion
Radicular pain following cervical spine surgery
Pain associated with peripheral vascular disease
Intercostal neuralgia, such as post-thoracotomy
Other peripheral neuropathic pain syndromes, such as those following trauma
Complex regional pain syndrome
Avulsive brachial plexopathy
Nociceptive axial pain following surgery
Central pain of nonspinal cord origin
Pain in spinal cord injury
Phantom pain/postamputation
Postherpetic neuralgia

Adapted from British Pain Society. Spinal cord stimulation for the management of pain: recommendations or best clinical practice; April 2009. www.britishpainsociety.org

INCLUSION AND EXCLUSION CRITERIA

Encompassed in the selection for SCS therapy, the anatomical, clinical, and psychosocial criteria must be considered.[15]

Among the anatomical criteria that will determine whether SCS therapy can be performed is the possibility to physically access the target along with the nervous system's ability to transmit the signal. Among the clinical criteria for SCS indication, classic practice deems that the patients who can benefit from SCS as a treatment for chronic pain are those with lack of response to conservative treatment modalities, no coagulation or immune system alterations, and no signs of infection. It should be noted that the presence of a demand pacemaker can pose a threat to the patient when implanting an SCS device. Implantation of a neurostimulator in the presence of a demand pacemaker is a real risk for the patient's life because the cardiac device may sense the neurostimulation signals and interpret them incorrectly. This could cause inhibition or variation of the cardiac stimulation, potentially sending a defibrillation shock. Although there have been advances in both systems, medullar as well as cardiological factors make this contraindication an extremely relevant one.

The psychosocial criteria are the most difficult to determine; they appear to be the most relevant for the maintenance of the treatment long term. The patient must understand, accept, and—above all—believe in the therapy (Tables 9.3 and 9.4).

To obtain the best result with this therapy, several basic prerequisites must be met:

- Professional motivation that allows for an extensive informative search about neurostimulation treatment and its practical repercussions
- Patient motivation for the treatment
- Realistic prospect about the possible outcomes

TABLE 9.3 Inclusion Criteria for Spinal Cord Stimulation
Age ≥ 18 y
Chronic pain with a duration of at least 6 mo
One of the following primary indications: • Chronic low back/leg pain • Complex regional pain syndrome • Failed back surgical syndrome • Neuropathic pain syndrome • Ischemic pain syndrome • Others (e.g., abdominal pain, pelvic pain, peripheral vascular disease)
Pain severity at least moderate, having a substantial impact on daily functioning and quality of life
Insufficient response to appropriate trials of medication and/or minimally invasive treatments and/or experiencing intolerable side effects of these treatments
No clear benefits of surgery expected

TABLE 9.4 Exclusion Criteria for Spinal Cord Stimulation (SCS)
Unwilling to have an implant
Unable to manage the device
Absolute contraindications for active treatment (e.g., unfit for undergoing SCS, pregnancy, spine infection, coagulation disorder)
Uncontrolled disruptive psychological or psychiatric disorder
Ongoing alcohol and drug misuse
Widespread pain that cannot be targeted by SCS

- Efficient diagnosis
- Central nervous system integrity
- Ineffective appropriate conservative and interventional treatment, and no surgical indication to treat the underlying pathology
- Positive psychological evaluation
- No indication of drug abuse–related problems
- No pending lawsuits or monetary compensation related to the pain issue
- Positive test phase

The absolute and relative contraindications in relation to the previously mentioned factors are listed in Table 9.5.

PREOPERATIVE PREPARATIONS

Preoperative preparations for this procedure, as with other surgical procedures, are important to decrease potential complications and improve results. As part of case preparation, comorbidities have to be considered to ensure the patient's safety and minimize risk. It is crucial to carefully plan all details of the surgery ahead of time to be able to execute the procedure safely and with reliability and to achieve the best results.

PREPROCEDURE ASSESSMENT

As with all surgeries, a well-taken clinical history and complete physical examination are mandatory so that possible intraoperative complications can be anticipated and prepared for. It is important to know the patient's health status regarding possible skin alterations that could generate complications, such as altered coagulation states and the intake of clotting-related drugs, heart disease, diabetes mellitus, dermatological problems, metal allergies, or allergy to any system component.

TABLE 9.5 Contraindications for Spinal Cord Stimulation[16]

Contraindications	Absolute	Relative
Anatomical	Pregnancy	Severe spondylosis
	Previous dorsal root entry zone lesions that will interfere with the implant procedure	Severe scoliosis
	Critical central stenosis that will interfere with the implant procedure	Significant fibrosis in the implant area
	Severe neurological deficit	
	Spinal instability progression	
Medical	Immunosuppression or another medical condition that does not allow the surgery	Active infection
		Implanted pacemakers or defibrillators
		Existence of another pain-related health issue
		Ongoing anticoagulation that cannot be stopped for procedure
Psychosocial	Drug abuse	Psychosocial lability or psychiatric issues in treatment
	Lack of social support	Secondary gain

Special preparation of the operating room (OR) is required to avoid the most feared complications of the procedure, which can be found in Table 9.6.

Radiology Studies

In a medullar stimulation case, the procurement and preparation of the patient's imaging studies is very important but often forgotten. Patients can present to practices with magnetic resonance imaging (MRI) and sometimes with X-rays of the painful area. On occasion, patients can present with myelography or computed tomography (CT) scans. However, in a few scenarios, patients present with a series of X-rays of the area where work is to be performed.

Planning the area where the implantation of the SCS leads are going to be placed is vital. For example, if the patient is going to undergo an implant in the thoracic area for postlaminectomy syndrome, it is recommended to take an X-ray of the dorsolumbar hinge (T11–L2) to visualize the anatomy of the area. If the patient is going to undergo an implantation in the cervical area, it is advised to have an X-ray study of the cervicothoracic hinge (C7–T4) to determine possible complications (Figs. 9.1A and 9.1B).

Patient Marking and Intrasurgery Preparations

This section contains essential information to perform the procedure adequately. Patient preparation in the OR is one of the most important factors for the correct performance and proper completion of the technique. Before beginning the procedure, we must remind the patients of the steps to take and their fundamental role in the preprocedure instructions, procedure success, and the recovery process. A visit to the patient's room with the collaborating technician is essential so that the patient meets and eventually recognizes the provider's and technician's voices in the OR when the intraoperative stimulation is done and if tonic stimulation is going to be performed. Patients must be placed on the operating table so that they are comfortable and can maintain the required posture for at least 60 minutes. For this reason, even though many texts recommend an abdominal support or pillow, our recommendation is to first do a radiological study of the patient to see if that is necessary. In some cases, the patient is put in a forced posture to decrease the physiological lordosis. This makes the patient maintain a more uncomfortable posture, hindering the patient's collaboration throughout the procedure.

As an example, from a case with postlaminectomy syndrome, the following markings are recommended before beginning the procedure:

1. Marking the patient´s most painful area (left/right leg/lumbar area; Fig. 9.2)
2. Final lead location (T8; Fig. 9.3)
3. Epidural space entry point (T12–L1; Fig. 9.4)
4. Entry in the skin to access the epidural space (L3; Fig. 9.5)
5. Marking the location of the permanent generator (Figs. 9.5–9.7)

TABLE 9.6 Preoperative Measures to Avoid Complications

Infection	Coagulopathy	Cardiac Risk	Diabetes Mellitus	Allergies
Preoperative disinfection with chlorhexidine	International normalized ratio (INR)	Careful evaluation with cardiology team	Primary care physician	Clinical history of allergies to the system's components
Intranasal mupirocine pommade	Prothrombin time/partial thromboplastin time (PT/PTT)	Discontinue tobacco use	Hemoglobin A1c (HgA1c)	
Antibiotic prophylaxis	Bleeding times			
Basic complete blood count (CBC)	Platelet function assay studies			
Urinalysis if at risk for urinary infection	Review drug intake			

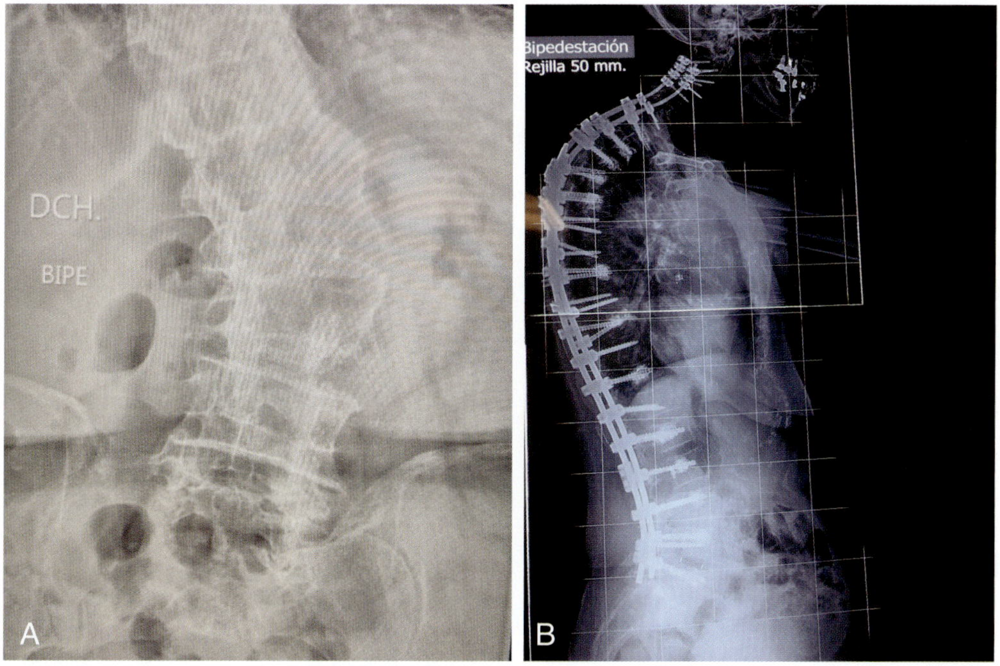

Fig. 9.1 Preoperative X-rays of the treatment area of a patient scheduled for neurostimulation. (A) Posteroanterior view of the lumbar area of a selected patient. (B) Lateral view of all spinal segments of a selected patient.

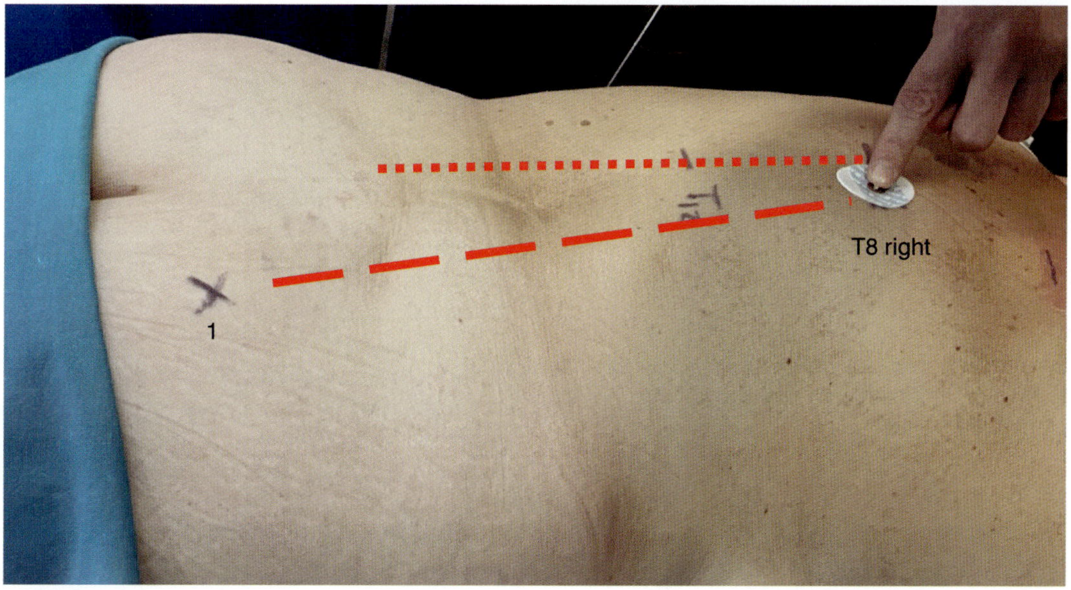

Fig. 9.2 1. Marking the patient's most painful area. 2. Marking the location where the tip of the leads will be, in this case, T8. Note that the marking is done with an ECG electrode in the painful side—in this patient, the electrode is placed on the right side. *Dotted line:* midline. *Discontinuous line:* limiting of the patient's painful area

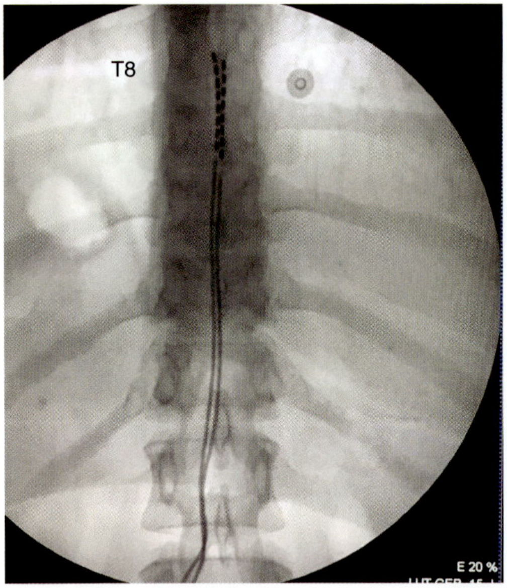

Fig. 9.3 An electrode is located at the T8 level on the right side, consistent with the patient's most painful area.

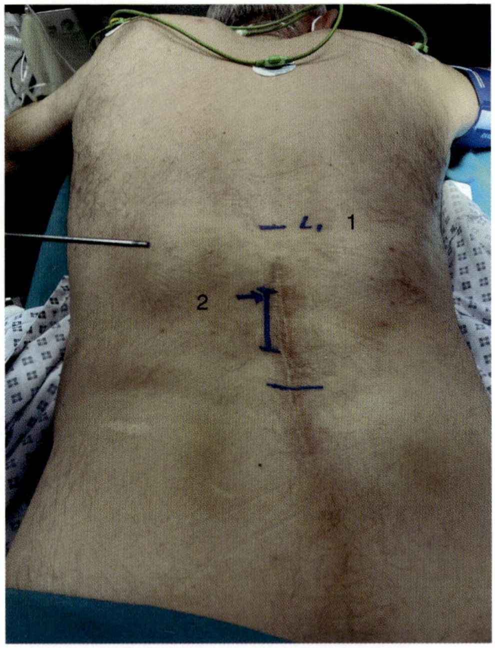

Fig. 9.5 Marking the entrance point to the epidural space (L1) by drawing an arrow on the skin. 1. Entry to the epidural space. 2. Entry in the skin to access the epidural space.

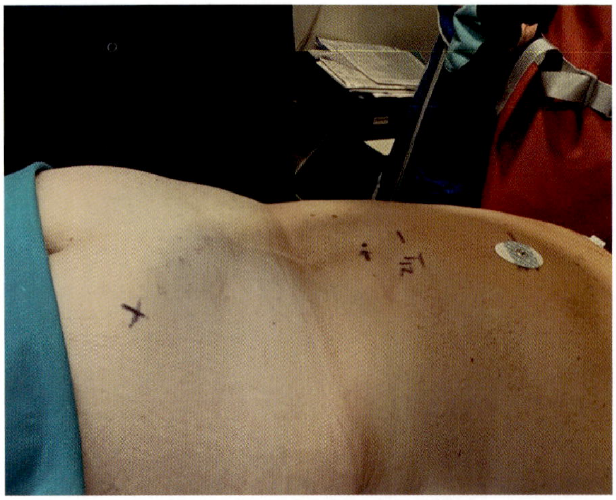

Fig. 9.4 Marking the entrance point to the epidural space, corresponding to L1. It is marked with an arrow.

Skill is needed with a C-arm in the process of locating the various structures. To be able to achieve a correct approach with no intraoperative delays, radiological views are very important and must be as well adjusted as possible. The most recommended view for this case is to have a clear vision of an equidistant line from the line made by the pedicles. The entry point on the skin is marked medial to the pedicle between the spinous process line and the pedicles line so that access to the epidural midline is more precise (Figs. 9.8A through 9.8F).

Puncture Technique

The puncture technique is a crucial part of the procedure. If this step is not performed correctly, the treatment will almost always fail.

It is important that the steps prior to this point are performed with precision so that the puncture is simpler. Also, it is key that, even though this is a vital part of the technique, the goal of implantation is to position the leads according to plan and not to perform an epidural.

Before beginning the procedure, the entry area (pedicle chosen for entry and the one above and below) is infiltrated with bupivacaine 0.5% as vasoconstrictor and lidocaine 2% to decrease surgical bleeding. Avoid overhandling which may cause a

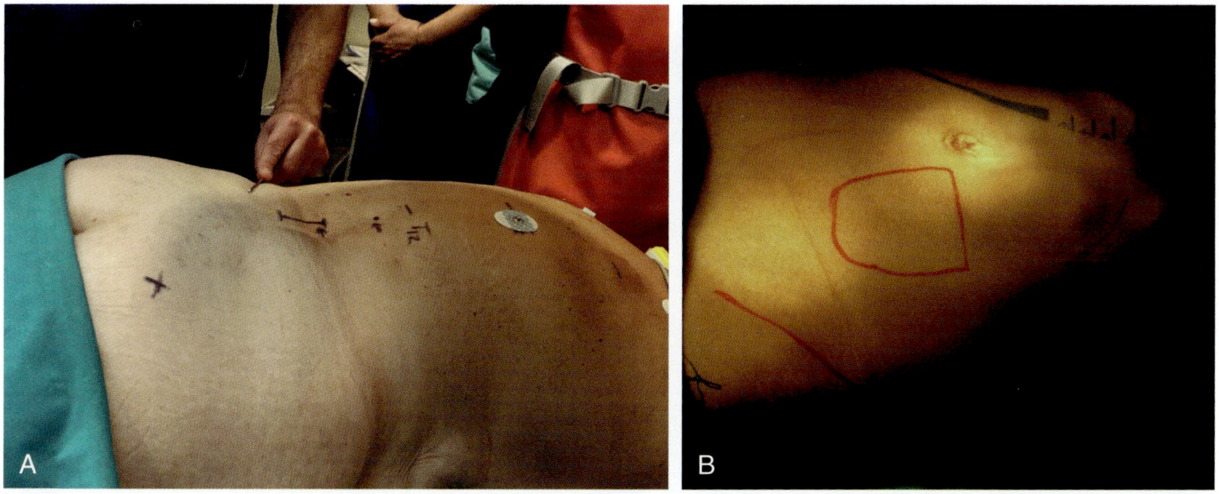

Fig. 9.6 (A) Marking the location of the permanent generator. Approximately the width of 2 fingers below the iliac crest in the gluteal area in case the implant is in the gluteal area. (B) Markings for the implant in the abdominal area. Draw a line from the anterosuperior iliac crest and another line following the last rib. Between them, draw the marking for the generator to its full scale.

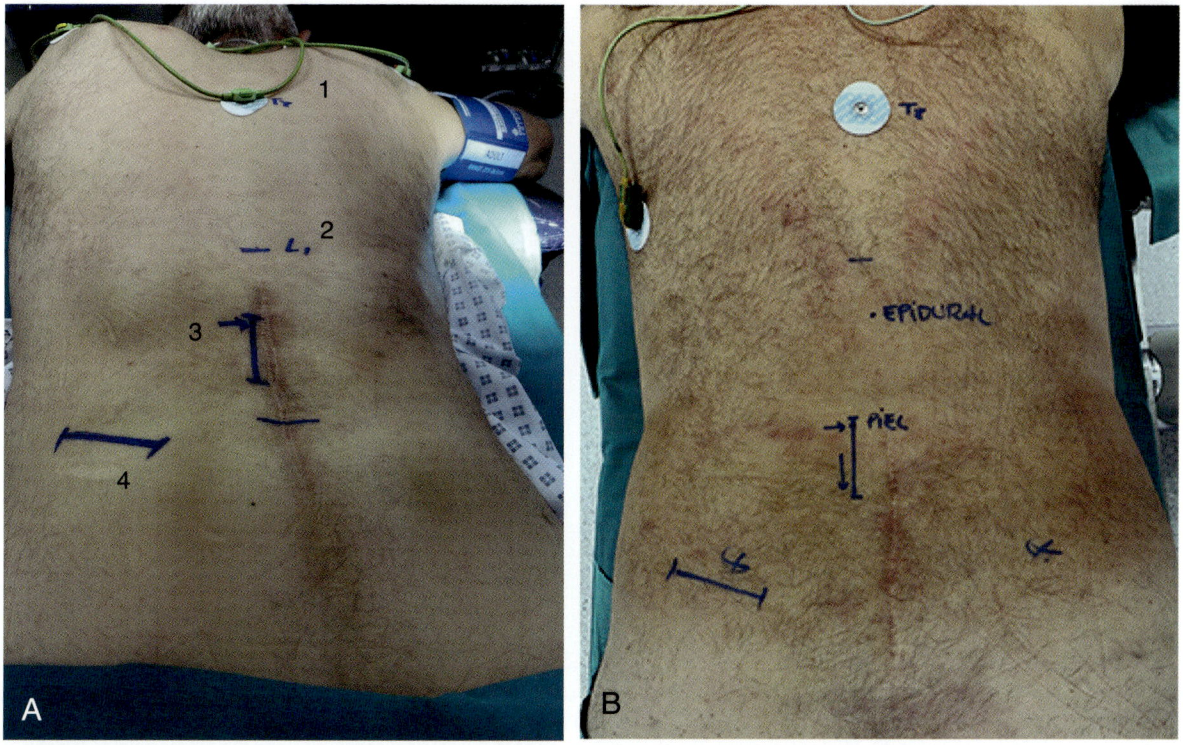

Fig. 9.7 (A) and (B) Complete the patient´s markings before beginning the procedure. 1. T8. Final location of the tip of the leads. 2. L1. Entry point to the epidural space. 3. Arrow—needle entry point. 4. Permanent generator´s implant area.

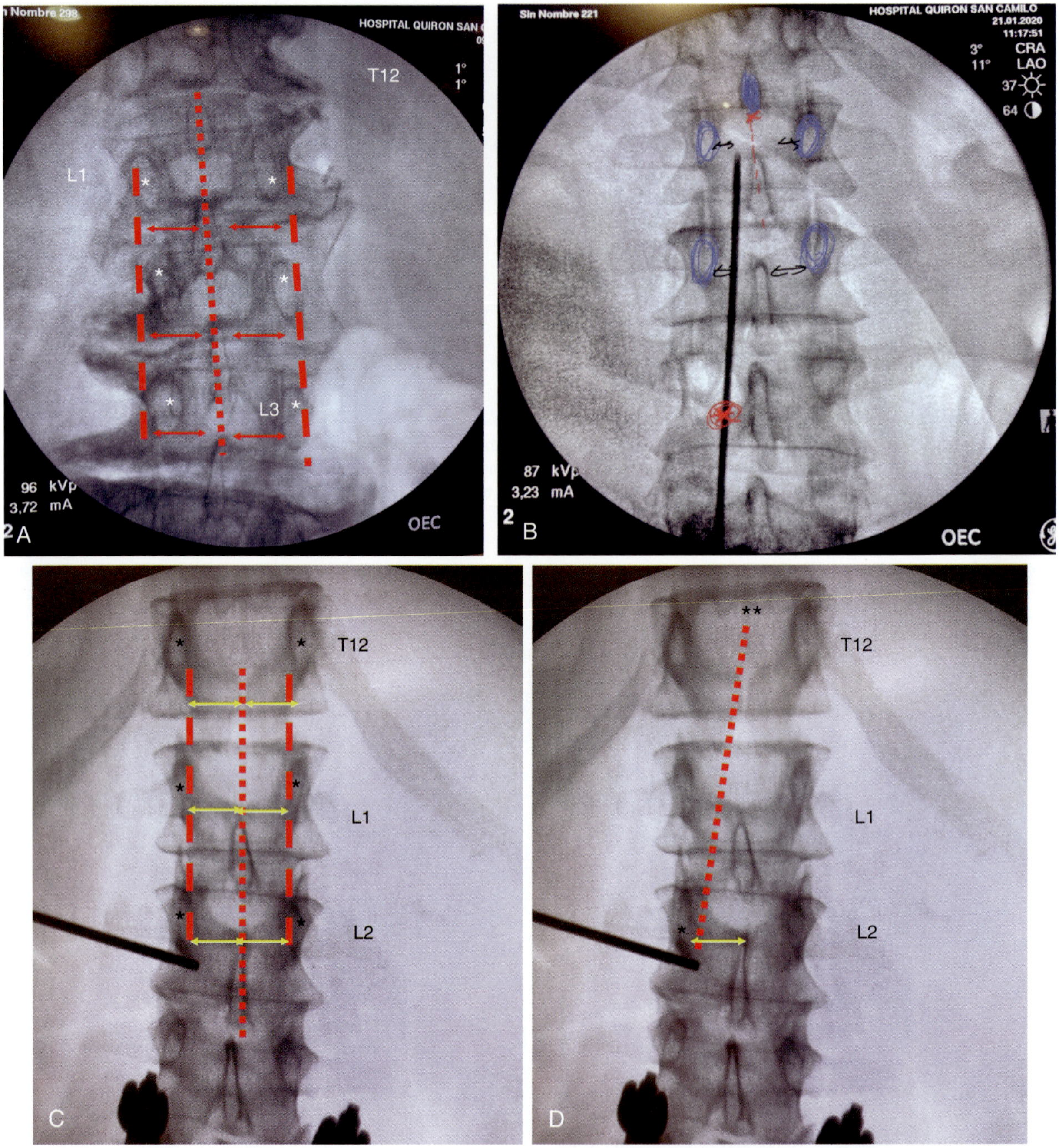

Fig. 9.8 (A) and (B) T12 is recognized. The chosen entry point to the epidural space is L1 and the access point to the skin will be L3. An imaginary line that connects the spinous processes is drawn (*dots*). Another is drawn connecting the pedicles on both sides (*asterisks*). It can be seen that the lines are equidistant at all levels. (C) T12 is recognized. The chosen entry point to the epidural space is L1 and the access point to the skin will be L3. An imaginary line that connects the spinous processes is drawn. Another is drawn connecting the pedicles on both sides. It can be seen that the lines are equidistant at all levels. (D) The entry point on the skin is marked medial to the pedicles in the area between the line of the spinous process and the line of the pedicle´s line. *, Pedicle; **, spinous process; *dotted line,* direction that needs to be taken to secure the desired target.

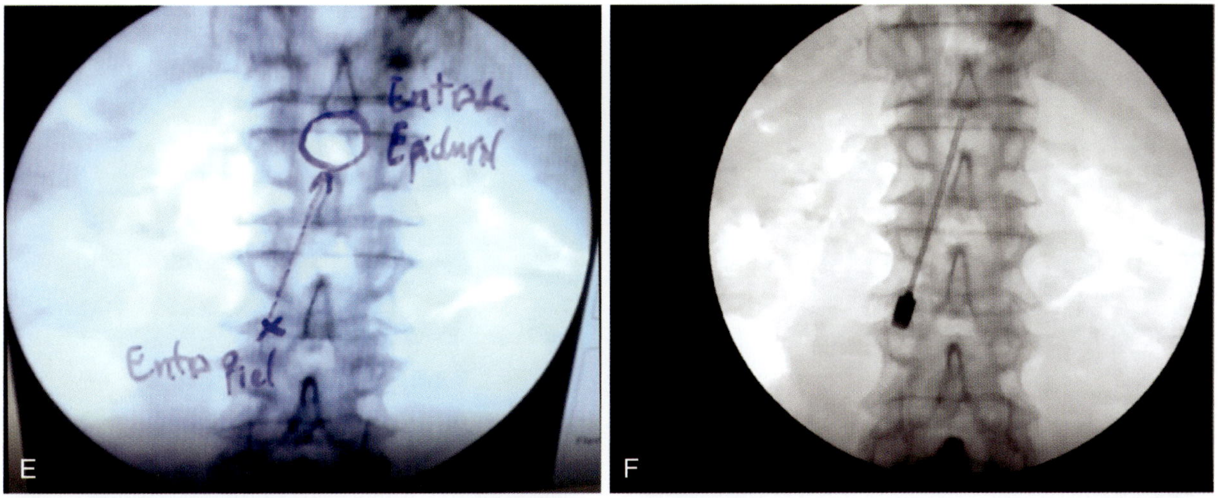

Fig. 9.8, cont'd (E) Case image with the patient's full markings over the X-ray. (F) Needle inserted in the skin taking the direction marked previously.

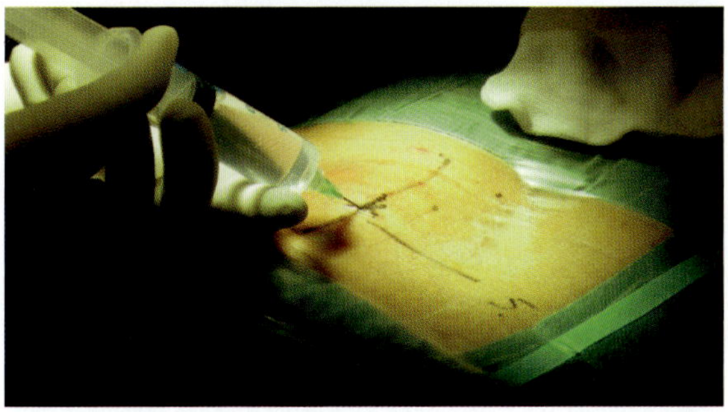

Fig. 9.9 The entry area is infiltrated with local anesthetic (entry at the pedicle level and one above and one below). It is important to infiltrate the area from the interspinous ligament up to the laminae in the direction the needle is going to take, as seen in the figure.

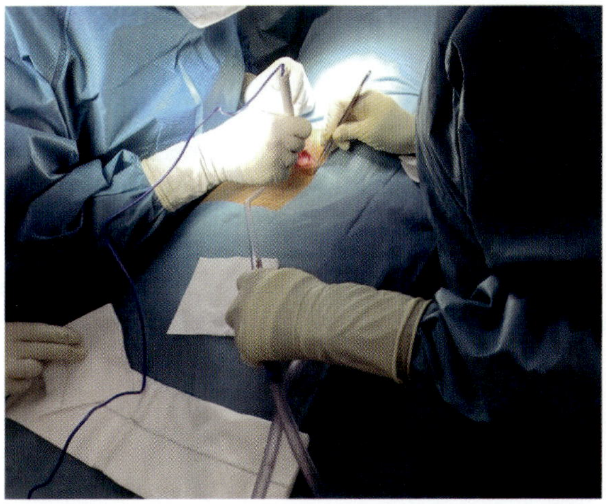

Fig. 9.10 Skin incision and hemostasis before proceeding to needle placement. Even though other technique modalities are described, skin incision before performing the epidural is recommended so that a surgical field with perfect hemostasis is achieved to avoid introducing pathogens into the epidural space, which can increase the risk of infection.

posterior hematoma in the puncture site and electrode anchoring zone. The area is first sterilized and prepared for surgical intervention (Fig. 9.9).

There are two equally valid techniques for implantation. In one technique, the surgical incision is made up to the fascia muscularis before finding the epidural space; in the other, the epidural space is first found and, after the electrode is positioned and a good paresthesia is obtained (covering the pain area), an incision is made in the skin to the fascial plane (Fig. 9.10). The advantages of the former technique over the latter are that finding the epidural space is easier and that there is a decrease in the risk of introducing pathogens from the skin into the epidural space, therefore decreasing the risk of infection.

The key to needle placement in this intervention is the angle of the needle in the entrance to the epidural space; this angulation must be around

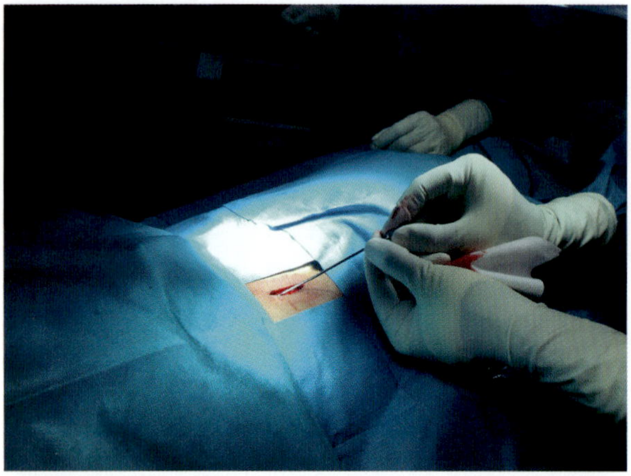

Fig. 9.11 The most important aspect of placing the epidural needle is the angle at which it is inserted into the epidural space, which must be about 30-degree angle. If 30-degree angle is not achieved, the needle must be reinserted more caudal.

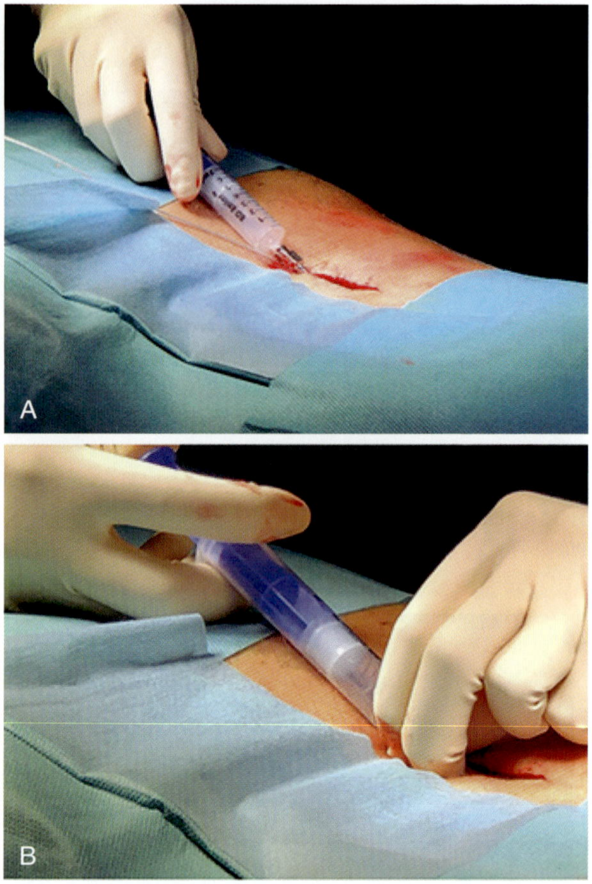

Fig. 9.12 (A) and (B) Loss-of-resistance technique with air. In performing the epidural, we recommend your usual practice technique, either loss of resistance with air or saline, or pending drop.

30 degrees. The needle incline will allow the provider to navigate the posterior epidural space without any difficulty (Fig. 9.11). When a greater angulation is used to reach the epidural space more easily, the navigation afterward is almost impossible, directing the lead to the anterior epidural space. The needle is advanced until it reaches the flavum ligamentum. At this point, the stylet is removed and the epidural space is then found with either a loss-of-resistance technique (air or saline) or with a pending-drop technique (Figs. 9.12A and 9.12B). As stated earlier, the tip of the needle must be placed in the midline at the spinous process level (Figs. 9.13 and 9.14A through 9.14C).

Lead Placement

Once the epidural space is found with the needle, the next step is to position the leads correctly in the posterior epidural space. Lead navigation in the epidural space depends on how the previous step is performed (Figs. 9.15 and 9.16). In current practice, the final placement of the leads will depend on the specific system chosen. In the patients who choose a system with tonic stimulation, a paresthesia that covers their pain area must be found (Figs. 9.17–9.20). If a high-frequency system is chosen, an anatomical

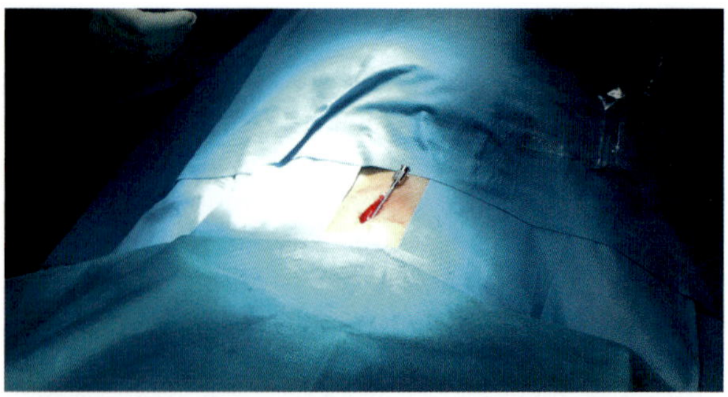

Fig. 9.13 The needle's final position in the epidural space. Note the angle of the needle. The most important aspect of navigating the posterior epidural space is to be able to reach the epidural space with an angle not superior to 45 degrees.

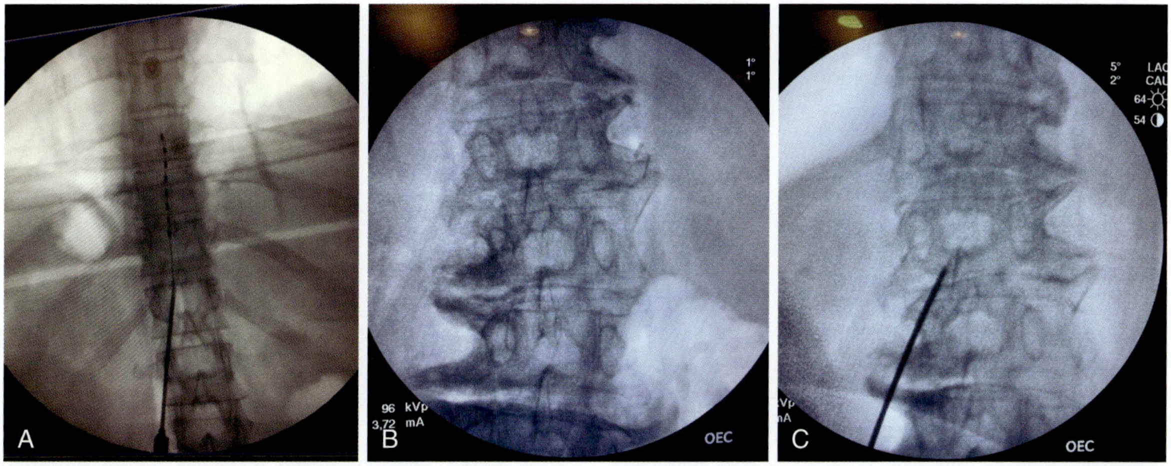

Fig. 9.14 (A through C) The needle's tip is in the midline at the spinous process level so that navigation is easier in that position to direct the lead to the patient's most painful area.

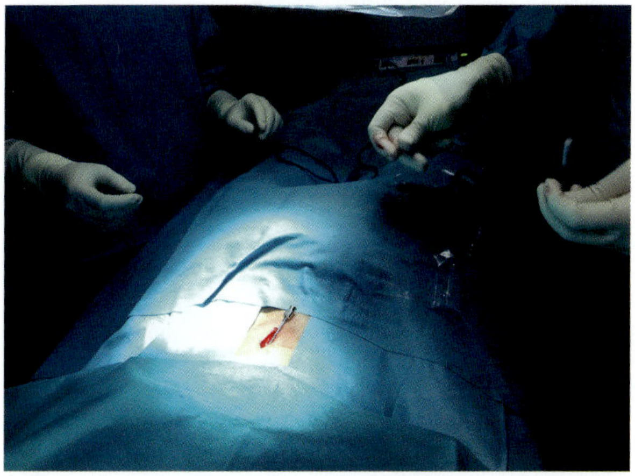

Fig. 9.15 Once the epidural space is found, the leads are placed in the selected area depending on the system chosen and the type of pathology.

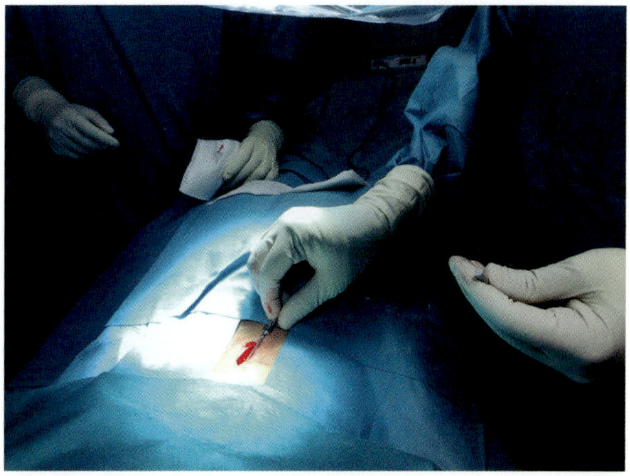

Fig. 9.16 To be able to navigate accurately, the hand placement in this figure is recommended. In this position, small movements of the hand with the stylet while advancing the leads with the other hand permit a correct placement of the leads.

positioning that covers part of T8 and part of T10 (Figs. 9.21A and 9.21B) is necessary. The number of leads implanted will depend on the patient's pathology (Figs. 9.22–9.24).

When lead navigation through the epidural space begins, it is important to consider the following for better mobility during navigation:

1. The needle's bevel: It can be positioned to the right or left depending on where lead placement is desired.
2. The lead stylet: There are curved and straight stylets that allow for correct movement of the leads in the epidural space—one can switch them while navigating to find the desired target.
3. The needle: Small needle movements can ease the correct placement of the leads in the desired target.

The key to correct navigation is correct needle placement in the epidural space. In some cases, fibrosis, stenosis, or anatomical alterations may contribute to difficult navigation. To avoid these issues, this

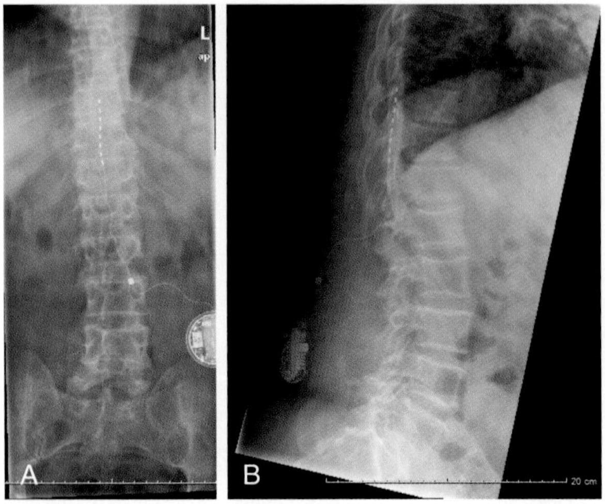

Fig. 9.17 (A) Final lead position in the posterior epidural space: posteroanterior X-ray image. (B) Final lead position in the posterior epidural space: lateral X-ray image.

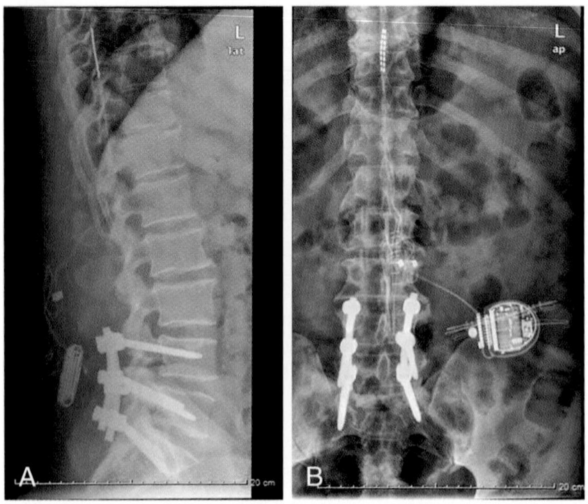

Fig. 9.18 (A) Final lead position in the posterior epidural space: posteroanterior X-ray image. (B) Final lead position in the posterior epidural space: lateral X-ray image.

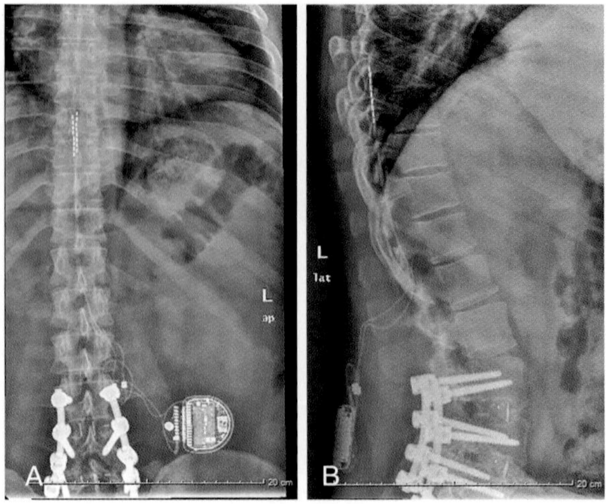

Fig. 9.19 (A) Final lead position in the posterior epidural space: posteroanterior X-ray image. (B) Final lead position in the posterior epidural space: lateral X-ray image.

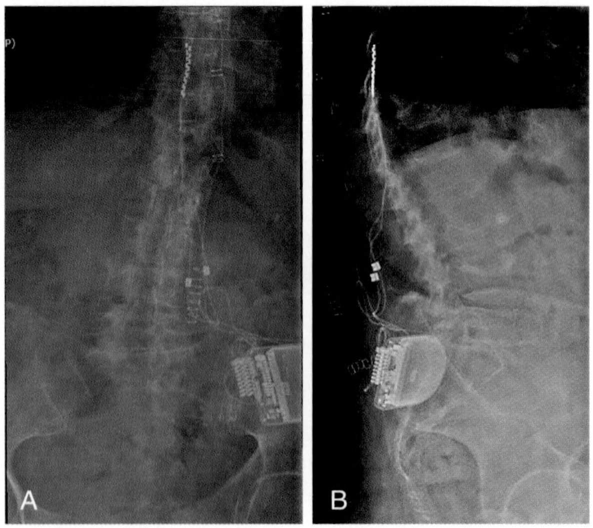

Fig. 9.20 (A) Final lead position in the posterior epidural space: posteroanterior X-ray image. (B) Final lead position in the posterior epidural space: lateral X-ray image.

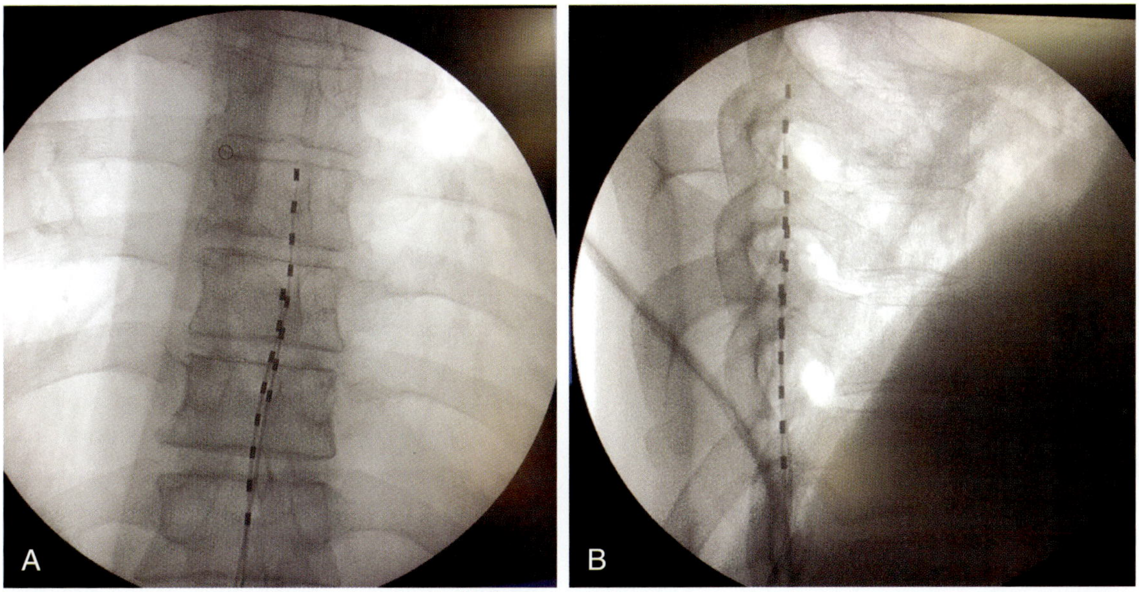

Fig. 9.21 Final lead position in the posterior epidural space, posteroanterior (A) and lateral (B) X-ray images. In this case, the placement is performed with anatomical cues without sensory mapping to obtain paresthesia. The leads cover T8 to T11.

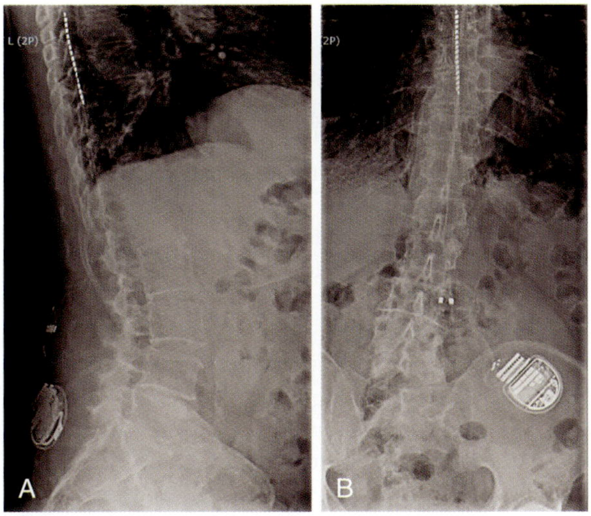

Fig. 9.22 (A) and (B) Complete implant with two 16-contact leads in posterolateral and lateral views in the posterior epidural space.

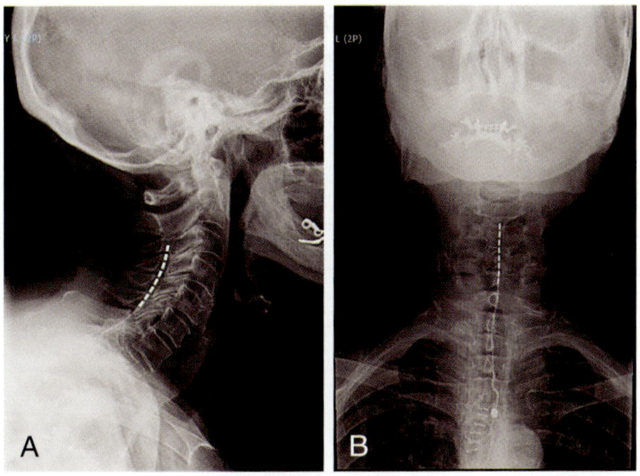

Fig. 9.23 (A) and (B) Cervical lead implant in the posterolateral and lateral views.

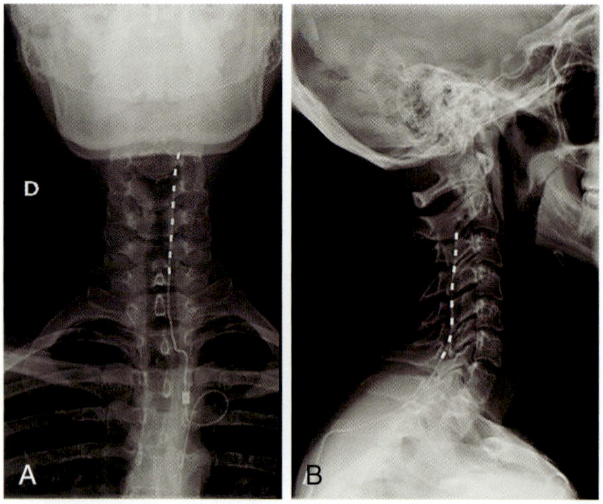

Fig. 9.24 (A) and (B) Cervical lead implant in the posteroanterior and lateral views.

procedure, which facilitates quality needle placement in the epidural space, as well as a previous study of the patient, are crucial.

When the leads are placed in the target (Table 9.7), an intraoperative stimulation must be done to check that the leads were placed in the correct area (Figs. 9.25A and 9.25B). At this point, a lateral X-ray scan must be performed to confirm the lead placement in the posterior epidural space (see Fig. 9.25A) and subsequently in a posterolateral view. Images are recorded for later verification of the lead placement during anchoring and tunneling.

TABLE 9.7 Sensory Mapping[19]

Painful Area	Cathode Location
Neck	C2
Shoulder	C2–C4 Under C4 paresthesia is not obtained in the shoulder
Hand	C5 and C6
Thoracic (unstable angina)	C3 and C5
Abdominal	T5 and T7
Thigh, anterior	T11–T12 (DRG L1–L3)
Thigh, posterior	T11–L1
Foot	L1 (DRG L5–S1)
Perineum	T11–L1 (DRG S3)
Lumbar	T8–T9
Gluteal	T11–L1

DRG, Dorsal root ganglion.

Anchoring

Next, the Touhy needle is removed. This is performed under direct X-ray view to check whether there is any lead migration in the epidural space and to relocate it correctly as needed. Finally, the lead stylet is removed. Then, lead anchoring to the muscular fascia is started.

There are different anchors depending on the manufacturer (Fig. 9.26), each of which has its own anchoring method. This next step is essential to avoid the most frequent complication of the procedure;[17] lead migration.

The main cause of lead migration usually is the movement of the lead during anchoring. In current practice, the new anchor systems have avoided this complication with devices that lock over the lead (e.g., the Swift-Lock anchor and Clik anchor, Figs. 9.26A and Fig. 9.27, respectively) or that trap the lead with pressure (Injex Bumpy anchor, Fig. 9.26C). Even with these advancements, the lead and the anchor still need to be attached to the fascia. It is important to differentiate between percutaneous leads and paddle leads. With the former, the leads will be attached to the fascia, whereas with the latter, the leads can be attached to the ligament. It is also important to follow the indications for each type of anchor and to never attempt anything outside of the manufacturer's recommendations to avoid complications such the one in Fig. 9.28.[18]

The anchor attachment must be permanent; therefore, nonabsorbable sutures are recommended. According to their synthetic origin, sutures can be classified as absorbable or nonabsorbable. Currently, all absorbable sutures are synthetic polymers; the most frequently used are polyglactin, polyglycolic acid, poliglecaprone, polydioxanone, polyglyconate, and polyhydroxybutyrate. The most frequently used nonabsorbable sutures are polyamide, polyester, polypropylene, and polybutester (Table 9.8). Absorbable

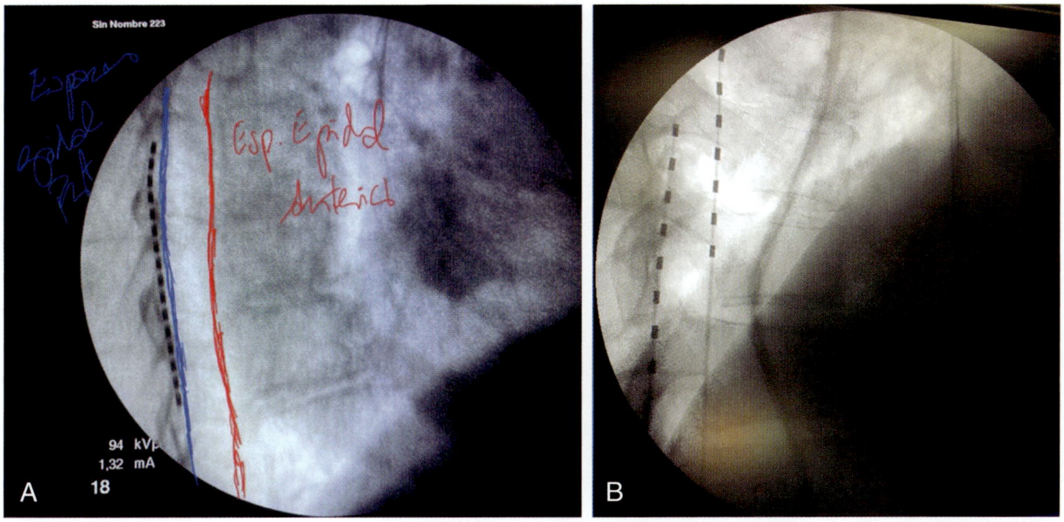

Fig. 9.25 (A) The lead is located in the posterior epidural space *(blue line)*. In all cases, the anterior epidural space *(red line)* should be avoided for the final location. (B) A lead is located in the posterior epidural space and another in the anterior epidural space.

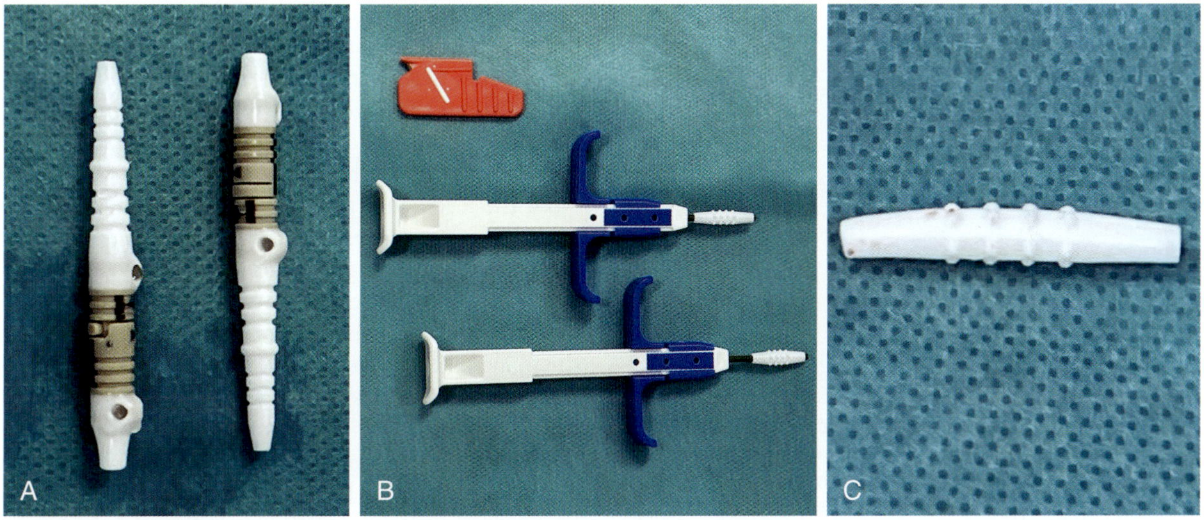

Fig. 9.26 Different anchors from the various commercial companies. (A) Swift-Lock anchor. (B) Injex dispenser tool. (C) Injex Bumpy anchor.

sutures are degraded by the body and do not need to be removed. Each suture has its own absorption time depending on its composition, structure, and covering. Nonabsorbable sutures are those that, due to their composition, are not degraded by the body and need to be removed. If they are not removed, the thread will become encapsulated during scarring and cause different body reactions.

At this point of the implantation, verification of lead placement must be done after handling the components of the implant. This is the reason that an image is taken after removing the needle and stylet.

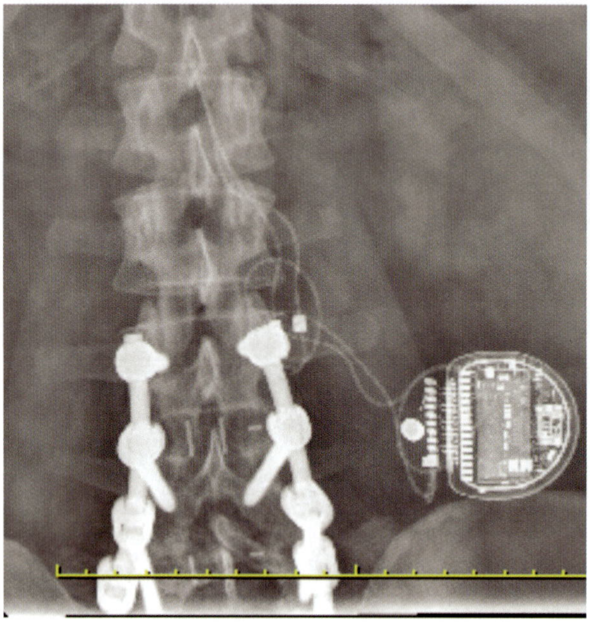

Fig. 9.27 Clik anchor radiological mark.

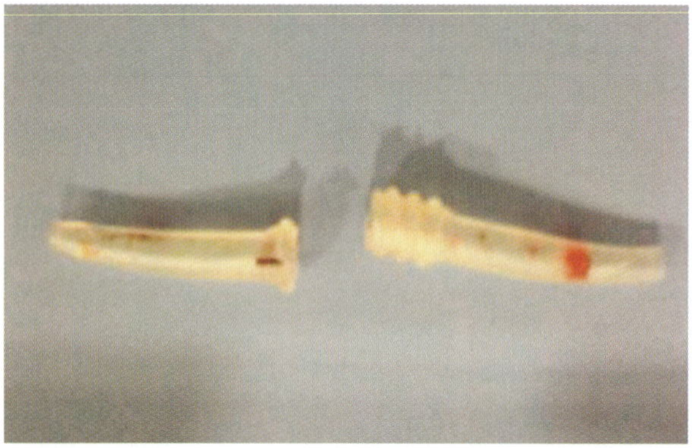

Fig. 9.28 In this picture we can see a fractured anchor after glue was used inside the anchor for better attachment to the lead; the result was the fracture of the lead and anchor. We strongly caution against using anything not recommended by the manufacturer.

When the anchoring is finished, a lead placement check is always performed to ensure that it is still in the correct place.

ANCHORING METHOD FOR THE CLIK ANCHOR (FIGS. 9.29–9.30)

In this type of anchor, which includes a sleeve with grooves and a wing on each side, an anchoring technique that decreases lead migration and eventual reoperation is proposed. To start, it is recommended to suture the anchor sleeve to the fascia with two stitches that encompass the junction between the two wings. A stitch to the fascia is then made and the needle is passed through the posterior part of the wing so that the stitch faces itself. This stitch is also performed on the other wing. This is broken down in the following steps:

1. Suture the anchor to the fascia with two stitches in the area between the wings.
2. Stitch in the fascia and posterior introduction in the wing.
3. Repeat this last stitch on the other side.

Tunneling

Tunneling, as with the procedures already addressed, should be performed with great care and, like much in medicine, there are tricks to obtain the best results (Fig. 9.31A and 9.31B). As shown before, different options exist to perform the technique. In this chapter, it has been recommended that the skin incision should be performed before finding the epidural space. In this case, we already have an epidural with a clean surgical field and complete hemostasis of the surgical area, and the leads anchored to the fascia. Now, the leads have to be tunneled, either to the skin in the context of a test phase (Figs. 9.32A and 9.32B) or to connect to the generator (Fig. 9.33).

It is essential to be careful at all times while tunneling and to monitor both the depth of the tunnel and the plane used so that the provider stays in the subcutaneous adipose tissue. To tunnel more easily, it is suggested that providers use their other hand as a guide to be more precise (Figs. 9.34A and 9.34B). On one hand, if muscle is tunneled, it can cause a major hemorrhage, whereas on the other hand, if the tunnel is too superficial, it can produce skin irritation and a possible erosion in the tunneled area that would necessitate its removal.

Tunneling in the high thoracic area for a cervical implant to the gluteal area has to be done in several steps to avoid this type of complication. If the tunneling is done in only one step, it may require patient sedation to avoid the pain of a surgical act that is traumatic and painful. This is also done to avoid

TABLE 9.8 Different Types of Nonabsorbable Sutures

Generic Name	Silk	Polyester	Polyamide (Nylon)	Polypropylene	Stainless Steel
Composition and structure	Natural Multifilament	Synthetic Multi/ monofilament	Synthetic Multi/ monofilament	Synthetic Monofilament	Synthetic Monofilament
Size (USP)	11/0 to 7	6/0 to 5	11/0 to 2	10/0 to 1	11/0 to 7
Capillarity	High	Medium	Medium/minimal	Minimal	Minimal
Tissue reaction	High	Moderate	Low	Low	Low
Tensile strength	Good	Very good	Very good	Good	Very good
Memoria	Low	Medium	High	High	Low
Uses	Skin anastomosis Vascular ligature Ophthalmology Digestive tract General surgery	Plastic surgery Vascular surgery Skin Orthopedic surgery Vascular prosthesis General surgery	Plastic surgery Nerve damage vascular surgery Microsurgery Orthopedic surgery General surgery	Dermatological and plastic surgery Fascias Nerves General surgery Abdominal wall Orthopedic surgery	Abdominal Wall Orthopedic surgery Neurosurgery Sternum closure

USP, United States Pharmacopoeia.

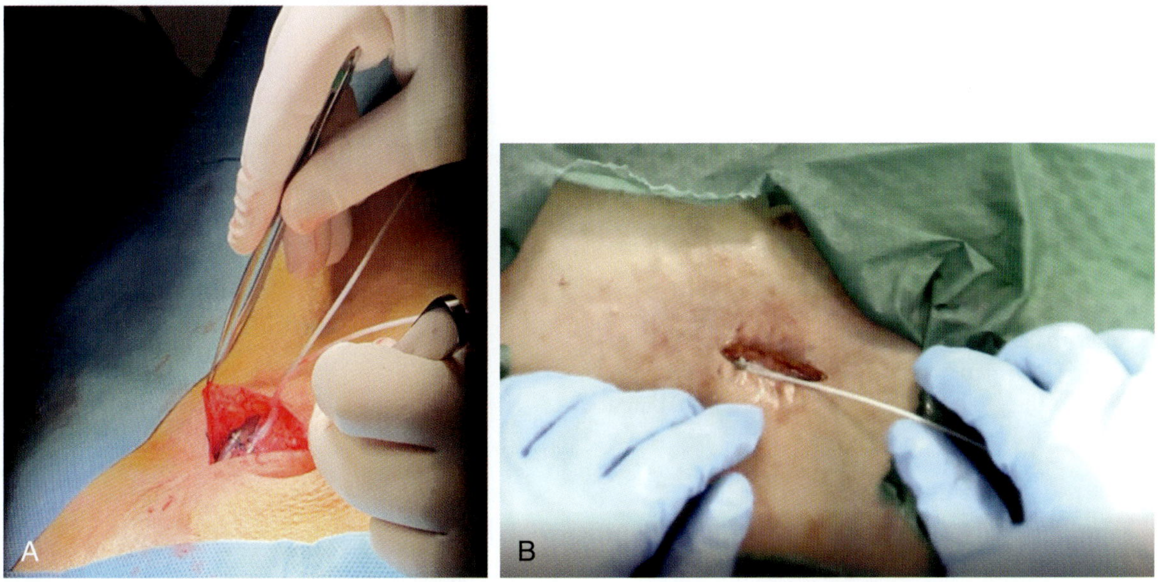

Fig. 9.29 (A) and (B) Anchoring to the fascia. One of the most important steps in this case is to completely introduce the anchor into the lead so that the anchor tip might even be within the fascia. This avoids a step that can facilitate an accidental lead fracture.

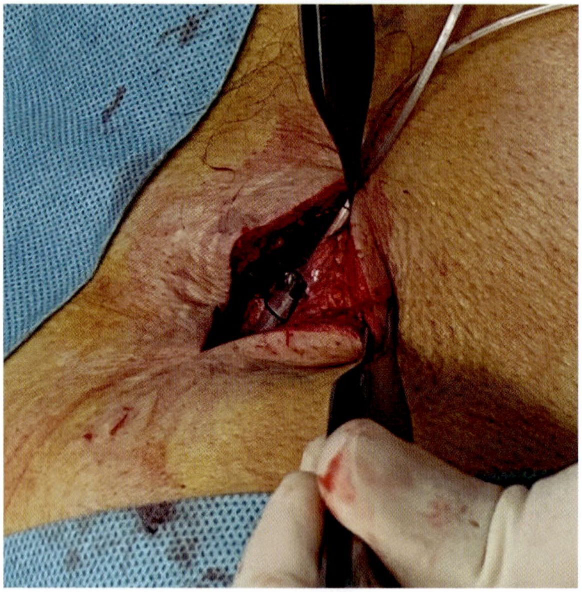

Fig. 9.30 In this case, we used a click anchor. It is recommended that two sutures surround the anchor between the wings and to posteriorly attach each wing with a stitch to the fascia, then pass the needle though the wing, inverting the needle so that the stitch faces itself.

patient movements that can cause complications or damage the system.

An important point of this section is how to pass the leads through to the desired area. To do so, the leads must go into the sleeve of the tunneling tool and be pulled through. Providers should not pull from the leads to avoid lead migration or other complications (Figs. 9.35–9.37).

Finally, to perform this task more easily, it is vital to remember that all of the tunneling shafts can be bent to conform to the patient's body depending on whether tunneling to the gluteal area or to the abdominal area or the flanks is needed.

Creating a Pocket

Creating a pocket is the last step of the procedure. However, that does not mean that it is any less important. As mentioned throughout the chapter, both marking and the case study must be done before

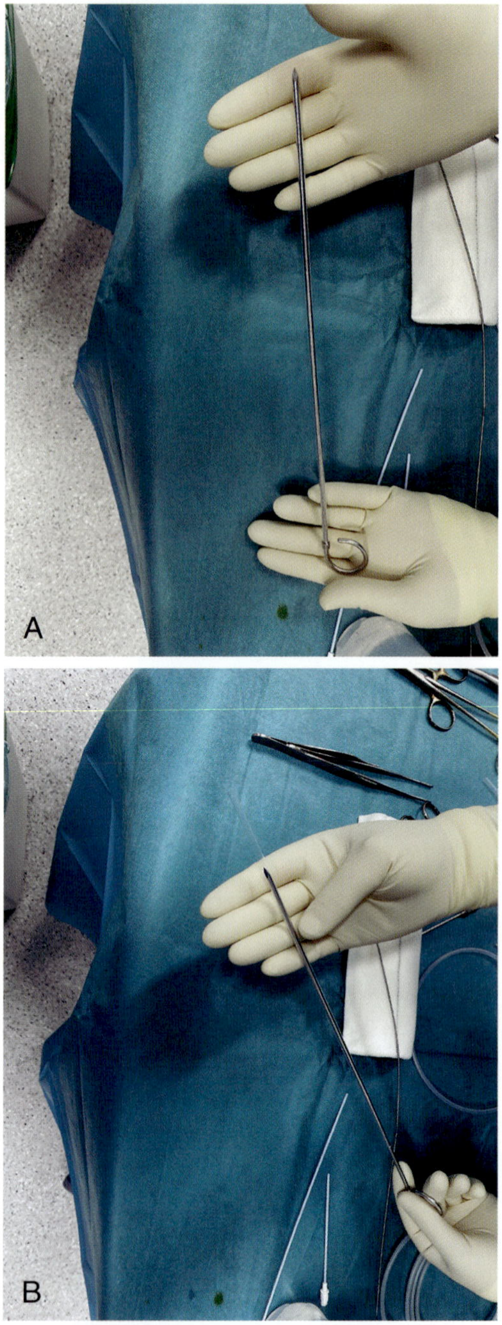

Fig. 9.31 (A) and (B) A tunneling tool that permits passing the leads from the implant area to the generator. All tunneling tools can be bent to facilitate tunneling and make the process less aggressive and atraumatic. On the right, we can see the sleeve of the tunneling tool.

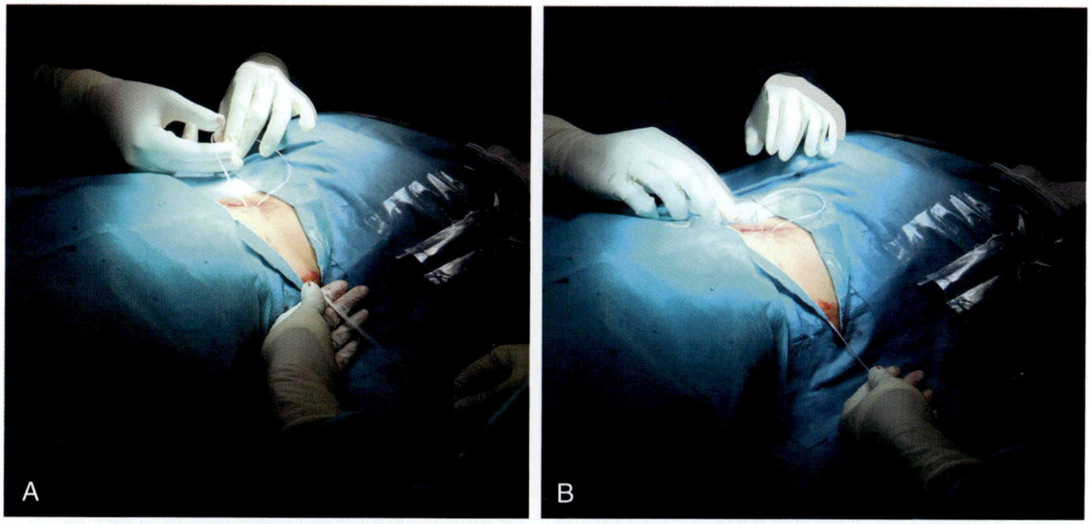

Fig. 9.32 (A) and (B) Tunnel the leads to the opposite side of where the final implant will be to perform the test phase. It is recommended to tunnel as far away as possible from the chosen site to decrease the risk of infection when performing the final implantation.

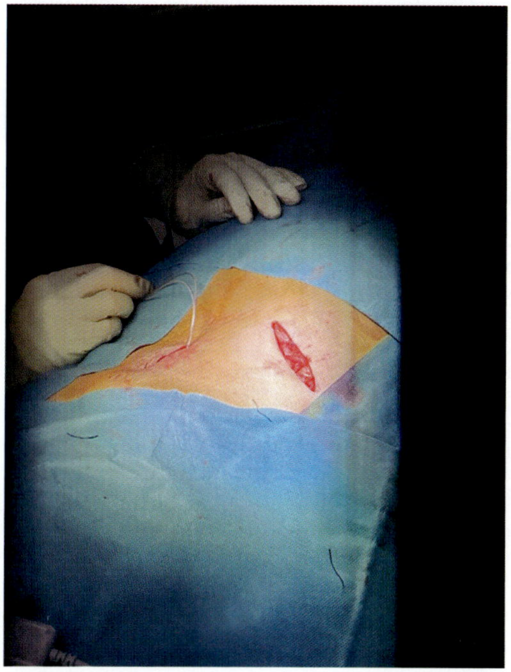

Fig. 9.33 The leads have been tunneled to connect to the generator or to the exterior if a phase test is going to be carried out. In this case, the pocket is ready so that the leads can be tunneled to it and then connected to the generator.

beginning the procedure. The position of the final implant must be discussed with the patient, taking into account their preferences and anatomy (Table 9.9). The type of generator chosen depends on each individual patient. If the generator is rechargeable, it must be located where it is possible to connect it to the charger. If the chosen generator is not a rechargeable system, the depth will be less important. In both cases, the technique must be carried out carefully to avoid pocket pain, which is a frequent complication with a difficult solution[20,21] (Figs. 9.38–9.40).

In general, the usual depth of the pocket is around 3 to 5 cm, but it is important to note that the pocket cannot be too superficial. If too superficial, the generator could erode the skin. If the pocket is too deep, it cannot connect.

The size of the pocket has to be adjusted to the size of the generator. If the pocket is not large enough, complications will be caused by decubitus. If the pocket is too big, the generator could rotate which can result in lead fracture due to constant rotating and, if the generator completely rotates, poor or no connection.

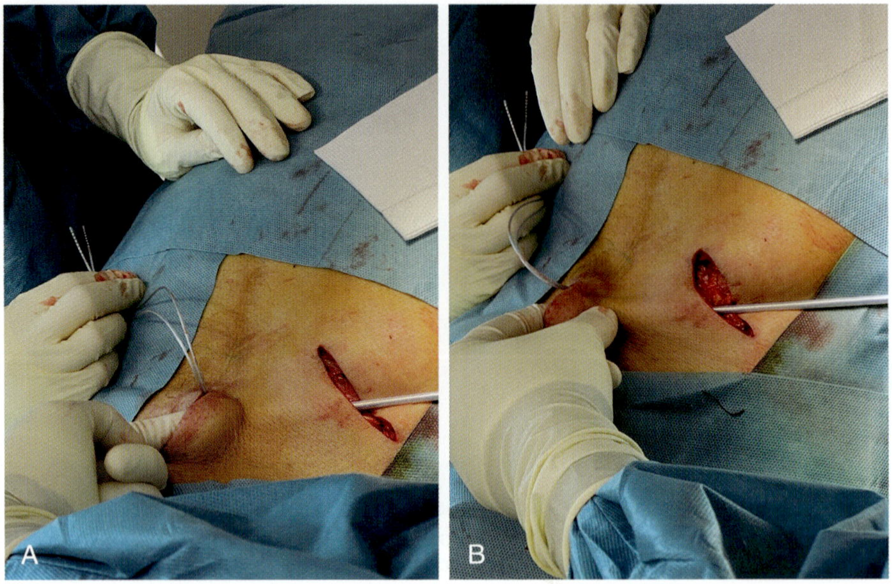

Fig. 9.34 (A) and (B) The tunneling technique is the same in both cases. The most important aspect of the procedure, as can be seen here, is to stay on the same plane and not be too superficial; for that, both hands are needed. The contralateral hand should always be placed in the area you want to reach with the tunneling tool in order to control both the depth of the tool and the plane you are in. This avoids the possible complications of this step—the tunnel will be neither too superficial nor too deep.

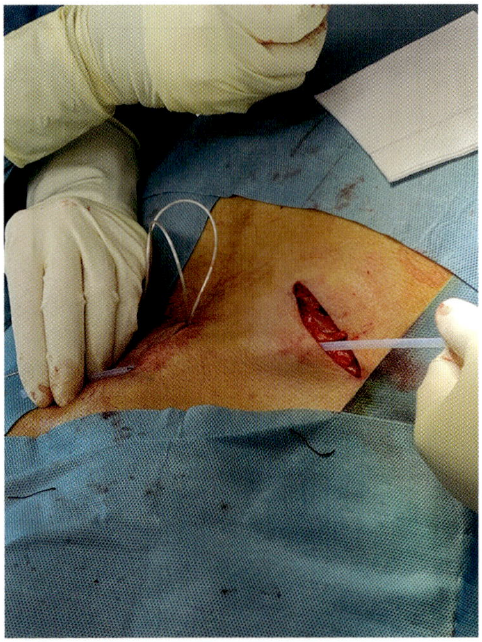

Fig. 9.35 Once the tunneling has been performed, remove the tunneling tool, leaving the sleeve to pass the leads to the pocket area.

TABLE 9.9 Pocket Location

Pocket location	Lead location
Gluteal area	Lumbar, thoracic, sacral, and caudal
Abdominal area	Lumbar, thoracic (if the leads are the same as in the trial phase)
Posterior flank	All
Spine implant site	Lumbar
Chest	Head, neck
Subpectoral	Children, cachectic
Extremities	Peripheral nerve stimulation
Axillar (T4)	Cervical, head and neck

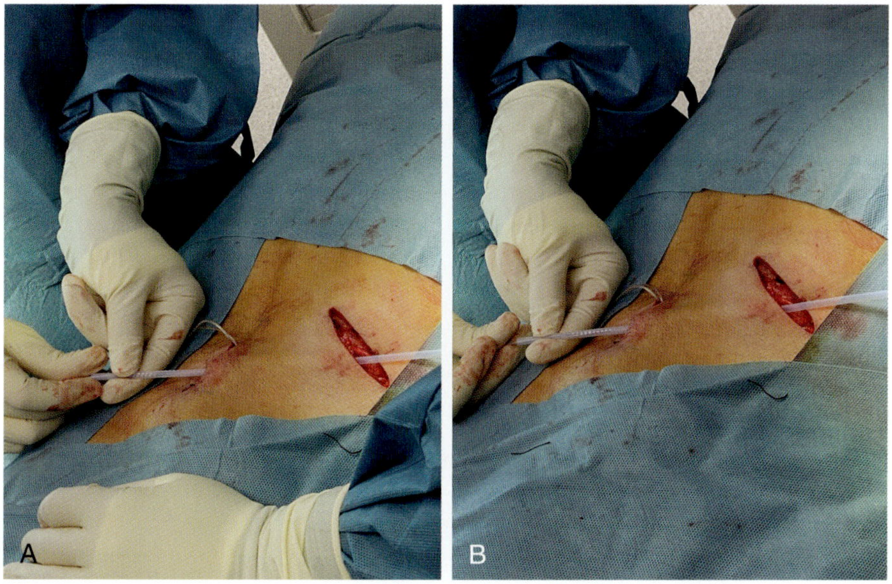

Fig. 9.36 (A) and (B) The leads are passed through the sleeve until they are visible on the other side. Once they can be seen, they are pulled through, pulling from the sleeve and avoiding pulling the leads and thus producing complications in the tunnelled lead.

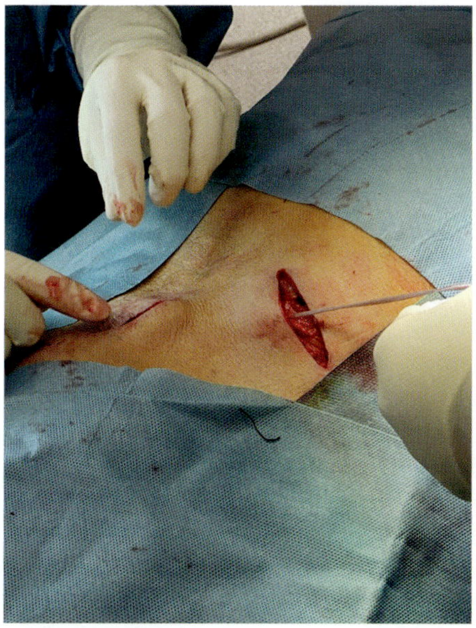

Fig. 9.37 Once the leads have passed through, a loop is made in the entry area of the leads and their length is adjusted so that another loop can be made in the pocket area to avoid lead migration complications.

The surgical technique can vary depending on the surgical team. Blunt dissection is recommended to avoid seroma creation and facilitate hemostasis, which prevents hematomas and possible future infections.

To summarize, although it may appear to be less important, providers must pay the same close attention to this step as they do during other aspects of the procedure, taking these important aspects into account:

1. depth and size of the pocket
2. avoiding seroma formation
3. careful hemostasis

After sizing the pocket in accordance with the system chosen to perform the implant, the electrodes must be connected to the generator ports and the impedances checked to see that they are working perfectly (Fig. 9.41).

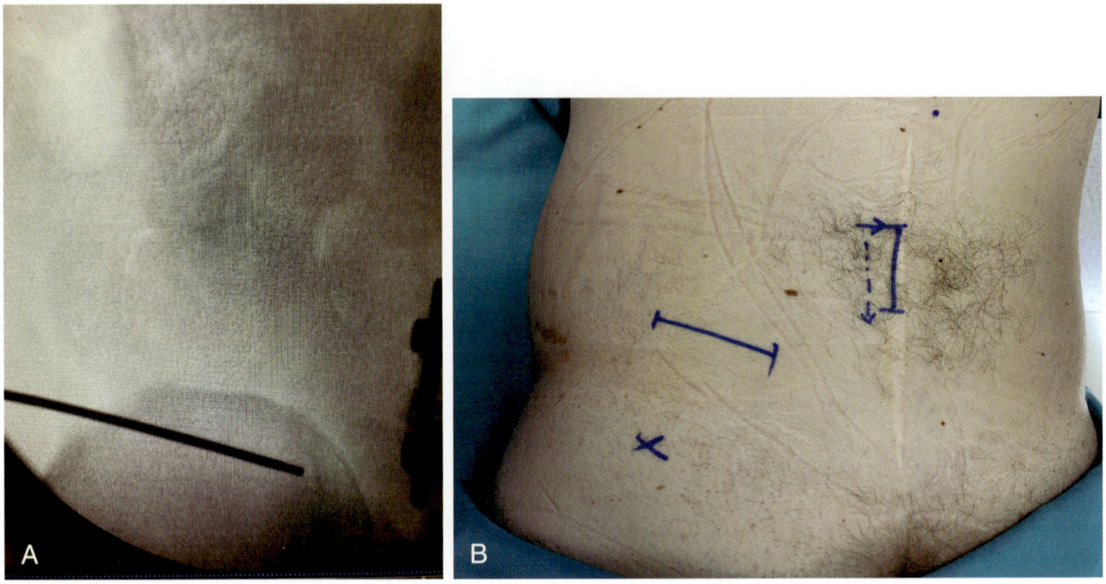

Fig. 9.38 (A) Marking of the location for the implant in the gluteal area using an anteroposterior X-ray view. (B) Marking of the location for the implant in the gluteal area. Note the direction of the incision: it has to be slightly angled instead of being completely perpendicular.

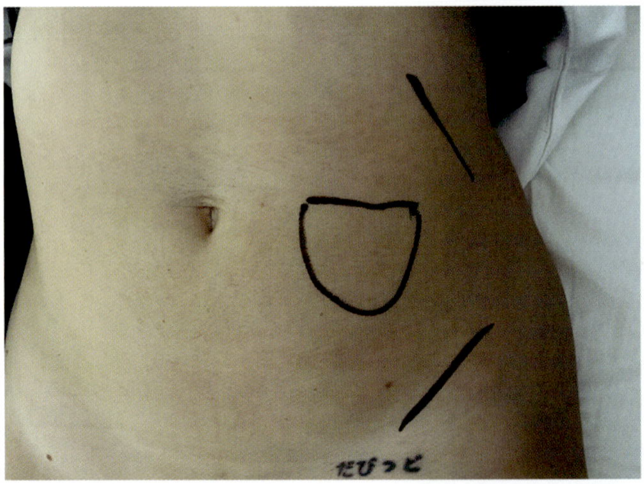

Fig. 9.39 Another frequent location used for pockets and final positioning of the generator is the abdominal area. In the abdominal area, avoid complications in the last rib (*top line*) and anterosuperior iliac crest (*bottom line*) and place the generator between them so that the generator will not stick the patient in the rib or crest in the sitting position.

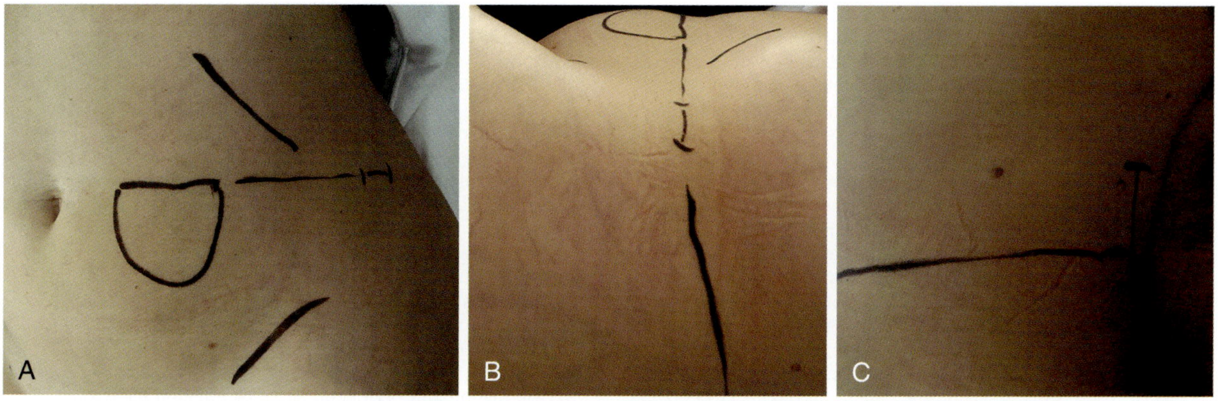

Fig. 9.40 (A) through (C). In this sequence, the markings for an abdominal implant can be seen. The last rib and the anterosuperior iliac crest will be marked as explained in the text and the direction to follow during tunneling from the electrode entry place will also be marked.

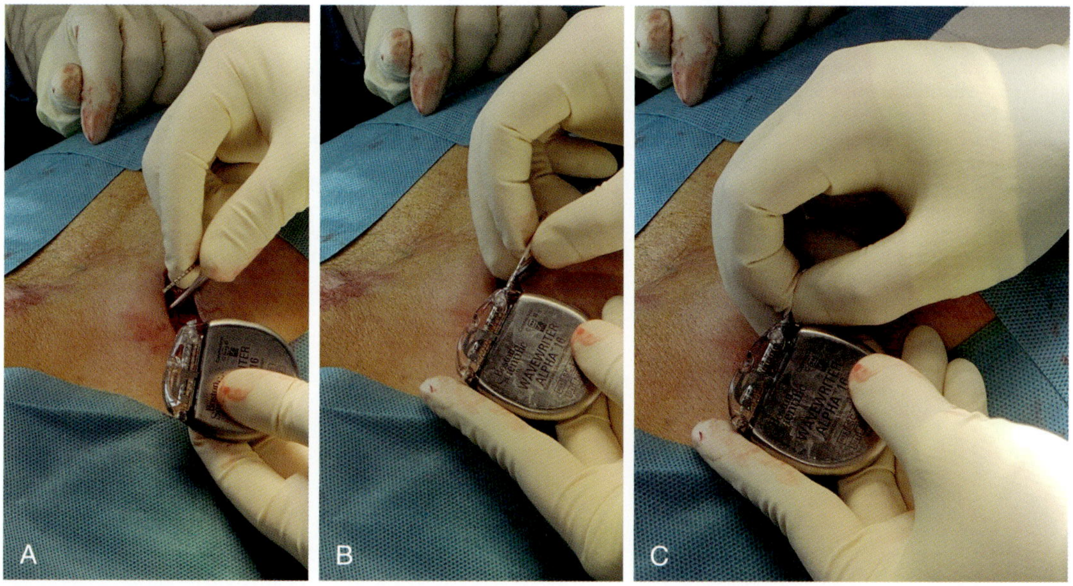

Fig. 9.41 (A) through (C). After creating the pocket according to the size of the system, the leads must be connected to the generator ports and the impedance must be checked to ensure correct functioning.

REFERENCES

1. Kapural L, Yu C, Doust MW, et al. Novel 10-kHz high-frequency therapy (HF10 Therapy) is superior to traditional low-frequency spinal cord stimulation for the treatment of chronic back and leg pain: the SENZA-RCT randomized controlled trial. *Anesthesiology*. 2015;123(4):851-860.
2. Deer T, Slavin KV, Amirdelfan K, et al. Success Using Neuromodulation with BURST (SUNBURST) Study: results from a prospective, randomized controlled trial using a novel burst waveform. *Neuromodulation*. 2018;21(1):56-66.
3. Kapural L, Yu C, Doust MW, et al. Comparison of 10-kHz high-frequency and traditional low-frequency spinal cord stimulation for the treatment of chronic back and leg pain: 24-month results from a multicenter, randomized, controlled pivotal trial. *Neurosurgery*. 2016;79(5):667-677. doi:10.1227/NEU.0000000000001418.
4. Russo M, Cousins MJ, Brooker C, et al. Effective relief of pain and associated symptoms with closed-loop spinal cord

stimulation system: preliminary results of the Avalon Study. *Neuromodulation*. 2018;21(1):38-47. doi:10.1111/ner.12684.
5. De Ridder D, Plazier M, Kamerling N, Menovsky T, Vanneste S. Burst spinal cord stimulation for limb and back pain. *World Neurosurg*. 2013;80(5):642-649.el. doi:10.1016/j.wneu.2013.01.040.
6. Thomson SJ, Tavakkolizadeh M, Love-Jones S, et al. Effects of rate on analgesia in kilohertz frequency spinal cord stimulation: results of the PROCO randomized controlled trial. *Neuromodulation*. 2018;21(1):67-76. doi:10.1111/ner.12746.
7. Cedeño DL, Smith WJ, Kelley CA, Vallejo R. Spinal cord stimulation using differential target multiplexed programming modulates neural cell-specific transcriptomes in an animal model of neuropathic pain. *Mol Pain*. 2020;16. doi:1744806920964360.
8. Kumar K, Taylor RS, Jacques L, et al. Spinal cord stimulation versus conventional medical management for neuropathic pain: a multicentre randomised controlled trial in patients with failed back surgery syndrome. *Pain*. 2007;132(1):179-188. doi:10.1016/j.pain.2007.07.028.
9. North RB, Kidd DH, Farrokhi F, et al. Spinal cord stimulation versus repeated lumbosacral spine surgery for chronic pain: a randomized, controlled trial. *Neurosurgery*. 2005;56(1):98-106; discussion 106-107. doi:10.1227/01.neu.0000144839.65524.e0.
10. Sharan AD, Riley J, Falowski S, et al. Association of opioid usage with spinal cord stimulation outcomes. *Pain Med*. 2017;19: 699-707. doi:10.1093/pm/pnx262.
11. Sanders RA, Moeschler SM, Gazelka HM, et al. Patient outcomes and spinal cord stimulation: a retrospective case series evaluating patient satisfaction, pain scores, and opioid requirements. *Pain Pract*. 2016;16:899-904. doi:10.1111/papr.12340.
12. Marshall B, Bland MK, Hulla R, Gatchel RJ. Considerations in addressing the opioid epidemic and chronic pain within the USA. *Pain Manag*. 2019;9(2):131-138. doi:10.2217/pmt-2018-0070.
13. Odonkor CA, Orman S, Orhurhu V, Stone ME, Ahmed S. Spinal cord stimulation vs conventional therapies for the treatment of chronic low back and leg pain: a systematic review of health care resource utilization and outcomes in the last decade. *Pain Med*. 2019;20(12):2479-2494. doi:10.1093/pm/pnz185.
14. British Pain Society. *Spinal Cord Stimulation for the Management of Pain: Recommendations for Best Clinical Practice*. April 2009. Accessed June 12, 2021. https://www.britishpainsociety.org/static/uploads/resources/files/book_scs_main_1.pdf.
15. Thomson S, Huygen F, Prangnell S, et al. Appropriate referral and selection of patients with chronic pain for spinal cord stimulation: European consensus recommendations and e-health tool. *Eur J Pain*. 2020;24:1169-1181. Available at: https://doi.org/10.1002/ejp.1562.
16. North RB, Wetzel FT. Spinal cord stimulation for chronic pain of spinal origin: a valuable long-term solution. *Spine (Phila PA 1976)*. 2002;27(22):2584-2591; discussion 2592. doi:10.1097/00007632-200211150-00035
17. Eldabe S, Buchser E, Duarte RV. Complications of spinal cord stimulation and peripheral nerve stimulation techniques: a review of the literature. *Pain Med*. 2016;17(2):325-336. doi:10.1093/pm/pnv025.
18. North RB, Recinos VR, Attenello FJ, Shipley J, Long DM. Prevention of percutaneous spinal cord stimulation electrode migration: a 15-year experience. *Neuromodulation*. 2014;17(7): 670-677. doi:10.1111/ner.12151.
19. Barolat G, Massaro F, He J, Zeme S, Ketcik B. Mapping of sensory responses to epidural stimulation of the intraspinal neural structures in man. *J Neurosurg*. 1993;78(2):233-239. doi:10.3171/jns.1993.78.2.0233.
20. Dietvorst S, Decramer T, Lemmens R, Morlion B, Nuttin B, Theys T. Pocket pain and neuromodulation: negligible or neglected? *Neuromodulation*. 2017;20:600-605. doi:10.1111/ner.12637.
21. Mehta SH, Hoelscher CM, Sharan AD, Thalheimer S, Wu C. Implantable pulse generator site may be associated with spinal cord stimulation revision surgeries. *Neuromodulation*. 2021;24: 1336-1340. doi:10.1111/ner.12976.

Chapter 10

Spinal Cord Stimulator Paddle Lead Trial Technique

Wendell Bradley Lake

Chapter Outline

Introduction

Spinal cord stimulation (SCS) is a well-established neuromodulation treatment for pain. Types of pain frequently treated by SCS include failed back syndrome, radiculopathy, neuropathic pain, chronic regional pain syndrome, and angina.[1] Patient selection, stimulator trial, and permanent stimulator implantation are all important steps in the SCS surgical process. Permanent implantation of a spinal cord stimulator with a paddle lead or percutaneous lead is covered elsewhere in this book. In this section, the nuances of the spinal cord stimulator paddle trial are described.

First, a general word about the trial process for spinal cord stimulators. A trial placement of a spinal cord stimulator lead is required prior to permanent implantation. The trial is required for insurance purposes and is also required to optimize lead location. In most scenarios, placement of a trial lead is standard of care and practitioners deviate from this protocol only if significant patient or surgical factors necessitate skipping the trial step.

Once the patient selection process is complete, the initial levels for lead placement are chosen. These are usually chosen based on the patient's description of pain. For example, if the plan is for traditional paresthesia-based stimulation coverage, lower spinal levels are chosen for pain in the more distal lower extremities and higher levels are chosen for pain symptoms in the more proximal lower extremities.[2] Of course, there have been significant changes in the stimulation paradigms offered and paresthesia-based stimulation is not always indicated in the case of high-frequency stimulation or burst stimulation. In these scenarios, the spinal levels chosen may be altered. The spinal level for trial lead location will be discussed in the anatomical considerations portion of this chapter.

The planned spinal level for the trial lead will dictate the method of trial lead placement. Most patients undergoing spinal cord stimulator trial lead placement have cylindrical leads placed in the epidural space. However, not all patients can undergo percutaneous trial lead placement safely. Common factors leading to this situation include epidural scarring and/or prior spinal instrumentation. In these cases, practitioners may have to resort to a spinal cord stimulator paddle lead trial. In this chapter, the anatomical considerations in placing a trial paddle lead are described along with the step-by-step process for paddle lead placement, how to manage complications, and general considerations.

Anatomical Considerations

Anatomical considerations related to paddle lead trial for SCS include spinal level determination and laminar anatomy relevant to laminectomy and paddle placement. First, spinal level determination is discussed since the level chosen dictates the laminar anatomy. Next, anatomy relevant to laminectomy and placement of the paddle lead is discussed.

The choice of spinal level is important when placing a spinal cord stimulator trial lead regardless of whether a paddle lead or cylindrical lead is used for a trial. Making a good choice of the spinal level for the trial may be even more important in the case of a paddle trial. This is because, due to the need for laminectomy during a paddle trial, the patient is under general anesthesia and, therefore, intraoperative testing cannot be performed to check paresthesia coverage. However, it must be noted that there is literature available on awake SCS paddle lead placement indicating favorable outcomes in appropriately chosen patients.[3]

When choosing the initial target spinal levels for an SCS lead trial the patient's pain symptomatology must be considered carefully. For patients with back pain and/or upper leg pain, one may consider centering the trial lead from approximately the mid-T8 vertebral body to the T9 to T10 disk space. For more distal leg pain, one may consider placing the lead from the T8 to T9 disk space down to the mid-T10 body or even down to the T10 to T11 disk space.[4] These recommendations hold true for paresthesia-based stimulation but may be modified somewhat for high-frequency nonparesthesia-based stimulation. Often, contacts used for high-frequency paresthesia-free SCS are in the T9 to T10 region.[5] Similar trial levels are relevant for burst stimulation paradigms.[6] In general, it is our practice to allow patients to trial both traditional paresthesia-based stimulation and higher-frequency nonparesthesia-based stimulation. Laminectomy for paddle trial in the cervical or thoracic level can also be performed for pain in the arms or chest but is much less common. Here, the spinal level corresponds much more closely with the expected pain level since spinal cord level and bony spinal level are very similar.

Once the spinal level has been chosen for the paddle lead trial, the relevant laminar and spinal anatomy can be discussed. To center a paddle lead for a trial at approximately the T8 to T11 level, it is generally necessary to perform a laminectomy at either the T10 to T11 or T11 to T12 level. In general, a small amount of the rostral spinous process is removed at the interspinous space. Then, the ligamentum flavum is opened with curettes and Kerrison punches. The inferior edge of the upper lamina and a portion of the superior edge of the inferior lamina are also resected with the Kerrison punch. Fig. 10.1 provides a schematic view of the lamina and laminectomy.[7]

Description of the Procedure

A spinal cord stimulator paddle lead trial begins with patient selection. Patients selected for this procedure fit the selection criteria of standard SCS trial patients but have significant risk for epidural scarring or other factors making percutaneous lead trial high risk, such as spinal stenosis, prior upper lumbar or lower to mid-thoracic instrumentation, or spinal surgery.[4] Once the patient has been selected, the procedure can be performed. The patient should be positioned prone on a

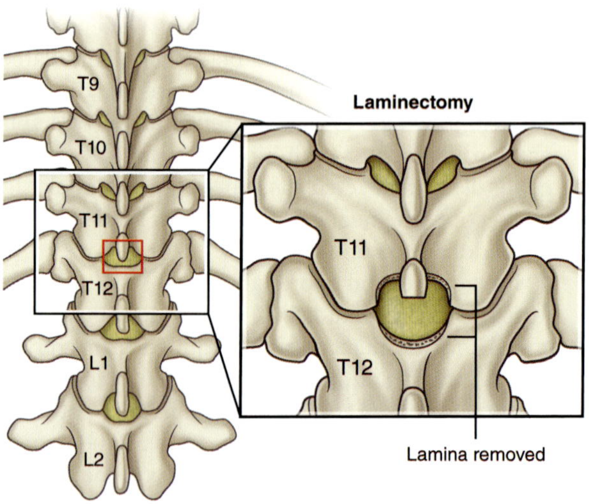

Fig. 10.1 Schematic diagram of the thoracic lamina. (A) Intact lamina. (B) Laminectomy. In general, only the lower 1/5 of the box drawn would be used for placement of a spinal cord stimulator trial. (Modified from Sun C, Chen G, Fan T, et al. Ultrasonic bone scalpel for thoracic spinal decompression: case series and technical note. *J Orthop Surg Res.* 2020; 15(1):309.

frame table. Allowing the patient's abdomen to hang free in a frame table reduces pressure in the epidural space. Fig. 10.2 demonstrates standard positioning.[2] Note that the internal pulse generator (IPG) incision site is marked out even though the IPG will not be placed at this time. This is to avoid tunneling the temporary wires to this area. Next, fluoroscopy is brought into the field to localize the area for the laminectomy. In general, the laminectomy is at the interspinous space at least one level below the site at which the most inferior trial contacts will reside. For example, if the paddle lead is to be centered over the T9 body and the inferior contacts will be at the upper edge of the T10 body, then the laminectomy will be the inferior portion of T10 and superior portion of T11.

Once the midline incision is created, the paraspinous muscles are reflected laterally with cautery (see Fig. 10.1A). The operative level is verified and self-retaining retractors are placed. The inferior portion of the lamina and spinous process is removed for the rostral level and the superior portion of the lamina for the caudal level is removed (see Fig. 10.1B). Once the laminectomy is done, the dura is dissected with care using a Woodson and then with a plastic dissector. The paddle lead is passed. The paddle lead used for paddle trials is the same as that used for permanent implants. Fluoroscopy is used to verify that the lead is midline and at the appropriate spinal levels. Fig. 10.3 shows a fluoroscopic image of an appropriately placed paddle lead.

After the paddle lead is placed, it is anchored to the fascia and interspinous ligament using the provided anchoring device. The lead is connected to thin temporary wires that are tunneled out of the skin away from the prospective site of the IPG. The wound is then closed in the standard fashion as described in Chapter 6. First, close the muscle and fascia, then the deep dermal layer, and, finally, the skin. The skin is normally closed using a nonabsorbable monofilament, such as nylon or prolene. Nonabsorbable sutures are used at this point because they have to be removed in 3 to 7 days at the conclusion of the trial period when the patient and clinician have determined that either the trial was unsuccessful and, therefore, the lead must be removed or the trial was successful and the lead needs to be connected to an IPG for permanent implantation.

Having presented the paddle lead implantation procedure, it is now useful to discuss the transition to a permanent lead or explant of the lead. A typical trial

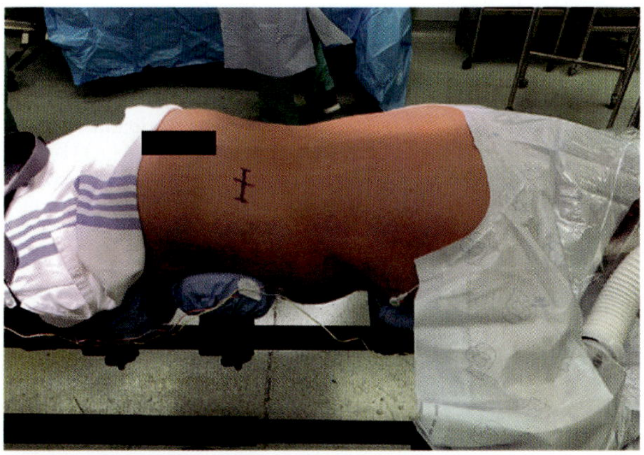

Fig. 10.2 Appropriate positioning for a paddle lead trial. Note that the prospective site and side for the internal pulse generator is marked out even though it is not to be placed at this time since the temporary wires will be tunneled away from the IPG incision site to reduce the risk of infection.

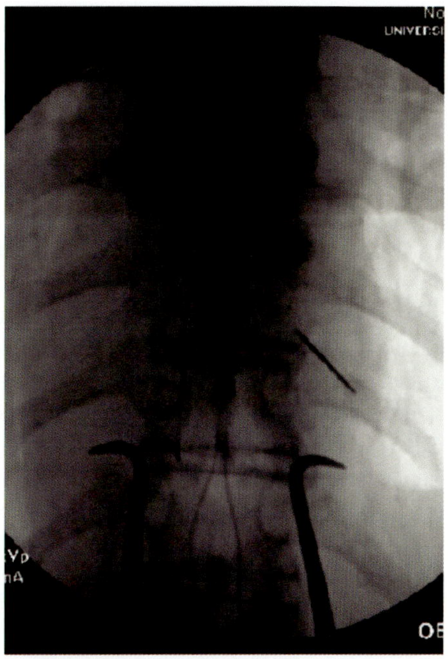

Fig. 10.3 Appropriate placement of a spinal cord stimulator paddle lead. Note that the lead is midline and at the appropriate spinal level.

period is 3 to 7 days. In the case of a paddle lead trial, the patient has to return to the operating room either for removal (unsuccessful trial) or IPG placement (successful trial). It is recommended to take a postoperative X-ray at the time of performing the transition to a permanent lead to ensure a stable position and to allow future comparison when the efficacy changes. To transition to a permanent implant, the back is prepped and draped with the tunneled temporary wires out of the field but accessible. The midline spinal incision is opened. The temporary wires connecting to the paddle lead are clipped internally; then, the assistant in the unsterile area pulls the remaining temporary wires from the skin. The temporary wires can then be disconnected from the paddle lead and the paddle lead is tunneled and connected to the permanent IPG as described elsewhere in this volume.

Intraoperative Complications

Several well-known complications can occur intraoperatively during spinal cord stimulator lead placement. The most common are epidural hematoma, cerebrospinal fluid leak, and inability to properly place the lead due to epidural scarring.

One of the most concerning, albeit rare, complications of spinal cord stimulator lead placement is epidural hematoma. This can be avoided to some degree by meticulous dissection and ensuring normal coagulation status. Some may consider intraoperative monitoring for early detection of neurological deficit. However, this generally is not considered standard of care.

Cerebrospinal fluid leak is a possible complication of either percutaneous lead placement or paddle lead placement by laminectomy.[8] In the case of laminectomy for paddle lead placement, an attempt should be made to close the leak primarily. Then, the practitioner has the option of carrying on with the procedure if the leak is well closed.

In some cases, the epidural space may be so scarred that even a paddle trial is very difficult. Often, the paddle can be partially placed. Some authors have advocated drilling a "trough" or narrow central laminectomy to facilitate direct onlay of the lead.[9]

General Considerations and Conclusions

SCS therapy may be a useful option to reduce pain in appropriately selected patients. Many patients undergoing SCS therapy have had significant spinal surgery and percutaneous SCS lead trials are not possible. In these patients, it is reasonable to consider SCS paddle trials. This offers patients the benefit of assessing the therapy prior to permanent implantation. Paddle lead trials require a laminectomy and, therefore, are more invasive than percutaneous lead trials. Nonetheless, a paddle lead trial can be safe and efficacious in appropriately selected patients with proper technique and attention to detail.

REFERENCES

1. Sitzman BT, Provenzano DA. Best practices in spinal cord stimulation. *Spine*. 2017;42(suppl 14):S67-S71.
2. Westrup AM, Conner AK. Percutaneous thoracic spinal cord stimulator placement. *Cureus*. 2021;13:e13916.
3. Vanhauwaert DJ, Couvreur T, Vandebroek A, De Coster O, Hanssens K. Conscious sedation using dexmedetomidine during surgical paddle lead placement improves outcome in spinal cord stimulation: a case series of 25 consecutive patients. *Neuromodulation*. 2021;24(8);1347-1350. doi:10.1111/ner.13124.
4. Lee JJ, Simpson RK, Dalm B. Permanent paddle-lead trial for spinal cord stimulation. *Cureus*. 2018;10:e2645.
5. Hagedorn JM, Layno-Moses A, Sanders DT, Pak DJ, Bailey-Classen A, Sowder T. Overview of HF10 spinal cord stimulation for the treatment of chronic pain and an introduction to the Senza Omnia™ system. *Pain Manag*. 2020;10(6):367-376.
6. Peeters JB, Raftopoulos C. Tonic, burst, high-density, and 10-khz high-frequency spinal cord stimulation: efficiency and patients' preferences in a failed back surgery syndrome predominant population. Review of literature. *World Neurosurg*. 2020;144:e331-e340.
7. Sun C, Chen G, Fan T, et al. Ultrasonic bone scalpel for thoracic spinal decompression: case series and technical note. *J Orthop Surg Res*. 2020;15(1):309.
8. Eldrige JS, Weingarten TN, Rho RH. Management of cerebral spinal fluid leak complicating spinal cord stimulator implantation. *Pain Pract*. 2006;6:285-288.
9. Pabaney AH, Robin AM, Schwalb JM. New technique for open placement of paddle-type spinal cord stimulator electrode in presence of epidural scar tissue. *Neuromodulation*. 2014;17:759-762; discussion 762.

Chapter 11

Spinal Cord Stimulator System Permanent Implant with Laminectomy for Paddle Lead

Wendell Bradley Lake

Chapter Outline

Introduction

As mentioned in other chapters, spinal cord stimulation (SCS) is a well-established neuromodulation treatment for pain. Types of pain frequently treated by SCS include failed back syndrome, radiculopathy, neuropathic pain, chronic regional pain syndrome, and angina.[1] Patient selection, stimulator trial, and permanent stimulator implantation are all important steps in the SCS surgical process. This chapter discusses permanent implantation of spinal cord stimulators with a paddle lead. Permanent SCS system implantation with percutaneous cylindrical leads is covered elsewhere in this volume.

Once a patient has been appropriately selected and a positive trial has concluded, the patient and practitioner may choose to move on to implantation of a permanent SCS system. At this point, implantation of a paddle lead or percutaneous cylindrical lead can be considered. In some cases, it is not possible to place a percutaneous cylindrical lead; these patients must have a laminectomy for permanent paddle lead implantation. These patients usually also underwent a paddle lead trial in most cases and, therefore, permanent SCS system implantation usually entails only placing the implantable pulse generator (IPG) and connecting it to the extant paddle lead. The paddle lead trial is discussed in another chapter in this volume. Alternatively, some patients who undergo a successful trial with a percutaneous lead will elect to have a paddle lead placed for their permanent implant. Reasons for electively choosing a permanent paddle lead vary but may include the need for lower-energy delivery, lower lead migration rate, and greater efficacy.[2,3] However, some authors have noted that migration rates for percutaneously placed leads may have declined in recent years and approach those of paddle leads placed via laminectomy.[4] If paddle lead placement via laminectomy is chosen for permanent implantation, it is important to counsel the patient on the recovery time following a laminectomy and the potential for increased postoperative pain when compared with percutaneously placed cylindrical leads.

In this chapter, the surgical nuances of permanent SCS implantation with a paddle lead are discussed along with anatomical considerations and intraoperative complication management and avoidance.

Anatomical Considerations

Anatomical considerations related to placement of a permanent spinal cord stimulator system with a paddle lead include laminar anatomy relevant to laminectomy and paddle placement.

The choice of spinal level is important when placing a spinal cord stimulator trial lead regardless of whether a paddle lead or cylindrical lead is used for a trial. Permanent SCS system placement with a paddle lead is generally performed under general anesthesia. However, some authors do describe laminectomy for paddle lead trial under sedation and local anesthetic, and their results appear favorable.[5]

When choosing the target spinal levels for a spinal cord stimulator lead trial, the patient's pain symptomatology must be considered. The chapter on paddle lead trials presents a detailed description of how to choose the levels for trialing patients with various pain symptomatologies as described by other authors.[6,7] When placing the permanent paddle lead for an SCS system, it is important to encompass the trial levels with the permanent lead. In particular, the area of the patient's preferred contacts must be covered, along with areas rostral and caudal, as much as possible. Intraoperative X-rays are taken at the time of trial lead placement and then prior to removal of the trial lead. This allows the practitioner to ensure coverage of the appropriate levels.

Once the spinal level has been chosen for the paddle lead, the relevant laminar and spinal anatomy can be discussed. In general, to center a paddle lead for a permanent implant, the laminectomy is performed one level caudal to the level of the vertebral body to be covered. For example, to center a lead on T10, a partial T10 to T11 laminectomy is performed. The practitioner must take care to allow sufficient lamina to remain such that the paddle lead is held in opposition to the cord. In general, a small amount of the rostral spinous process is removed at the interspinous space. Then, the ligamentum flavum is opened with curettes and Kerrison punches. The inferior edge of the upper lamina and a portion of the superior edge of the inferior lamina are also resected with the Kerrison punch. Fig. 11.1 provides a schematic view of the lamina and laminectomy.[8]

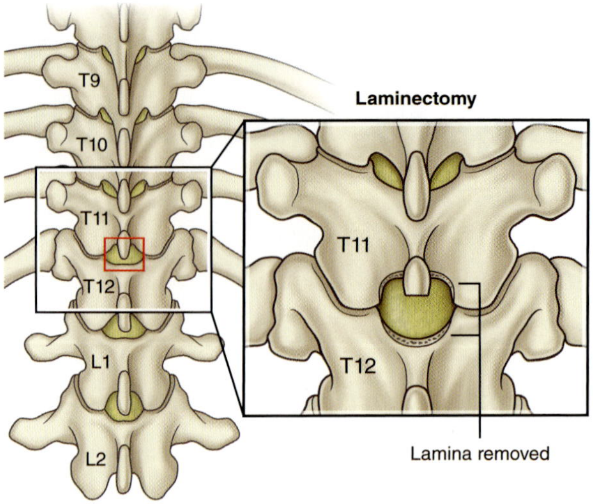

Fig. 11.1 Schematic diagram of the thoracic lamina. (A) Intact lamina. (B) Laminectomy. In general, only the lower 1/5 of the box drawn would be used for placement of a spinal cord stimulator trial. (Modified from Sun C, Chen G, Fan T, et al. Ultrasonic bone scalpel for thoracic spinal decompression: case series and technical note. *J Orthop Surg Res.* 2020; 15[1]:309.)

Description of the Procedure

Patients undergoing permanent SCS system implantation with a paddle lead generally fall into two categories. One category is those patients who have undergone trial with a paddle lead, usually due to epidural scarring or other factors precluding trialing with a cylindrical percutaneous lead. The other category is patients who have undergone trial with percutaneous cylindrical leads but now elect for permanent SCS implantation with a paddle lead because of a perceived increase in efficacy or reduced lead migration rate. The surgical procedure for permanent SCS system implantation differs for each of these scenarios and will be discussed in turn.

In the first case, the paddle lead is already implanted per Chapter 10 on paddle lead trials. The lead is externalized with temporary wires tunneled through the skin and the permanent SCS wires are coiled under the midline incision and anchored into place. In this scenario, the practitioner positions the patient on a frame table prone as demonstrated in Fig. 11.2.[9] The position for the IPG incision is marked out (this is usually on the side opposite to where the temporary wires are tunneled and penetrate the skin). The temporary lead wires are then trimmed at the skin with a pair of sterile scissors. A post-positioning X-ray is compared with the post-trial lead placement radiograph to ensure appropriate positioning of the lead.

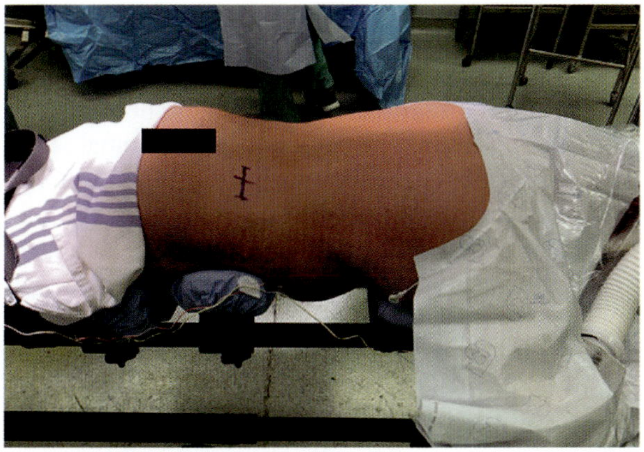

Fig. 11.2 Appropriate positioning for a paddle lead trial. Note that the prospective site and side for the implantable pulse generator (IPG) is marked out even though it is not to be placed at this time as the temporary wires will be tunneled away from the IPG incision site to reduce the risk of infection.

This step is crucial because the permanent lead has to encompass the lead area found to be efficacious during the trialing process. The back, including the midline incision site and the prospective IPG site, is prepped and draped in a sterile fashion. The IPG site should be chosen toward the least painful side if applicable and one should ensure that the selected incision site is away from the waist band and will not conflict with the use of a wheelchair if the patient is wheelchair bound.

The IPG site is anesthetized and opened. Using cautery, dissection is carried out down to whichever is least, the level of the fascia or down to the depth appropriate for IPG placement per the manufacturer's recommendations (usually < 2 cm). A word of caution is relevant in treating obese patients. In these patients, a large subcutaneous fat layer may make it difficult to adequately anchor the IPG. In general, the IPG pocket should be no larger than to accommodate the IPG. If the pocket is too large, it may increase postoperative pain and can allow the IPG to flip, thus damaging the lead.

Once the pocket is created, it is covered with a moist lap. The preexisting midline incision is then opened. Careful dissection reveals the lead wires coiled beneath the fascia and anchored to the spinous processes. The remnant of the temporary wire is disconnected from the paddle lead using the necessary screwdriver. The paddle lead tails are tunneled to the IPG incision site with care not to dislodge the paddle lead. The paddle lead tails are inserted into the IPG and secured with the driver. The IPG is anchored in place with nonabsorbable suture and lead impedances are verified. Finally, an X-ray is performed to ensure no shifting of the paddle lead and to provide a point of reference for future programming. Incisions are closed in layers as described in Chapter 6 of this volume. The exit site for the temporary wires is closed with steri-strips. Fig. 11.3 provides a typical final radiographical image of an IPG and paddle lead for a permanent SCS system implantation.

Now, the second scenario is described, in which a paddle lead permanent SCS system implantation is being done for a patient who underwent trialing with cylindrical percutaneous leads. In cases such as this, the patient usually has already had the trial leads removed. We recommend that the lead insertion sites should be allowed to heal fully before undergoing additional surgery. The patient is positioned on the frame table prone with careful padding as depicted in

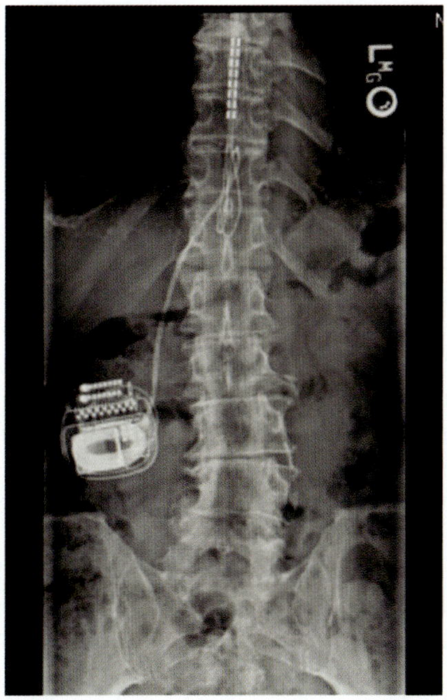

Fig. 11.3 Appropriate placement of a spinal cord stimulator paddle lead with an implantable pulse generator. Note that the lead is midline and at the appropriate spinal level.

Fig. 11.2.[9] A midline incision is marked out and an IPG incision is marked out. The back is prepped. We initially create the incision for the IPG as described earlier and place a lap sponge over the site to cover it while we work on the laminectomy.

Next, fluoroscopy is brought into the field to localize the area for the laminectomy. The practitioner examines the post-trial radiographs to ensure that placement of the permanent paddle lead will be at the correct level. Using fluoroscopy, the correct incision site is marked. In general, the laminectomy is at the interspinous space at least one level below the site at which the most inferior trial contacts will reside. For example, if the paddle lead is to be centered over the T9 body and the inferior contacts will be at the upper edge of the T10 body, then the laminectomy will be the inferior portion of T10 and superior portion of T11.

Laminectomy proceeds as described in Chapter 10 of this volume. Once the midline incision is created, the paraspinous muscles are reflected laterally with cautery (see Fig. 11.1A). The operative level is verified and self-retaining retractors are placed. The inferior portion of the lamina and spinous process is removed for the rostral level and the superior portion of the lamina for the caudal level is removed (see Fig. 11.1B). Once the laminectomy is done, the dura is dissected with care using a Woodson and then with a plastic dissector. The paddle lead is passed. The paddle lead used for paddle trials is the same as that used for permanent implants. Fluoroscopy is used to verify that the lead is midline and at the appropriate spinal levels. Fig. 11.3 shows a fluoroscopic image of an appropriately placed paddle lead.

After the paddle lead is placed, it is anchored to the fascia and interspinous ligament using the provided anchoring device. The paddle lead tails are then tunneled to the IPG pocket. The lead is sequentially connected to the IPG and secured using the driver. As described earlier, the IPG is anchored using nonabsorbable suture. Impedances are tested and a final radiograph is done to ensure correct positioning of the paddle lead. The wound is then closed in the standard fashion as described in Chapter 6. First, close the muscle and fascia, then the deep dermal layer, and, finally, the skin. The skin is closed using a nonabsorbable or absorbable monofilament.

Intraoperative Complications

Several complications can occur intraoperatively during spinal cord stimulator placement. These include infection, epidural hematoma, cerebrospinal fluid leak, and inability to properly place the lead due to epidural scarring.

One of the most concerning, albeit rare, complications of spinal cord stimulator lead placement is epidural hematoma. This can be avoided to some degree by meticulous dissection and ensuring normal coagulation status. Some may consider intraoperative monitoring for early detection of neurological deficit but this is not generally considered standard of care.

Infection is one of the more common complications for any implantable device. SCS infection occurs in 2% to 10% of patients in some literature studies, with the most common organism being *Staphylococcus aureus*. Lead type is not a risk factor for infection with percutaneous leads and paddle leads placed by laminectomy having similar infection rates. Staging the procedure between the trial and the permanent implant may be associated with a lower infection rate.[10] To minimize infection rate preincision, antibiotics are given and sterile technique is maintained.

Cerebral spinal fluid leak is a possible complication of either percutaneous lead placement or paddle lead placement by laminectomy.[11] In the case of laminectomy for paddle lead placement, an attempt should be made to close the leak primarily. Then, the practitioner has the option of carrying on with the procedure if the leak is well closed.

In some cases, the epidural space may be so scarred that even placing a paddle lead is very difficult. Often, the paddle can be partially placed. Some authors have advocated drilling a "trough" or narrow central laminectomy to facilitate direct onlay of the lead.[12]

General Considerations and Conclusions

SCS therapy offers a useful option for chronic pain in appropriately selected patients. In some patients, it is appropriate to carry out a permanent SCS system implantation with a paddle lead if an efficacious trial has been completed. Placement of a permanent SCS system with a paddle lead through the use of appropriate surgical technique has an acceptable safety profile and a complication rate now higher than that of percutaneous lead placement. Additional studies are necessary to determine whether SCS systems with paddle leads offer any definitive benefits over percutaneous cylindrical leads.

REFERENCES

1. Sitzman BT, Provenzano DA. Best practices in spinal cord stimulation. *Spine*. 2017;42(suppl 14):S67-S71.
2. North RB, McNamee JP, Wu L, Piantadosi S. Artificial neural networks: application to electrical stimulation of the human nervous system. *Neurosurg Focus*. 1997;2:e1.
3. Villavicencio AT, Leveque JC, Rubin L, Bulsara K, Gorecki JP. Laminectomy versus percutaneous electrode placement for spinal cord stimulation. *Neurosurgery*. 2000;46:399-405; discussion 405-406.
4. Gazelka HM, Freeman ED, Hooten WM, et al. Incidence of clinically significant percutaneous spinal cord stimulator lead migration. *Neuromodulation*. 2015;18(2):123-125, discussion 125.
5. Vanhauwaert DJ, Couvreur T, Vandebroek A, De Coster O, Hanssens K. Conscious sedation using dexmedetomidine during surgical paddle lead placement improves outcome in spinal cord stimulation: a case series of 25 consecutive patients. *Neuromodulation*. 2021;24(8):1347-1350. doi:10.1111/ner.13124.
6. Lee JJ, Simpson RK, Dalm B. Permanent paddle-lead trial for spinal cord stimulation. *Cureus*. 2018;10:e2645.
7. Hagedorn JM, Layno-Moses A, Sanders DT, Pak DJ, Bailey-Classen A, Sowder T. Overview of HF10 spinal cord stimulation for the treatment of chronic pain and an introduction to the Senza Omnia™ system. *Pain Manag*. 2020;10(6):367-376.
8. Sun C, Chen J, Fan T, et al. Ultrasonic bone scalpel for thoracic spinal decompression: case series and technical note. *J Orthop Surg Res*. 2020;15(1):309.
9. Westrup AM, Conner AK. Percutaneous thoracic spinal cord stimulator placement. *Cureus*. 2021;13:e13916.
10. Esquer Garrigos Z, Farid S, Bendel MA, Sohail MR. Spinal cord stimulator infection: approach to diagnosis, management, and prevention. *Clin Infect Dis*. 2020;70:2727-2735.
11. Eldrige JS, Weingarten TN, Rho RH. Management of cerebral spinal fluid leak complicating spinal cord stimulator implantation. *Pain Pract*. 2006;6:285-288.
12. Pabaney AH, Robin AM, Schwalb JM. New technique for open placement of paddle-type spinal cord stimulator electrode in presence of epidural scar tissue. *Neuromodulation*. 2014;17:759-762, discussion 762.

Chapter 12

Dorsal Root Ganglion Stimulator Trial

Shiv Patel, Nathanael Leo, and Sayed Emal Wahezi

Chapter Outline

Introduction

Dorsal root ganglion (DRG) stimulation was introduced in Europe in 2011 and in the United States in 2016.[1] The DRG encompasses cell bodies for primary cell neurons thought to be the primary modulator site for chronic pain disorders.[2] As a result, modulation of the DRG may be an effective treatment in patients with focal pain syndromes.[2,3] DRG stimulation differs from traditional spinal cord stimulation (SCS) devices mainly by the placement and type of energy delivered by the leads. SCS leads are placed juxtaposed to the dorsal column, but DRG stimulator leads are placed adjacent to the DRG.

Anatomical Considerations

- Magnetic resonance imaging (MRI) of the spine (at target stimulation level) should be evaluated prior to a DRG stimulator trial to ensure no significant neuroforaminal stenosis (Figs. 12.1 and 12.2).
- The starting level and approach will differ depending on the level of stimulation (L3 or higher vs. L4/L5 vs. sacral). In Fig. 12.3, note that the starting point for L3 DRG is the contralateral pedicle two levels below whereas the starting level for L4 or L5 is the sacroiliac joint at approximately the S1 level.
- The steeper approach necessary for L4 and L5 DRG targets increases risk of dural puncture.

Procedural Steps

1. Patient positioning: Lying prone. Bolster at the lower pelvis to reduce lumbar lordosis (Fig. 12.4).
2. Confirm the correct level of target stimulation with an anteroposterior (AP) view of the spine.
3. Place a marker on the contralateral pedicle two levels below the target DRG (Fig. 12.5).
4. The needle should enter the epidural space at the midline interlaminar space one level below the DRG target. Anesthetize the tract with a local anesthetic, then introduce the needle at the marked site. The needle should be advanced anteriorly and medially without crossing the midline. See Fig. 12.6 for needle trajectory in the AP view.
5. The depth of the needle can be confirmed periodically in the lateral view (Fig. 12.7). Once the needle is engaged in the interspinous ligament, a loss-of-resistance syringe can be attached to the needle.

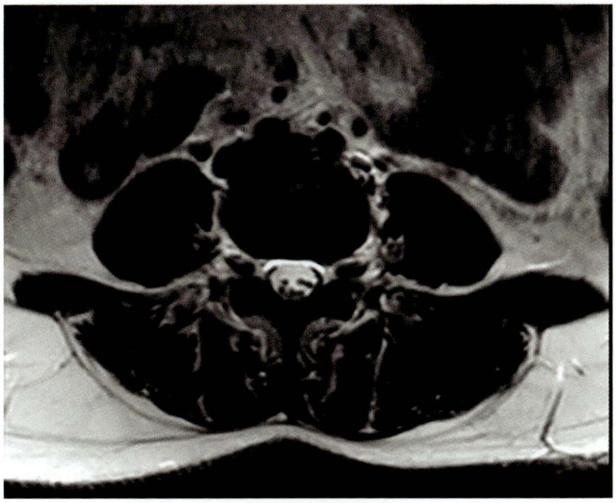

Fig. 12.1 Magnetic resonance imaging scan of the lumbar spine in axial view displaying no neuroforaminal stenosis.

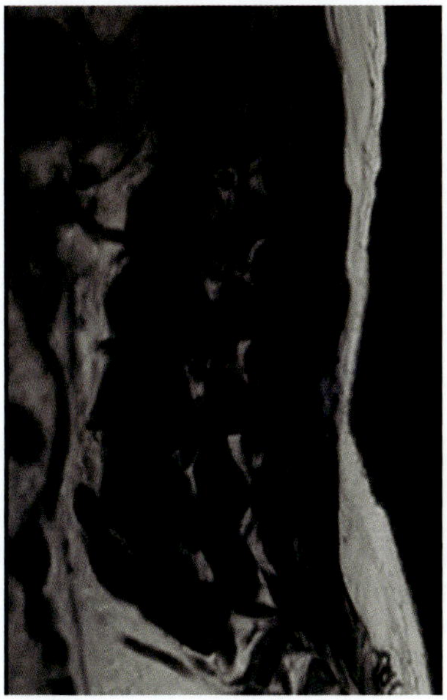

Fig. 12.2 Magnetic resonance imaging scan of the lumbar spine in sagittal view displaying no neuroforaminal stenosis.

6. Once the epidural space is accessed, insert the preloaded sheath into the needle. Prior to introduction of the sheath, ensure that the tip of the lead is protruding from the end of the sheath. Advance the lead from the sheath to ensure that it is in epidural space

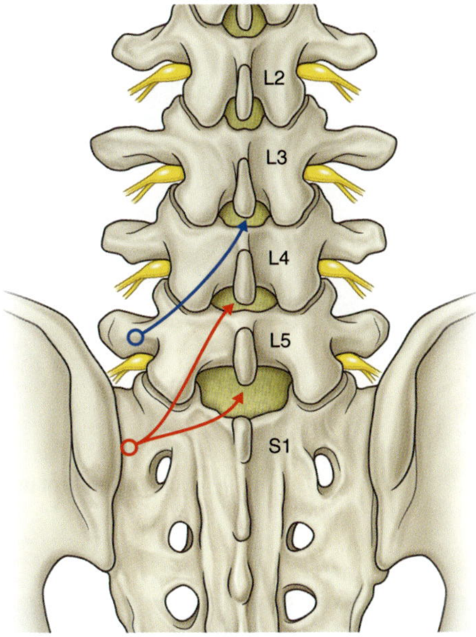

Fig. 12.3 Posterior view of the lumbosacral spine. *Green* indicates starting point for L3 dorsal root ganglion (DRG), *blue* indicates starting point for L4 and L5 DRGs, and *red* indicates starting point for S2 DRG.

(Figs. 12.8 and 12.9). Once confirmed, retract the lead into the sheath.

7. Confirm that the tip of the needle remains midline and the newly introduced sheath continues to advance toward the intended DRG level by returning to the AP view.
8. Advance the sheath toward the target foramen and contact the inferior aspect of the pedicle at the target level (Fig. 12.10).
9. Replace the lead with a guidewire, as the guidewire can penetrate the neuroforaminal ligaments with greater ease than the lead. With the guidewire remaining in the sheath, advance the sheath past the pedicle and through the foraminal ligaments.
10. The guidewire/sheath complex is in the correct position when the tip of the guidewire has passed beyond the lateral border of the pedicle and a subtle texture change is felt to indicate that the neuroforaminal ligaments have been breached (Fig. 12.11).
11. Replace the guidewire in the sheath with the lead (Fig. 12.12).

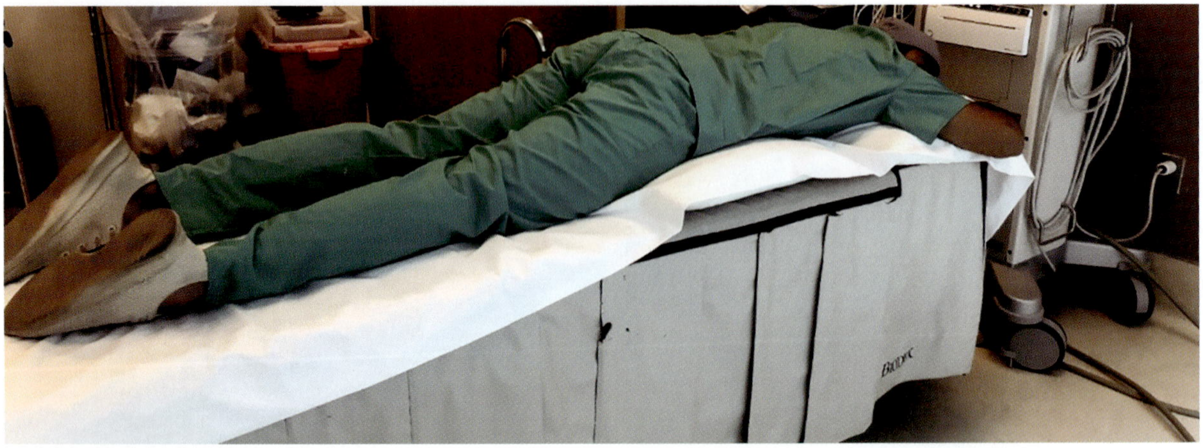

Fig. 12.4 Patient positioning for dorsal root ganglion stimulator.

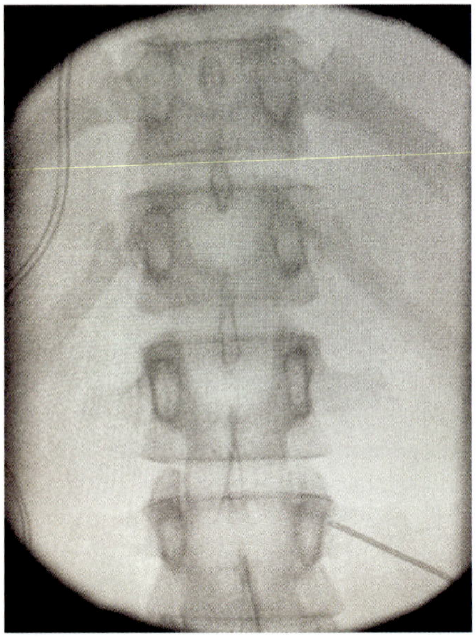

Fig. 12.5 The "marker" is at the right L2 pedicle with the target dorsal root ganglion at left T12 in anteroposterior view.

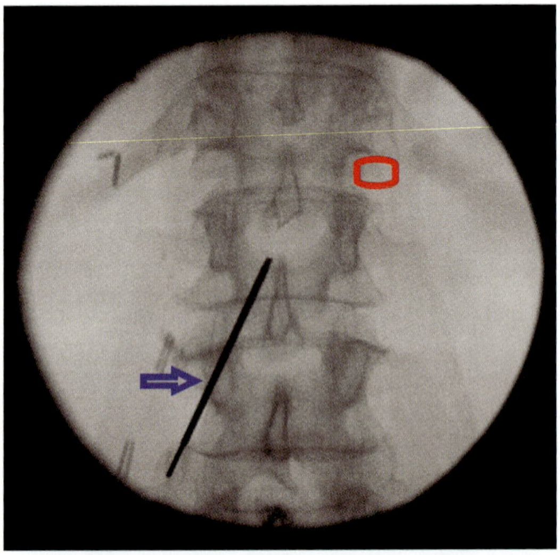

Fig. 12.6 Anteroposterior view of advancement of the needle toward the midline epidural space (T12–L1 interlaminar space). The *red circle* indicates the target dorsal root ganglion (right T12) and the *blue arrow* indicates the needle entry point at the contralateral pedicle two levels below the target.

12. A lead restrain relief loop will be necessary to reduce the risk of lead migration. The instructions are as follows (Fig. 12.13):
    a. While slowly advancing the lead, retract the sheath from the lead until the tip of the sheath (*blue arrow*) is at the tip of the needle. The lead tip (*orange arrow*) should not advance or retract during this process. Rotate the needle to the 12 o'clock position and advance the lead into the epidural space (should see an inverted U-curve start to take shape, see image 12.13).
13. Rotate the needle to the 3 o'clock position (if target DRG on the right) or 6 o'clock position (if target DRG on the left) and advance lead

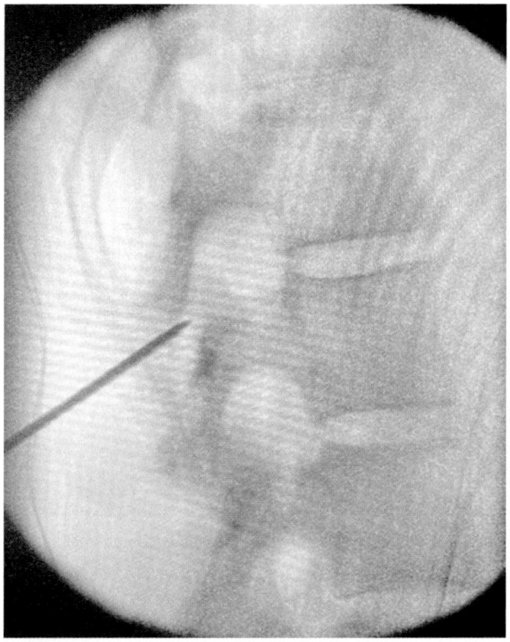

Fig. 12.7 A lateral view provides safety with regard to depth of needle placement while advancing into the epidural space.

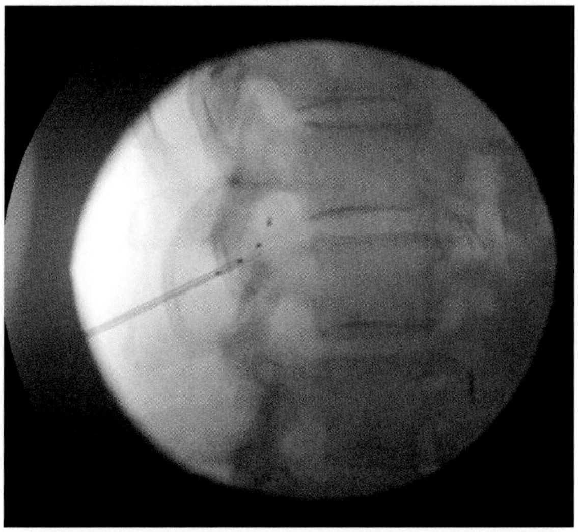

Fig. 12.8 Lateral view of initial lead placement. Note that leads are in the posterior epidural space.

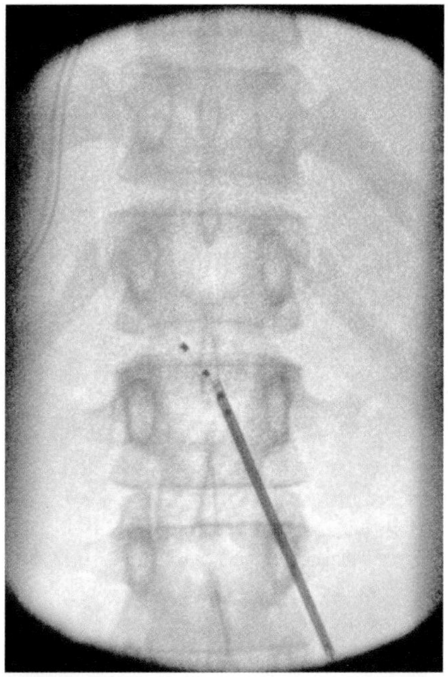

Fig. 12.9 Anteroposterior view shows initial lead placement in epidural space and advancing toward intended dorsal root ganglion (target is left T12 DRG).

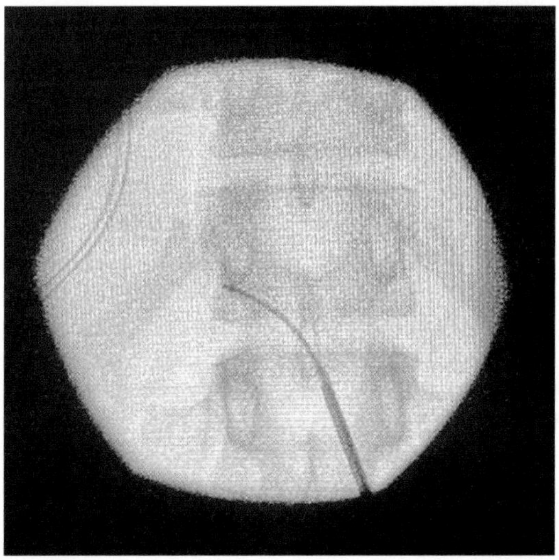

Fig. 12.10 In anteroposterior view, make contact with the inferior aspect of the pedicle at the target level (target is left T12 dorsal root ganglion).

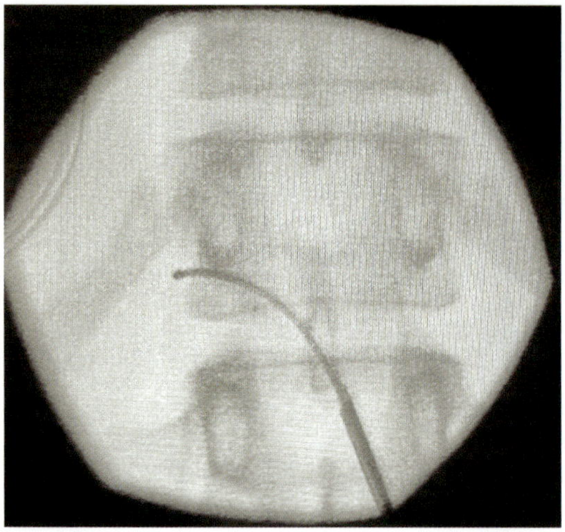

Fig. 12.11 Advancement of the sheath past the inferior border of the pedicle and through the intraforaminal space in the anteroposterior view.

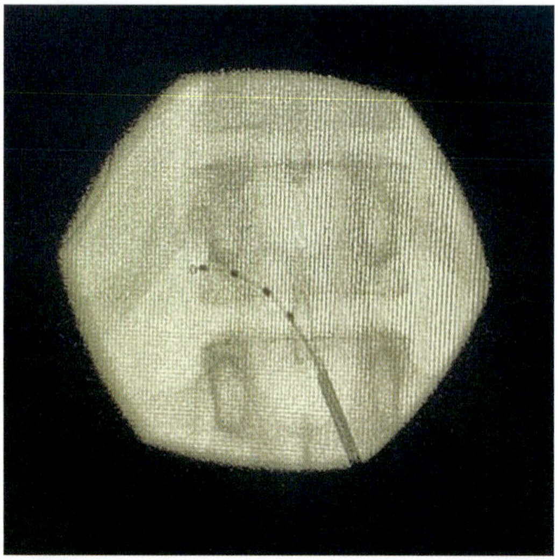

Fig. 12.12 Leads contacting the dorsal root ganglion in the anteroposterior view. Note that, ideally, more leads should pass through the intraforaminal space if possible.

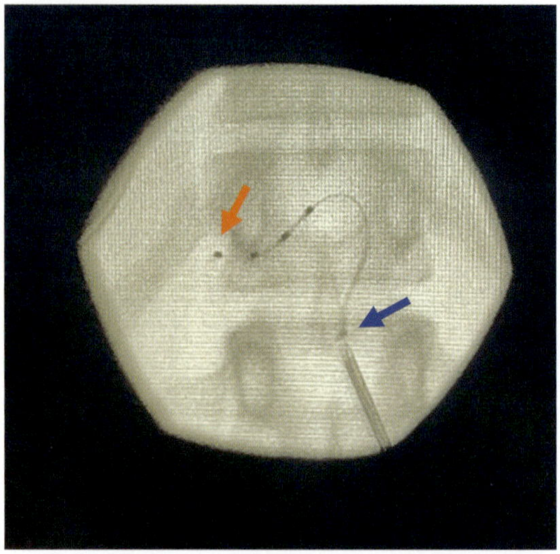

Fig. 12.13 Initial loop placement in the anteroposterior view.

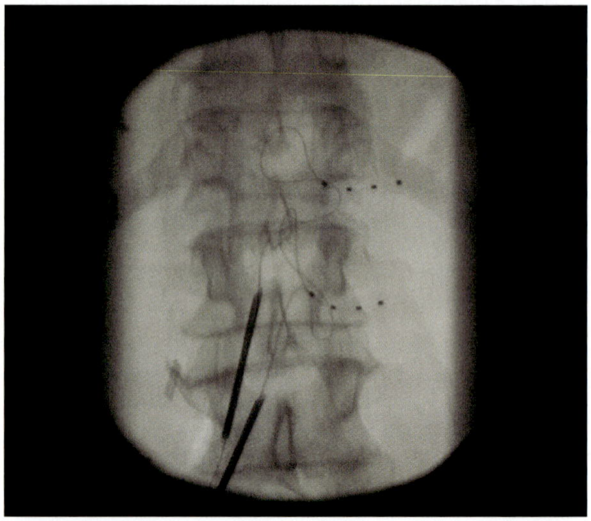

Fig. 12.14 Final loop in the anteroposterior view.

without advancing the sheath to create the inferior loop (Fig. 12.14). Confirm that the lead tip has not moved during the loop creation process.

14. Confirm that the lead and loop remain in the posterior epidural space by the lateral view (Fig. 12.15).
15. Remove the sheath, needle, and stylet. Be careful not to retract the leads. Confirm that leads have not moved after removing (Fig. 12.16). Anchor the leads to the skin with sutures or bandages. Apply gauze and an occlusive dressing.

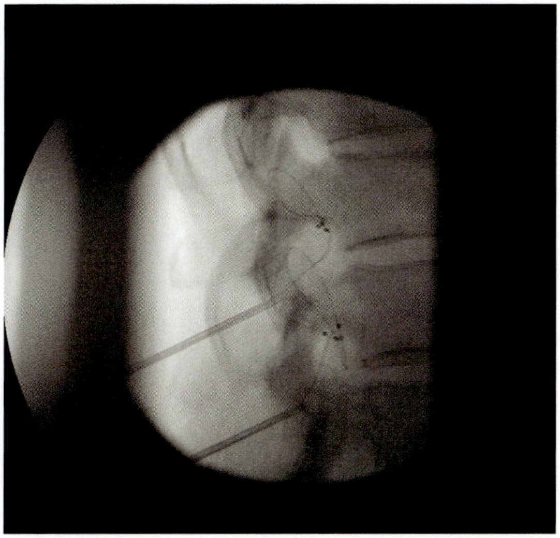

Fig. 12.15 Final loop, lateral view. Note that leads and loop remain posterior.

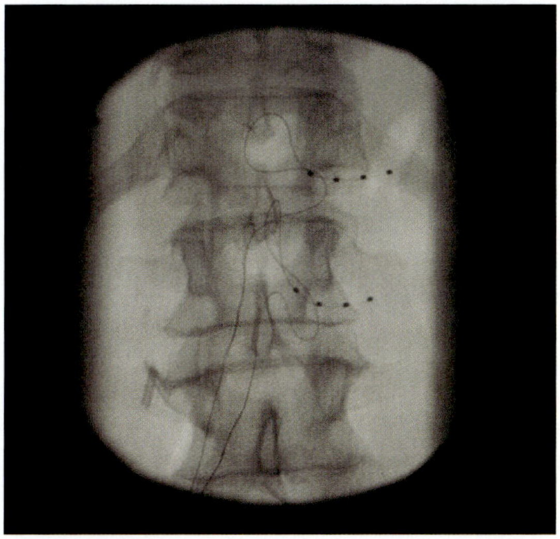

Fig. 12.16 Confirmation of loop and lead placement after needle, stylet, and sheath removal.

Placement of Sacral Dorsal Root Ganglion Stimulator

PROCEDURAL STEPS

1. Steps 1 and 2 are the same in the previous section. Note that fluoroscopy may require cephalad tilt to best visualize the sacral foramen.
2. Mark the target foramen (Fig. 12.17).
3. Introduce the needle at the site of the marker (Fig. 12.18). Use the lateral view to check the depth of the needle.
4. Ensure that the needle bevel is facing caudal and insert the preloaded sheath. Prior to insertion, confirm the tip of the lead protruding from the end of the sheath. Feed the sheath through

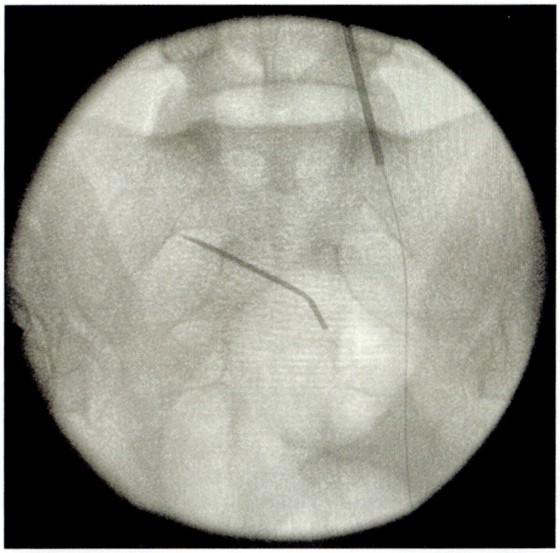

Fig. 12.17 Anteroposterior view with cephalad tilt with marker on the left S1 foramen.

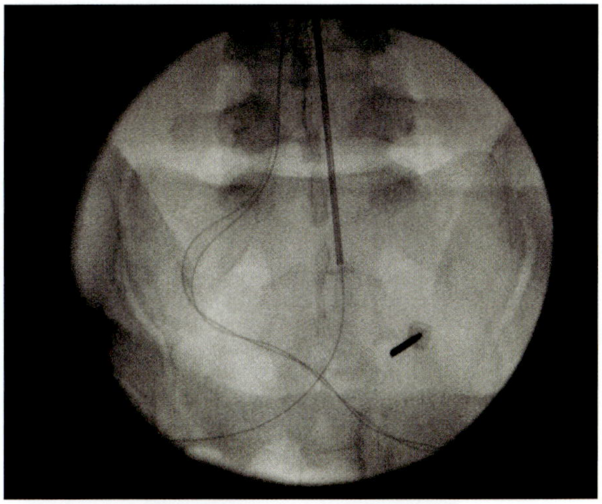

Fig. 12.18 Placement of needle for right S2 dorsal root ganglion in anteroposterior view with the beam at caudal-cranial tilt.

the sacral foramen and retract the sheath. The goal is to get two to three contacts within the sacral canal (Fig. 12.19).

5. Unlock the sheath and retract to the distal tip of the needle. Retract the needle, sheath, and stylet to just outside the posterior sacrum.
6. Turn the needle and sheath cranial, retract the stylet 6 inches, and feed the lead to create a superior loop (Figs. 12.20 and 12.21).

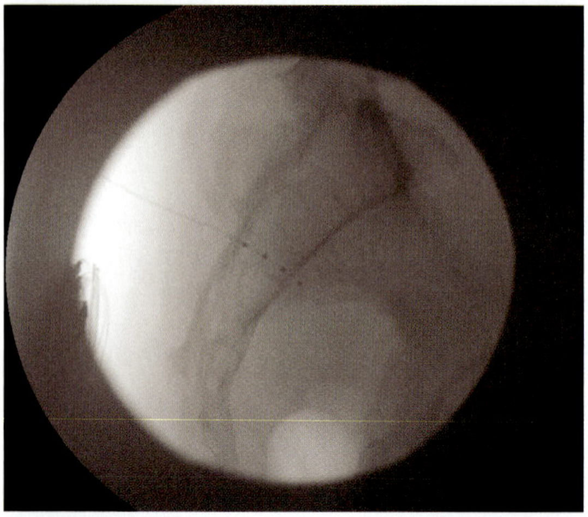

Fig. 12.19 Lead position for S2 dorsal root ganglion stimulator in the lateral view.

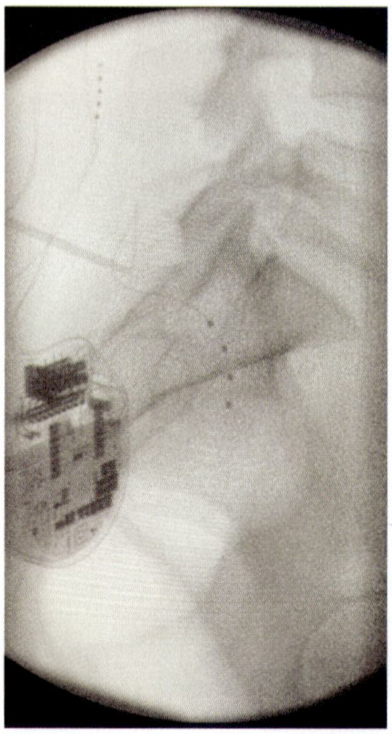

Fig. 12.20 Superior lead restrain loop in the lateral view.

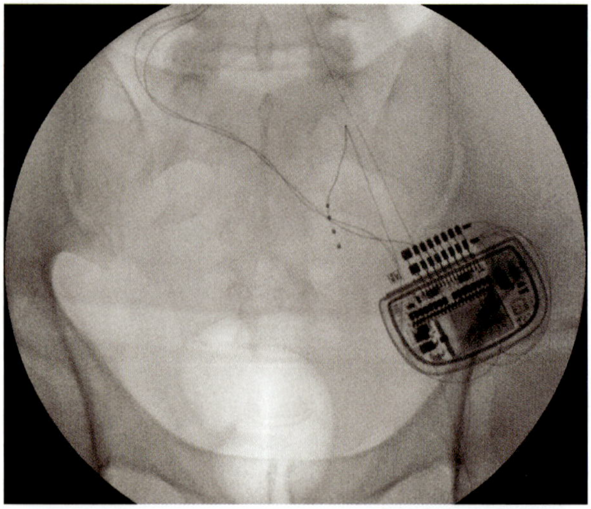

Fig. 12.21 Anteroposterior view confirming sacral dorsal root ganglion placement with superior strain relief loop after needle removal.

7. Retract the sheath to the needle and rotate the needle and sheath caudal. Feed the lead to create an inferior loop if possible.
8. Repeat steps 15 and 16 for the DRG stimulator from the previous section.

Procedural Complications

DURAL PUNCTURE

The process of placing a DRG stimulator lead requires entrance into the epidural space. Once access is obtained, a specialized sheath is tunneled within the epidural space, advancing toward the foramen of choice. Finally, the DRG stimulator lead is then advanced through this sheath until it is placed over the targeted foramen. During this process, the dura is at risk for puncture due to the extensive manipulation that may be required for proper placement of the lead. Puncturing of the dura sac may result in development of a puncture headache as well as CSF leak into the wound. Traditional risk factors for a dural puncture are associated with sex (11.1% female vs. 3.6% male), age (11.0% 31–50 years of age vs. 4.2% others), and previous history of postdural puncture headache. The incidence of dural puncture has been estimated at 0% to 0.3%.[4] Patients who experience a postdural puncture should be monitored for signs and symptoms. More commonly, this includes development of a postdural puncture headache characterized as a positional headache, diplopia, tinnitus, neck pain, or photophobia. Strategies to reduce the risk of development of postdural puncture headache include bed rest and/or prophylactic epidural blood patch. If symptoms persist, surgical exploration should be considered.

NEUROLOGICAL SYMPTOMS

Neurological injury is a serious complication that can arise from DRG stimulator lead placement. This can result from inadvertent trauma caused by needle puncture, sheath navigation, and final lead positioning. Neurological symptoms include new or worsened symptoms involving numbness, paresthesias, weakness, or pain. The physician should remain vigilant when neurological symptoms are reported, as 50% of neurological complications are associated with surgical intervention. A safe approach is to keep patients awake to allow for verbal feedback during painful sessions of the procedure, such as neuroforaminal interrogation.[5] This will serve to mitigate the risk of nerve damage. If a patient has progressive pain and/or weakness after the procedure, a computed tomography (CT) scan should be performed as soon as possible to rule out epidural bleed. If an epidural bleed is ruled out, the leads should be removed and an MRI scan should be performed to evaluate for conus injury (if the thoracolumbar or high lumbar interspace was interrogated) or peripheral nerve root injury (at the level of DRG stimulator placement).

INFECTION

Infection is a common cause for explantation of the entire system. There is evidence to suggest that technique and number of device components (additional leads, up to 4) specifically required for DRG stimulator placement could alter the risk of infection. In addition, the dura normally serves as a barrier to the central spread of infection; thus, an increased risk of dural puncture may increase the likelihood of infection.[6] Potential risk factors for infection include diabetes, poor functional status, malnutrition, obesity, autoimmune disorder, high-dose steroid use, decubitus ulcers, preexisting infection, and poor hygiene. Infection prevention techniques include administration of prophylactic antibiotics, adequate skin preparation, meticulous attention to sterile techniques in the operating room, and adequate wound hemostasis.[7]

Device-Related Complications

Similar to traditional spinal cord stimulation (SCS), device-related complications from DRG stimulation are not uncommon. A survey of the Manufacturer and User Facility Device Experience (MAUDE) found that lead migration was the most frequently reported complication.[6] Decreasing lead migration rates is key to minimizing reoperation and improving the effectiveness of DRG stimulation.

Typically, the leads are secured with strain relief loops within the epidural space rather than the traditional method of anchoring and strain relief loops. This method may be a more frequent cause of lead migration, especially for sacral lead stimulation. Reprogramming is often attempted to salvage the leads that have migrated. Ultimately, however, revision is often necessary.

Additionally, the creation of a strain relief loop may actually increase lead damage. In order to create the strain loop, more length is required for appropriate formation, which increases the number of potential damage sites. Lead damage may occur both during insertion and removal. When difficulty is encountered during lead removal, deliberate lead cutting is sometimes warranted but ostensibly results in retained segments in the epidural space. Similarly, damage to the sheath used for lead placement sometimes results in a retained segment.

Lead migration rates vary greatly between studies, likely owing to implanter experience, different definitions of "migration," varying clinical contexts of the therapy, and differing clinical practices.[8]

REFERENCES

1. Hagedorn JM, Demian PS, Scarfo KA, Engle AM, Deer TR. Proclaim™ DRG Neurostimulator System for the management of chronic, intractable pain. *Pain Manag.* 2020;10(4):225-233. doi:10.2217/pmt-2020-0010.
2. Vuka I, Marciuš T, Došenović S, et al. Neuromodulation with electrical field stimulation of dorsal root ganglion in various pain syndromes: a systematic review with focus on participant selection. *J Pain Res.* 2019;12:803-830. doi:10.2147/JPR.S168814.

3. Deer TR, Levy RM, Kramer J, et al. Dorsal root ganglion stimulation yielded higher treatment success rate for complex regional pain syndrome and causalgia at 3 and 12 months: a randomized comparative trial. *Pain*. 2017;158(4):669-681. doi:10.1097/j.pain.0000000000000814.
4. Kumar K, Wilson JR, Taylor RS, Gupta S. Complications of spinal cord stimulation, suggestions to improve outcome, and financial impact. *J Neurosurg Spine*. 2006;5(3):191-203.
5. St. Jude Medical. *Axium™ Neurostimulator System. Clinical Implant Experience Summary*. Available at: https://www.accessdata.fda.gov/cdrh_docs/pdf15/P150004d.pdf. Accessed May 19, 2021.
6. Sivanesan E, Bicket MC, Cohen SP. Retrospective analysis of complications associated with dorsal root ganglion stimulation for pain relief in the FDA MAUDE database. *Reg Anesth Pain Med*. 2019;44(1):100-106. doi:10.1136/rapm-2018-000007.
7. Eldabe S, Buchser E, Duarte RV. Complications of spinal cord stimulation and peripheral nerve stimulation techniques: a review of the literature. *Pain Med*. 2016;17(2):325-336. Available at: https://doi.org/10.1093/pm/pnv025.
8. Kumar K, Buchser E, Linderoth B, Meglio M, Van Buyten JP. Avoiding complications from spinal cord stimulation: practical recommendations from an international panel of experts. *Neuromodulation*. 2007;10(1):24-33.

Chapter 13

Dorsal Root Ganglion Stimulation—Implant

Joseph Hanna, Ramsey Saad, and Nabil Sibai

Chapter Outline

Anatomy

The dorsal root ganglion (DRG) plays a key role in relaying sensory information from the peripheral nervous system to the central nervous system (i.e., a gatekeeper role). It comprises a collection of pseudo-unipolar neurons surrounded by glial cells. The DRG is located bilaterally at the distal end of the dorsal root in the anterolateral epidural space. The DRGs of L1 to L4 lie within the intervertebral foramen. The DRG of L5 in the majority of cases lies inside the foramen whereas in the minority of cases, it lies intraspinal. The DRG of S1 is mostly intraspinal.[1,2] Refer to Fig. 13.1 for details.

Selection Criteria[3]

Given its precise coverage of painful areas, DRG stimulation is particularly appreciated in the management of complex regional pain syndrome (CRPS) and groin pain. The best indications for DRG stimulation seem to be dermatome-specific pain syndromes such as postherniorrhaphy pain, postthoracotomy pain, postradiation neuropathy, postmastectomy/breast surgery pain, posttraumatic foot pain, CRPS, and postherpetic neuralgia. Placing leads in nonadjacent spinal levels results in broader coverage (Table 13.1).

Effective Dorsal Root Ganglion Stimulation Lead Combinations for Various Pain Locations[4]

For the back, the most impactful DRG location will be T12. Optimal lead combinations can be T12, L1, L2 > L5, and S1. For the buttock area, coverage can be obtained with L2 with the possible combination of T12, L1, L2 > T12, and S1. The pelvic area can be covered optimally by S2 with the possible addition of L1 (bilaterally for bilateral pain). T12 appears to

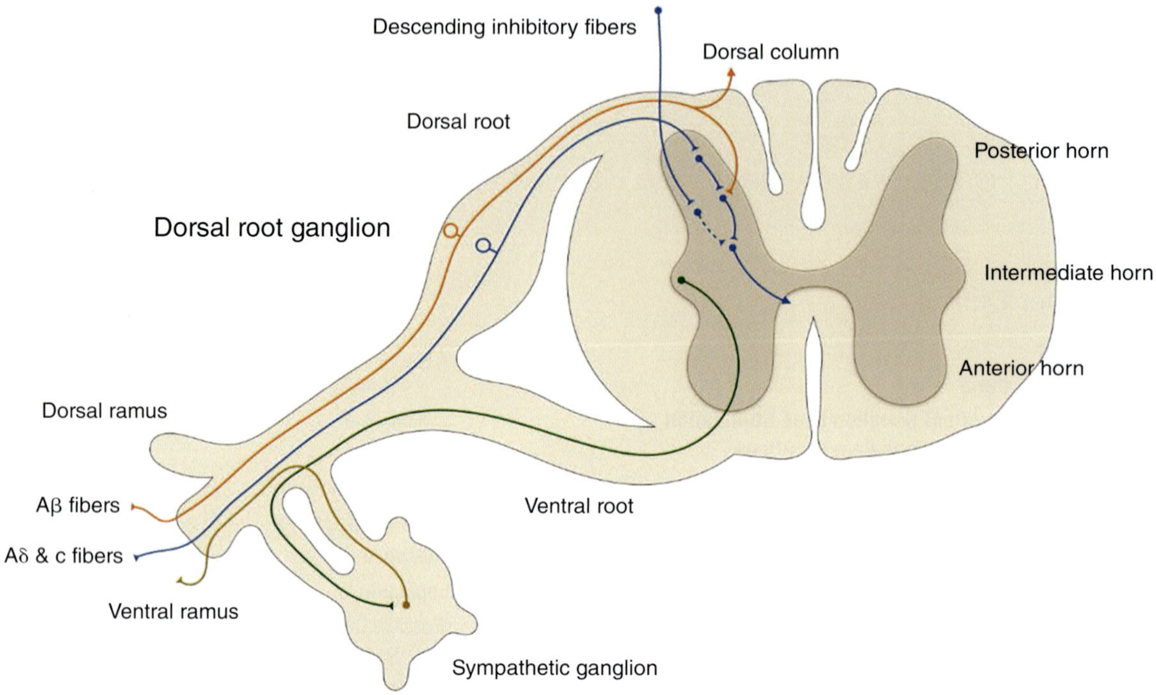

Fig. 13.1 Anatomy of the dorsal root ganglion.

TABLE 13.1 Selection Criteria for Dorsal Root Ganglion (DRG) Stimulation
Absence of aberrant opioid use disorder
Absence of psychiatric or psychological comorbidities (untreated or uncontrolled)
Appropriate and realistic understanding of risks and benefits of DRG stimulation therapy
Absence of bleeding diathesis
Absence of site infection or signs of systemic infection
Appropriate indication, mainly dermatome-specific pain syndrome (e.g., complex regional pain syndrome)
Successful trial, with > 50% pain reduction and improved functionality

be the most impactful location for the groin with the possible combination of T12, L1 and L2 > T11, T12 and L1 = T11, T12. The knee is usually covered by the L4 DRG with a possible combination of both L3 and L4. Finally, the foot is mostly S1 with the optimal lead combination of L5, S1, and L4 (if ankle pain is present).

Technique

EQUIPMENT

From Fig. 13.2, we can identify 3 pieces of equipment:

1. 14-gauge epidural needle (4.5 or 6 inch)
2. Delivery sheath (big curve vs. small curve, 22 cm in length) with lead stabilizer and side port

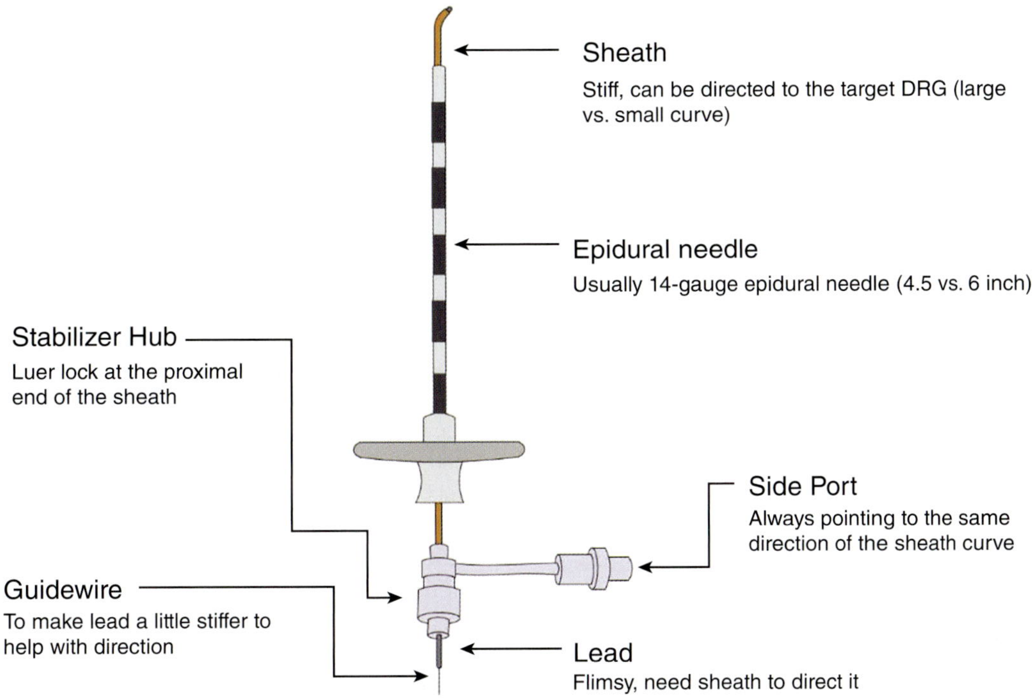

Fig. 13.2 Equipment for dorsal root ganglion stimulation. *DRG*, Dorsal root ganglion.

3. Lead with stylet wire inside (SlimTip). Trial and implant leads are available (either 50 or 90 cm in length, 1 mm in diameter with 4 cylindrical electrodes, each 1.25 mm). For implant leads, lead extension is available (50 cm in length and 5.7 mm in diameter).

The kit includes another guidewire that can placed instead of the lead in the sheath, which can be simulated to the lead blank that comes with spinal cord stimulation (SCS) kits. Refer to Fig. 13.2 for details.

Another important point to note is that the side port of the sheath points in the same direction as the tip of the sheath, which is how we know where the curve of the sheath is pointing throughout the procedure.

Steps of the Implant

PREOPERATIVE

At this point, the patient should have gone through a successful trial with >50% pain improvement and decided to proceed with the implant. Details of the procedure, along with risks and benefits, should be discussed with the patient and a consent form signed. Discussion about the site of battery implant should have taken place so that patient knows where it will be implanted. It is mostly done at the waistline at the side of the patient's preference, well below the iliac crest. The patient is asked to take a shower using chlorhexidine the day before the procedure and maintains NPO status (nothing by mouth) for at least 8 hours except for medications. Anticoagulation guidelines should be followed meticulously given that DRG stimulation is considered to be a high-risk procedure. A critical step is to review the procedure notes as well as X-ray images saved from the trial as they will be used as a guide for the actual implant. Few practitioners will have these images available in the operating room (OR) during the implant as reference. Verify with the patient the location of the pocket for the impulse generator. Once the site is determined, mark the proposed skin incision with a permanent marker while the patient is in the sitting position. Once the patient is ready to be wheeled to the OR, antibiotics should be started. These include cefazolin 2 to 3 g intravenously (IV); if allergic to penicillin or cephalosporins, clindamycin 900 mg IV can be used instead. If the patient has a history of methicillin-resistant *Staphylococcus aureus* (MRSA), consider vancomycin 1 g IV. Antibiotic timing is as follows: cefazolin or clindamycin should be administered within 30 minutes before actual incision and vancomycin within 1 hour.

INTRAOPERATIVE

Positioning

The patient is then transferred to the OR and placed in the prone position. After verifying the patient's name, surgical site, and procedure, the surgery can proceed. Usually, the procedure is performed under IV sedation, as testing should be performed at the end of the procedure in which the patient should effectively participate. Some providers prefer to proceed with conscious sedation (using minimal doses of midazolam and fentanyl) while mainly depending on sufficient local anesthetic usage, whereas others prefer deep IV sedation (propofol infusion). It is preferred that sedation is done under the supervision of an anesthesiologist to ensure patient safety, especially if IV deep sedation is chosen. Another approach is under general anesthesia, including securing the airway, in which the patient is not responsive to painful stimuli. Some have advocated electrophysiological neuromonitoring in this scenario as a means of detecting nerve injury.

The patient's mid- and lower back is then prepped with alcohol 2 or 3 times and sterile drapes are applied. It is important for the patient's back to be as straight as possible to facilitate epidural needle placement. Placement of a pillow(s) under the patient's abdomen can help in achieving that goal. Using C-arm fluoroscopy, the superior endplate of the targeted DRG should be squared. Once this is performed, the skin entry point can be planned.

Lead Placement

Ideally, we prefer the entry point to be 2.5 to 3.0 pedicles below and on the contralateral side of the targeted DRG. A straight line should be able to connect the skin entry point, epidural entry point, and targeted pedicle in a 6 o'clock position (Fig. 13.3). Plan for the epidural space entry point to be midline almost in the upper half of the interlaminar space. The skin entry point and the anticipated epidural needle track should be anesthetized. Then, using anteroposterior and lateral fluoroscopy, the 14-gauge epidural needle available in the DRG kit is advanced cautiously until it is felt to be engaged in the ligamentum flavum. At this point, loss-of-resistance technique is used until the epidural space is entered, preferably midline and in the upper half of the interlaminar space, as previously mentioned. Keep the tip of the sheath pointed dorsal (in the 12 o'clock position) upon entry of the needle in the epidural space. In Fig. 13.4, the *first white line* indicates the tip of the lead and sheath entering the epidural space. The *second white line* is if using a 6-inch needle. Refer to Figs. 13.3 and 13.4 for details.

Prior to removing the trocar from the epidural needle, it is important to ensure that sheath loaded with the lead is ready (with the lead tip just protruding out of the sheath) and the stabilizer hub is tightened (Luer lock at proximal end of sheath). The trocar of the epidural needle is then removed and the sheath loaded with the lead is advanced under live anteroposterior (AP)-fluoroscopy towards the 6 o`clock position of the targeted pedicle. As the sheath approaches the pedicle, rotate the epidural needle bevel as well as sheath 45 degrees to be pointing toward the targeted pedicle (Fig. 13.5A). Please note that the curve of the sheath should be pointing in the same direction as the epidural needle bevel at all times—if one changes, the other has to change as well (Fig. 13.5B). Once the sheath lands on the inferior border of the pedicle, a trial should be done to further advance the sheath to pop through the intraforaminal ligaments (Fig. 13.5C). Care should be taken not to kink the sheath. If this happens, the sheath should be withdrawn and replaced. Note that a kink in the sheath will not appear on fluoroscopy—it will be evident only when trial to advance the lead through the sheath fails repeatedly, with resistance felt with each attempt. Injecting saline from the sheath side port for lubrication will not help this situation. Once the sheath is withdrawn, the kink can be felt manually. Given no sheath kinks, if resistance is encountered, one maneuver that can be tried is to replace the lead with a guidewire, which is stiffer and can help create a path for the lead. Remember to unlock the stabilizer hub if removing the lead and

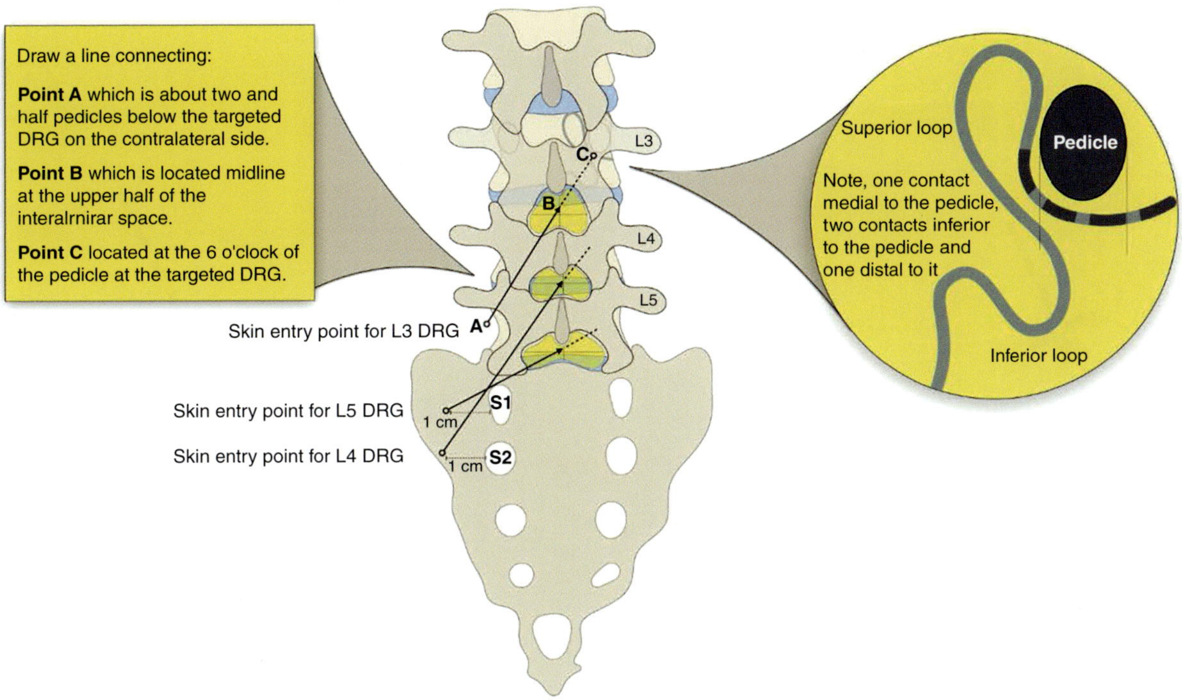

Fig. 13.3 Skin entry points for different target dorsal root ganglions (DRGs).

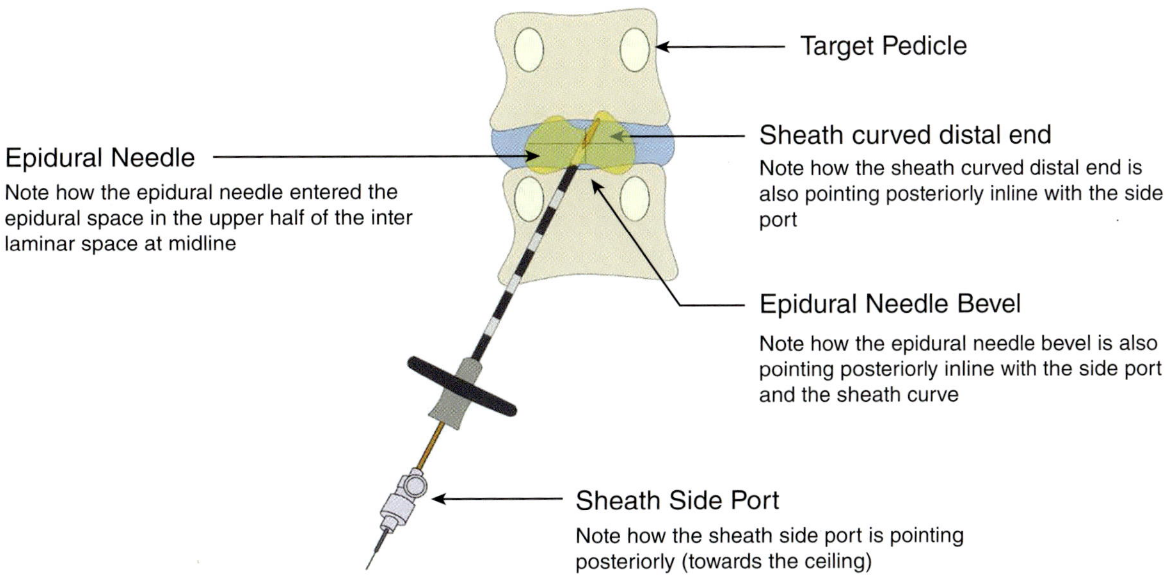

Fig. 13.4 Epidural needle after epidural space has been accessed.

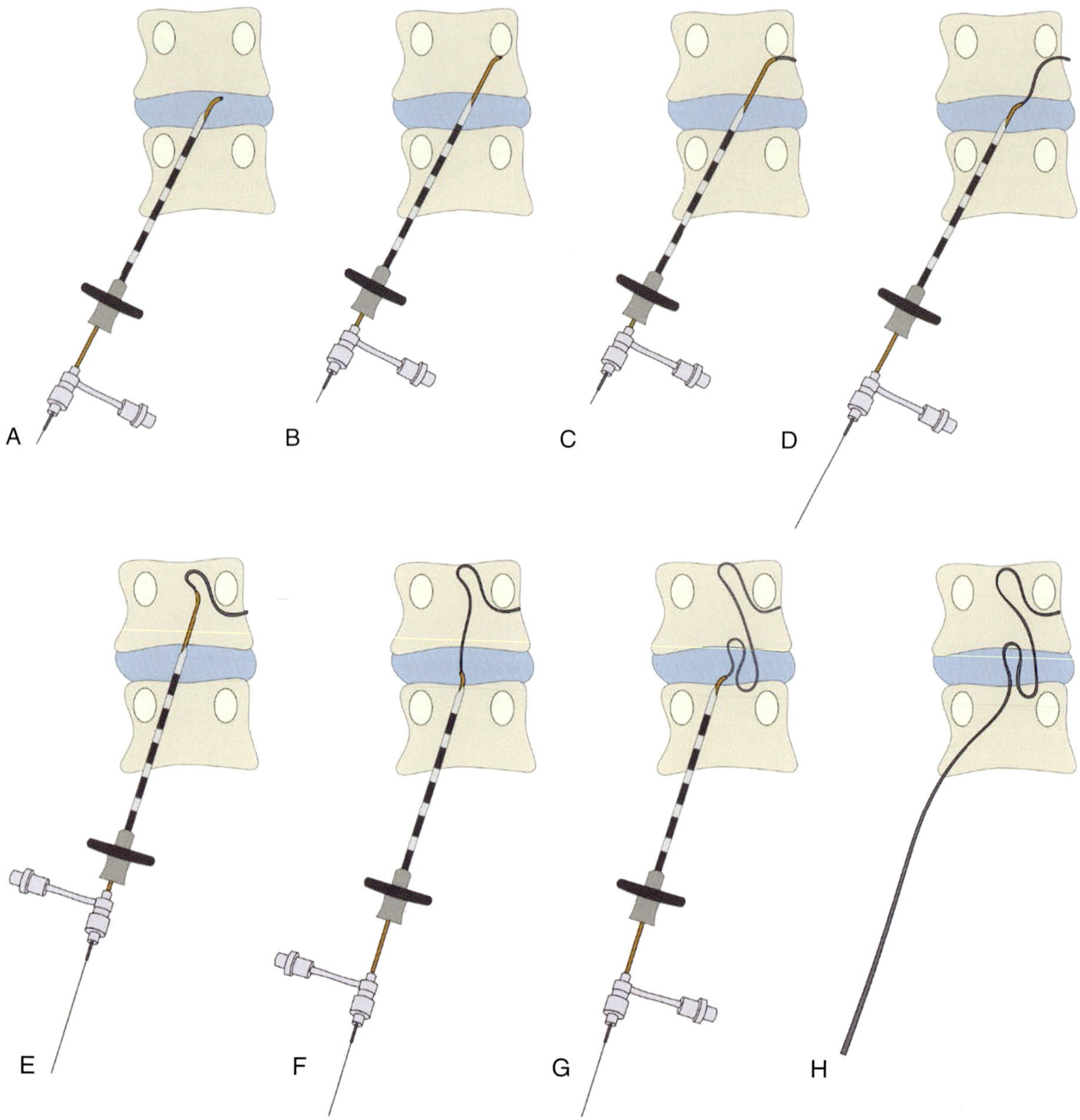

Fig. 13.5 (*A*) through (*H*) Steps for deploying dorsal root ganglion stimulation lead.

introducing the guidewire. Once the sheath pops through, the lead is advanced through the foramen and the sheath is retracted to about halfway between the tip of the epidural needle and the tip of the lead (Fig. 13.5D). Note that the tip of the sheath is radiopaque.

Creating Loops

The next stage is to work on getting the lead into the appropriate position, with one contact distal to the pedicle, two contacts inferior to the pedicle, and the last one medial to it. Then, create the loops, both superior and inferior, which is the alternative of anchoring in SCS.

Once the sheath is midway between the epidural needle and tip of the lead, both the epidural needle and sheath are rotated 45 degrees back so that the sheath curve is facing posteriorly. Sometimes, both epidural needle and sheath will need to be rotated further than that. After that, the lead guidewire is withdrawn about 2 inches to make the lead flimsy. If needed, withdraw the lead further to make sure that the distal contact is just lateral to the pedicle. The next step is to work on creating the superior loop. To accomplish this, the interventionist should start advancing the lead through the sheath, which will start to go up and bend, forming the superior loop given its "flimsy" consistency. If redirection is needed, this can be accomplished by undergoing some sheath advancements or maneuvers, which can be helpful (Figs. 13.5E and 13.5F). Once the superior loop is done, the sheath is retracted back to the tip of the epidural needle and both are rotated about 90 degrees toward the side of the targeted DRG (Figs. 13.5F and 13.5G). If needed, withdraw the guidewire from the lead to make sure that it is flimsy. At this point, the lead is advanced, forming the inferior loop. Refer to Figs. 13.5 A to H for details.

Confirming Lead Position (Posterior in the Foramen)

Once the loops are created, the procedure at the DRG is concluded. An especially important step is to get a lateral X-ray to ensure that the lead is in the posterior part of the foramen. Otherwise, the lead must be withdrawn and the procedure must be restarted from the beginning (Fig. 13.6). At this point, some providers will elect to do testing to ensure appropriate coverage of painful areas with no motor stimulation. If lateral X-rays show the lead to be in an acceptable position with successful testing, the sheath is then withdrawn carefully under live AP fluoroscopy followed by the epidural needle, while every caution is taken to keep the lead in place (see Fig. 13.5H). Note that some providers elect to keep the epidural needle in place to protect the lead during the tunneling step. Refer to Fig. 13.6 for details.

Sacral Leads

Accessing the S1 epidural space should be straightforward. The dorsal S1 foramen can be visualized with cephalad as well as ipsilateral tilt.[5] The amount of tilt varies from one person to another. After local anesthetic infiltration of the skin and track, introduce the epidural needle aiming for the lateral aspect of the foramen. After the epidural needle is in the foramen (evident on the lateral view; Fig. 13.7), the lead

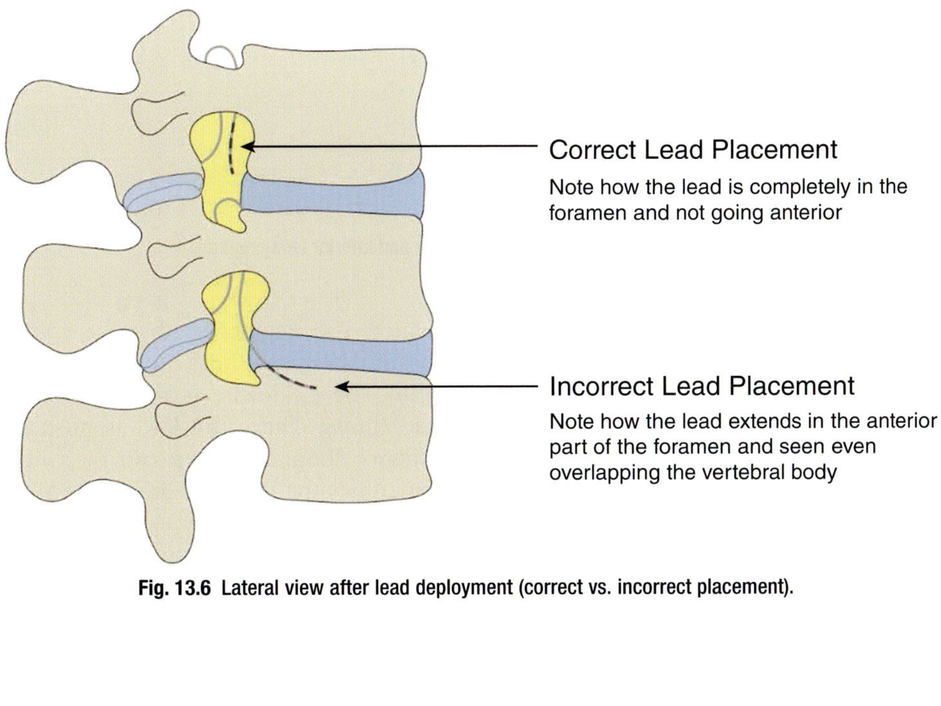

Fig. 13.6 Lateral view after lead deployment (correct vs. incorrect placement).

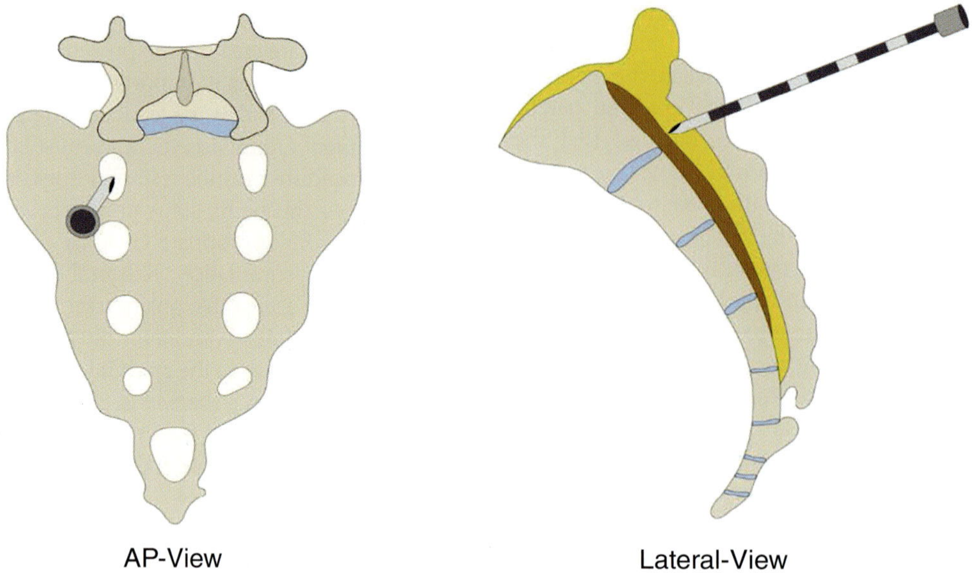

Fig. 13.7 S1 lead placement. *AP*, Anteroposterior.

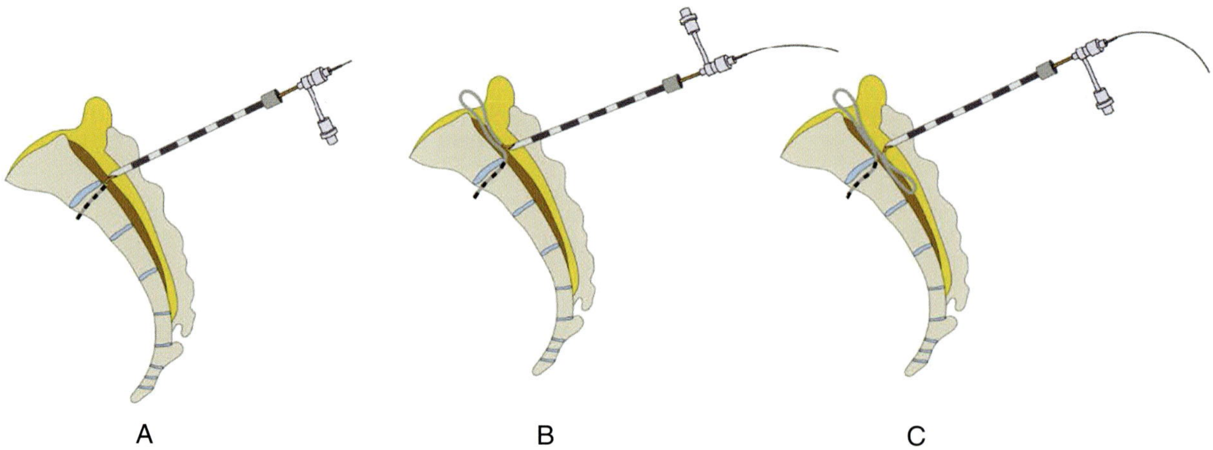

Fig. 13.8 S1 lead placement—superior and inferior loop creation.

is passed with the help of the sheath through the foramen. Once it pops through, the hub stabilizer is unlocked and the lead is pushed through the ventral foramen till one contact is outside the ventral aspect of the sacrum. The sheath is then retracted back while the lead is held in place (pull/push method) till the sheath curve is almost close to the epidural needle tip (Fig. 13.8A). It is now time to create the superior loop. Both sheath and needle are rotated 180 degrees so that the epidural bevel and sheath curve are both pointing superiorly. At this point, the guidewire is retracted back to make the lead flimsy. Then, the lead is pushed, creating the superior loop. This step can be a little difficult, as sometimes the lead will only go anterior and not superior. This may require some manipulation of both the sheath and lead till the lead goes superior while making sure that only one contact is anterior to the ventral aspect of the sacrum on the lateral view (Fig. 13.8B). Once a satisfactory superior loop is created, both the epidural needle and sheath are rotated 180 degrees again so that both are pointing inferiorly (Fig. 13.8C). The lead is then pushed, creating the inferior loop. Once achieved, the sheath followed by the needle are removed while the lead is kept in place. Refer to Figs. 13.7 and 13.8 for details.

Programming

After lead placement, programming is done with a handheld mobile device. The following table shows median values of programmed parameters from the ACCURATE study.

Parameters	*Median values (ACCURATE study)*
Amplitude	575–687.5 μAmp
Frequency	20 Hz
Pulse width	300 μs
Impedance	< 3000 ohms

Stimulating above 1 mV is normally not tolerated and indicates poor placement in most settings. If any motor contractions occur, the lead is likely in the ventral aspect of the foramen—thus, stimulating the ventral root—and should be repositioned. The location of the DRG may be more lateral in relation to the foramen in the lower lumbar spine and may be more medial in the foramen as leads are placed in the upper lumbar spine. This may impact programming.

The following are a few unique approaches to programming the DRG relative to dorsal column stimulation.

1. Sub-mAMP amplitudes are often sufficient to provide the therapeutic benefit since the DRG is an intradural structure surrounded by a minimal volume of cerebrospinal fluid.
2. Low pulse widths (200–300 μs) are preferred because narrower pulse widths tend to maximize the width of the therapeutic window.
3. Simple bipolar arrays can achieve optimal activation of the DRG without the need of complex programming.
4. Unlike SCS, patient movement does not produce significant changes in stimulation intensity

Pocket Creation

The last step is the creation of the pocket, implanting the implantable pulse generator (IPG), tunneling, and connecting the lead to the IPG. Although the location varies, the DRG IPG is typically implanted in the posterior lateral flank below the Scarpa's fascia. The IPG is often implanted on the same side as the lead entry. A transverse incision is created and the ideal pocket should be 120% to 130% of the generator volume. The skin is incised using a sharp scalpel. The subcutaneous pocket is then created using blunt dissection (using surgical scissors in an opening rather than a closing or cutting motion works effectively). Keep in mind a few critical points while creating the pocket:

1. The IPG can cause pain and irritation if placed superficially or placed close to a bony prominence.
2. The IPG may be unable to communicate with telemetry if placed too deep.
3. Hemostasis is critically important; a hematoma or seroma can cause wound dehiscence and/or infection, which may require surgical exploration.
4. Avoid cautery near the surface of the skin.
5. Prior to closing the wound, the pocket should be irrigated aggressively.
6. Lead coiling above the IPG can cause pain and erosion.

Tunneling

After the pocket creation is completed, a tunneling device is extended within the subcutaneous tissues between the epidural entry point and the pocket. Care must be taken to continuously palpate the tip of the tunneling device as it is being advanced to ensure that the depth of the subcutaneous track is neither too deep nor too shallow. The lead is then advanced through the tunnel toward the pocket. Once accomplished, the tunneling device is withdrawn. Now, with the lead(s) in the pocket, it is connected to the IPG. Any excess lead is coiled and placed behind the IPG within the pocket. This loop allows for patient movement without placing tension on the distal lead and causing it to be pulled from the epidural space. The skin incision is then closed in two layers: a series of interrupted subcutaneous sutures to securely close the fascia overlying the IPG within the pocket followed by a skin closure using suture or staples.[6] No anchoring method is needed; the superior and inferior loops within the epidural space are the alternative for anchoring. Refer to Fig. 13.9 for details.

Postoperative

The patient is then transferred to the postanesthesia care unit for further testing and adjustment of the DRG stimulator programming. The patient is usually instructed to follow up in 1 week for a wound check and postoperative X-ray to check on the lead(s) positioning.

COMPLICATIONS[4]

As with all other spine pain procedures, the risk of complications is present. These are some of the expected risks of the procedure plus maneuvers implemented to try reducing their incidence.

1. *Nerve injury secondary to needle puncture or lead/sheath trauma.* This can be avoided with preprocedure imaging, landmarks, appropriate angle, gentle technique, and patient conversation. The physician implant manual explicitly warns physicians with the statement, "The patient must be awake and conversant during portions of the procedure to minimize the likelihood of nerve damage."[7]
2. *Dural puncture/cerebrospinal fluid leak secondary to inadvertent dural puncture by the big 14-gauge needle.* Risks can be reduced by using a shallow angle and loss-of-resistance technique with lateral fluoroscopic images.
3. *Lead migration—most likely happening secondary to lack of proper strain relief and not piercing the ligaments.* To avoid, provide proper S-loop strain relief, making sure that the sheath went through the foraminal ligaments during lead insertion.
4. *Lead fracture, which usually happens at the ligament or anchor. Modification of needle and tunneling angles as well as anchoring method may help decrease the risk of lead fracture.*
5. *Lead retention at time or removal or revision.* Attempt to remove under fluoroscopy if resistance is encountered. If retained, consult neurosurgery. There is usually no need for removal unless it is causing nerve impingement.
6. *Pocket pain due to shallow implant, body habitus, or frequent recharging.* Avoid by making sure that the

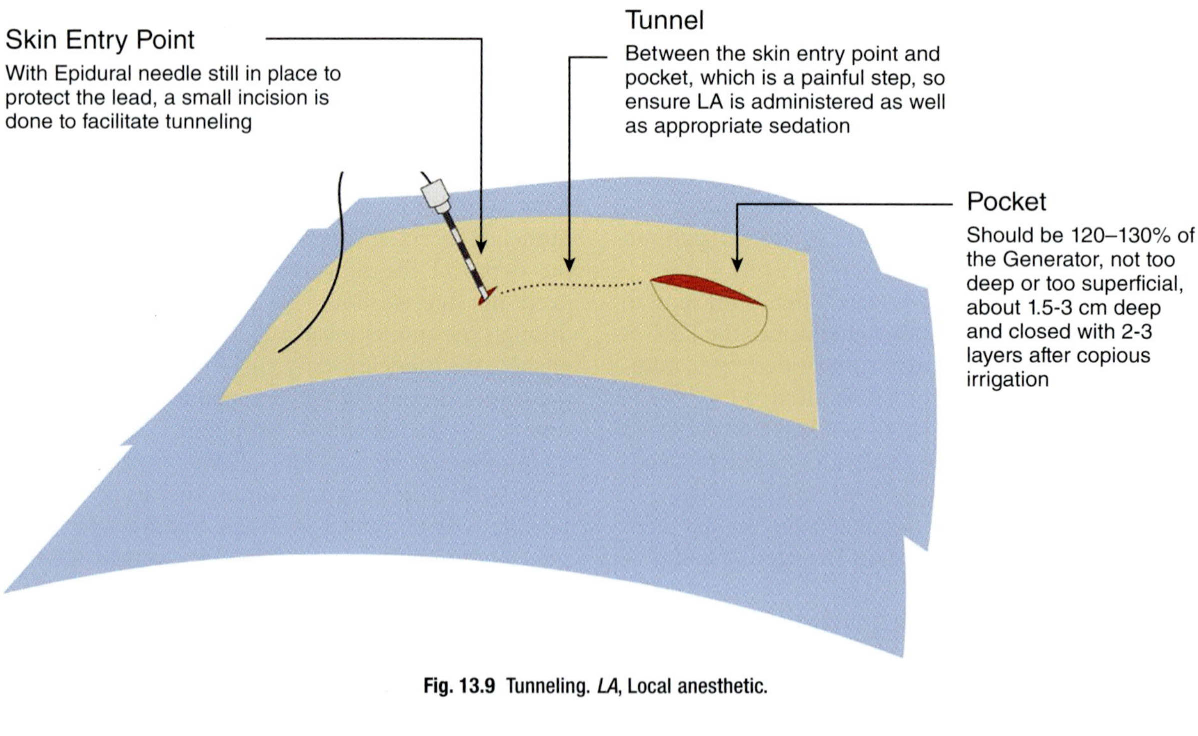

Fig. 13.9 Tunneling. *LA*, Local anesthetic.

battery is implanted at the proper depth. If feasible, use a nonrechargeable device. Pay attention to the patient body habitus and contour prior to implantation to plan for the appropriate area for pocket creation and battery implantation.

Possible Complications of DRG Trials/Implant[8]

In summary, complications may be device related, such as lead migration, erosion through skin, lead and/or sheath damage, connection failure, and malfunction in addition to difficulty with insertion or removal. Procedural complications include neurological symptoms such as numbness, paresthesias, weakness and pain, dural puncture, infection (which may range from infection at the generator site to epidural abscess requiring neurosurgical intervention), and epidural hematoma. Serious adverse events include epidural abscess, meningitis, seizure, asystole/cardiac arrest, stroke, and neuraxial hematoma, which may require admission to long-term rehabilitation and could be complicated by deep venous thrombosis and the need for laminectomy/decompression surgery. Death could even be caused by the procedure. Other risks may include IPG site pain in addition to inappropriate stimulation or overstimulation. Complications that require repeat surgery may also range from explant (removing all implanted components) to revision (removing any implanted component).

Conclusion

DRG stimulation can be specifically helpful in the management of pain secondary to CRPS as well as dermatome-specific pain syndromes. As with any implantable device, patient selection and attention to detail are paramount in order to achieve optimal results.

REFERENCES

1. Van Buyten JP. Dorsal root ganglion stimulation. In: Benzon HT, Raja SN, Liu SS, Fishman SM, Cohen SP, eds. *Essentials of Pain Medicine*. 4th ed. Elsevier; 2018:683-692.e1.
2. Hansen JT. Spinal Cord. In: Delaney CP, ed. Netter's Clinical Anatomy. Philadelphia: Elsevier; 2014. 3rd ed.
3. Deer TR. *Atlas of Implantable Therapies for Pain Management*. New York, NY: Springer; 2011.
4. Deer TR, Pope JE, Lamer TJ, et al. The Neuromodulation Appropriateness Consensus Committee on best practices for dorsal root ganglion stimulation. *Neuromodulation*. 2019;22(1):1-35. doi:10.1111/ner.12845.
5. Stone JB, Berkwits L, Baez-Cabrera LD, Furman MB. S1 transforaminal epidural steroid injection. In: Furman MB, ed. *Atlas of Image-Guided Spinal Procedures*. 2nd ed. Elsevier; 2018:185-191.
6. Rathmell JP. *Atlas of Image-Guided Intervention in Regional Anesthesia and Pain Medicine*. 2nd ed. Philadelphia: Wolters Kluwer Health; 2011.
7. St. Jude Medical. *Axium™ Neurostimulator System. Clinical Implant Experience Summary*. Available at: https://www.accessdata.fda.gov/cdrh_docs/pdf15/P150004d.pdf. Accessed December 23, 2017.
8. Sivanesan E, Bicket MC, Cohen SP. Retrospective analysis of complications associated with dorsal root ganglion stimulation for pain relief in the FDA MAUDE database. *Reg Anesth Pain Med*. 2019;44(1):100-106. doi:10.1136/rapm-2018-000007.

Chapter 14

Medial Branch Neurostimulator Trial

Kenneth J. Fiala, Joshua M. Martens, and Alaa Abd-Elsayed

Chapter Outline

Introduction

Chronic back pain can significantly impact and reduce a person's quality of life.[1,2] Chronic lower back pain has also been shown to have a societal impact along with the personal impact due to the cost of its management.[3] Thus, it is in our best interest not only for the patient but for society to help manage these patients' pain well. Treatment options for lower back pain can include physical therapy, medications, nonsurgical interventions, and surgical interventions. Minimally invasive interventions include acupuncture, exercise, functional restoration, low-level laser therapy, massage, progressive relaxation, traction, and more.[4] Interventions found to have a moderate net benefit for the treatment of lower back pain include acetaminophen, nonsteroidal antiinflammatory drugs, skeletal muscle relaxants, superficial heat, acupuncture, physiological therapy, exercise therapy, interdisciplinary rehabilitation, spinal manipulation, opioids and tramadol, brief individualized educational interventions, benzodiazepines, massage, and yoga.[4] Although there are many nonsurgical treatment modalities for back pain, for a subset of patients who do not find relief with these, procedural modalities may be the best choice to help alleviate their pain. The existing nonopioid procedural options for chronic lower back pain include open surgery, permanently implanted neurostimulation, and radiofrequency ablation.[5] A previous study of percutaneous peripheral nerve stimulation (PNS) of medial branch nerves (MBNs) as a treatment for chronic lower back pain found there to be a 50% or more pain reduction in 67% of participants.[5] Several PNS systems have been used for stimulating the medial branches. This chapter describes the procedure of percutaneous PNS in general as a trial performed before the permanent implantation of a PNS system for chronic low back pain.

Anatomical Considerations

SKELETAL ANATOMY

A lumbar vertebra has a large vertebral body with a short and thick spinous process that extends perpendicularly from the body and two transverse processes extending laterally from the vertebral arch, which is composed of bilateral pedicles that connect the arch to the vertebral body.[6] Each vertebra contains two superior and two inferior articular processes, which further come into contact with the inferior and superior articular processes of adjacent vertebrae, respectively.[6] The facet, or zygapophyseal, joint is where these adjacent processes meet.[6] Additional processes can be found on the larger aforementioned processes of each vertebra. The accessory process originates from the dorsal surface of the transverse process, near

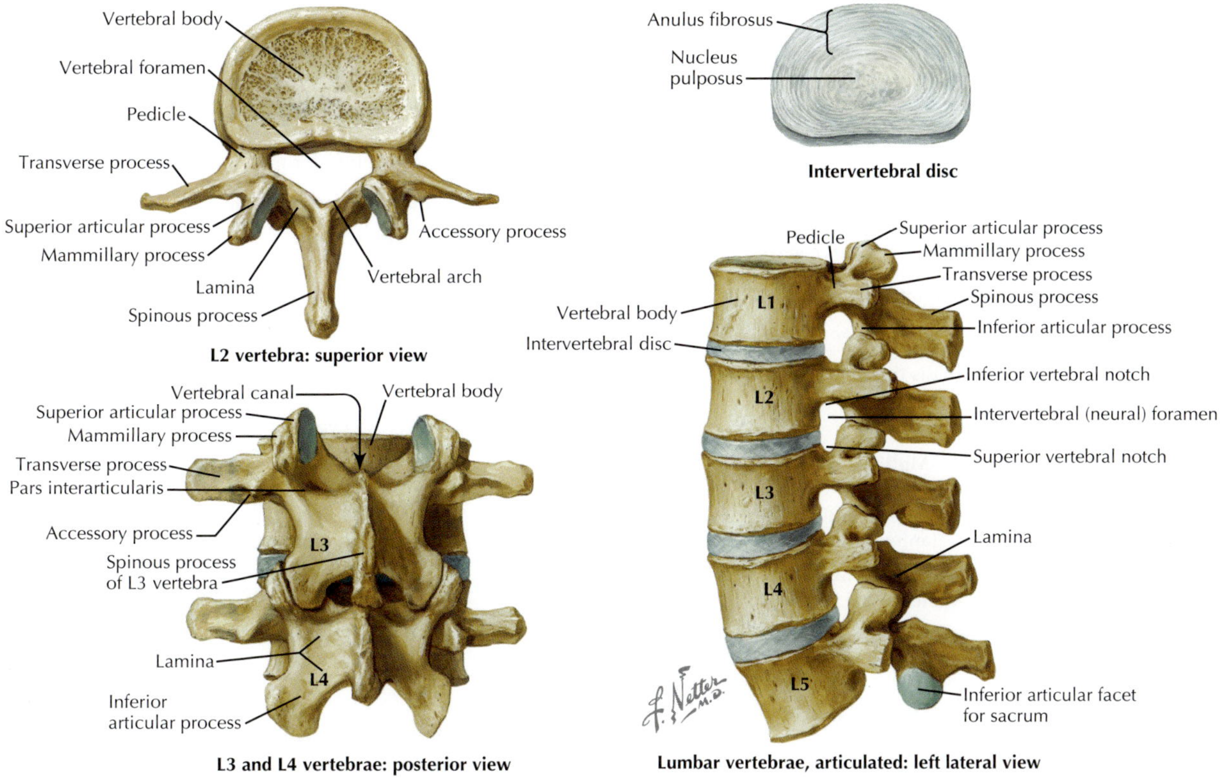

Fig. 14.1 Skeletal anatomy considerations. Bony anatomy of the vertebra. (From Overview of skeletal anatomy. In: Ward PJ, ed. *Netter's Integrated Musculoskeletal System: Clinical Anatomy Explained!*. Elsevier; 2022.)

its junction with the superior articular process.[6] The mamillary process is a smaller prominence that originates from the dorsolateral surface of the superior articular process itself.[6] An understanding of the skeletal anatomy of the lumbar spine is important for guiding needle and lead placement toward the multifidus and intertransversarii muscles (Fig. 14.1).

MUSCULATURE

The lumbar multifidus, the primary target of the ReActiv8 system (Mainstay Medical, MN) and other systems, has three sets of fibers: deep, intermediate, and superficial. The deep fibers span two vertebral segments and function tonically. These fibers are the most important for stabilization and proprioception of the lower back.[7] Intermediate and superficial fibers function tonically, span three to five levels and are primary responsible for lumbar rotation.[7] Because deep fibers are the primary drivers of low back stabilization, it is important that intervention targeting an increase in lumbar multifidus action extends deep enough to reach these fibers.

The lumbar intertransversarii muscles are another group of fibers that lie proximal to device leads and assist in confirmation of correct lead placement. These muscles are divided into lateral and medial groupings, with lateral intertransversarii running from the superior to inferior border of the lumbar transverse processes and the medial intertransversarii running from the transverse processes to mammillary process of lumbar vertebrae (Fig. 14.2).[8] Together, these muscle groupings assist with lateral flexion of the spine. Stimulation of these muscles during confirmatory testing may occur as they are also innervated, in part, by the dorsal rami of lumbar spinal nerves.[9] The lumbar intertransversarii muscles serve as a key landmark for lead placement.

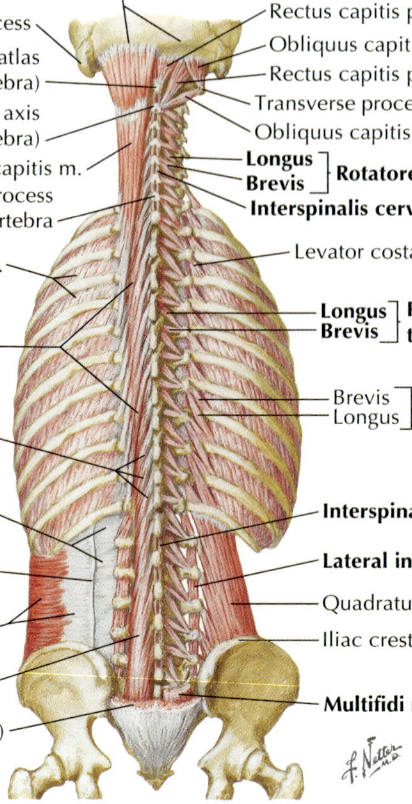

Fig. 14.2 Musculature considerations. Muscles of the back: deep layers of the posterior neck and back. *m(m)*, Muscle(s). (From Cleland JA, Koppenhaver S, Su J. Thoracolumbar spine. In: Cleland JA, Koppenhaver S, Su J, eds. *Netter's Orthopaedic Clinical Examination.* 4th ed. Elsevier; 2022:137–212.)

NEURAL ANATOMY

The MBN, which innervates the lumbar multifidus targeted by the neurostimulator implant, is a derivative of the dorsal rami that arise from the spinal nerves at the level of each lumbar intervertebral disc. The MBN lies against the bone at the junction of the transverse process and superior articular process and runs caudally and dorsally through the fibro-osseous canal formed by the superior articular process, dorsal surface of the transverse process, and accessory process.[6] After exiting the canal, the MBN runs medially and caudally along the caudal surface of the facet joint, traveling within fibrous and adipose tissue between the multifidus muscle and lamina, ultimately branching to the interspinalis muscle, multifidus muscle (entering through the muscle's deep fibers), and the ligaments and periosteum of the vertebral arches (Fig. 14.3).[6]

Description of Procedure

The procedure is conducted in a procedure room or an operating room (OR) setting, aiming for the MBNs at the desired vertebral level. Placement of the percutaneous leads can be aided with ultrasound or fluoroscopy.

1. The patient is put in the prone position for the procedure to access the MBNs. The prone position creates easier access because, after the medial branch of the dorsal ramus exits the

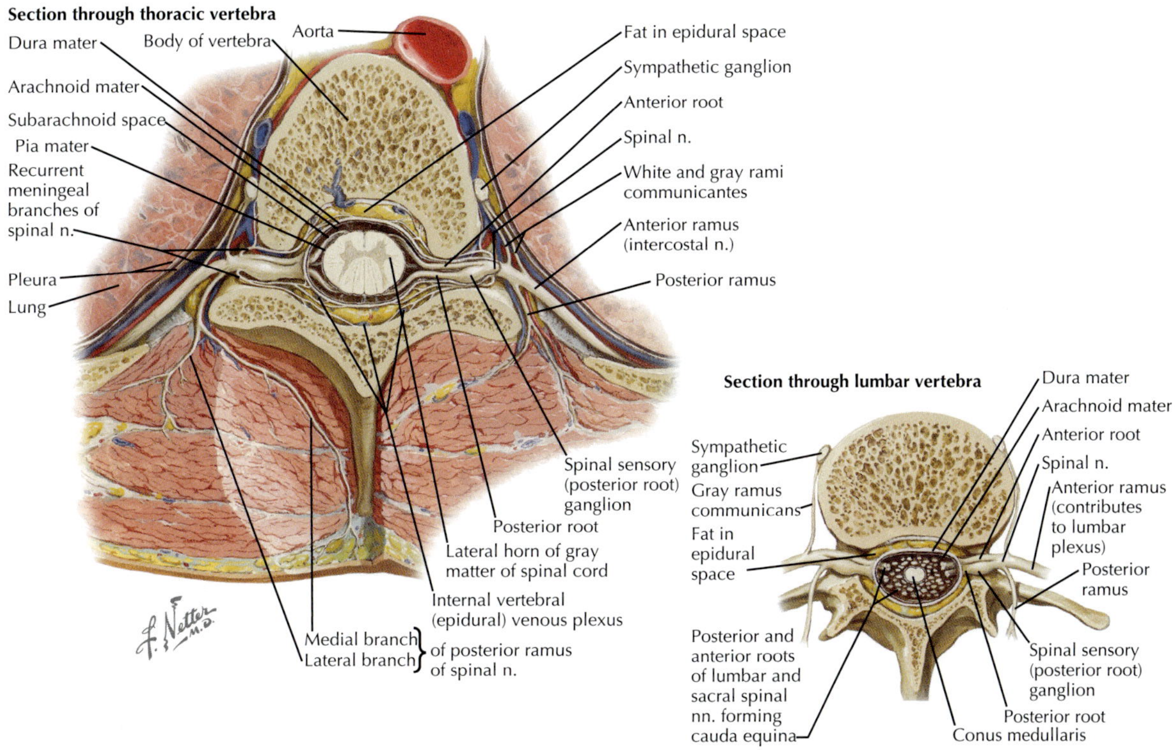

Fig. 14.3 Neural considerations. Spinal nerve origin: cross sections exit of spinal nerves. *n*, Nerve. (From Innervation of the muscle compartments. In: Ward PJ, ed. *Netter's Integrated Musculoskeletal System: Clinical Anatomy Explained.* Elsevier; 2022.)

fibro-osseous canal, it runs along the caudal surface of the facet joint, within the fibrous and adipose tissue between the multifidus and lamina.[6]

2. The needle/needle introducer is then inserted at or near a 90-degree angle and approximately 2 cm lateral from the midline.
3. Either ultrasound or fluoroscopy is used to guide PNS lead placement medial and inferior to the facet joint approximately 0.5 to 1 cm away from the targeted nerve.
4. Confirm activation of multifidi muscles. To analyze whether there is the intended activation of the multifidus muscles, a sensation over the region of pain is confirmed and ultrasound can be performed for visualization.
5. Securing leads. Once both multifidus muscles are determined to be stimulated as desired, the needle introducer is removed. The percutaneous leads are left in place and are surgically glued into place and connected to a wearable stimulator.
6. Programming. The programming is set up to stimulate the multifidi cyclically for many hours throughout the day. The trial duration can vary; for example, Gilmore et al. performed a 1-month trial[10] and Deer et al. did a 60-day trial[5] when analyzing the effect of percutaneous PNS. Gabriel and Ilfeld's article on acute postoperative pain management with percutaneous PNS had an expert opinion stating that the leads were safe to be in situ for up to 60 days.[11] The key to programming the stimulator is that the activation of both multifidus muscles is comfortable for the patient.

General Considerations

Before permanent implantation of a PNS is completed targeting MBNs to treat chronic back pain, a trial is performed[12] to assess the efficacy of a permanent procedure. There are two main reported types of trials:

percutaneous PNS with a wearable device to be followed by permanent implant or a nerve block with local anesthetic to be followed by a temporary PNS implant. Implantation without trial has been also reported in some studies. As the field of pain management continues to develop and progress, more procedures, medications, and lifestyle alterations are coming to light that are aiding in the treatment of lower back pain.

Percutaneous nerve stimulation has been shown to help in the pain management after ambulatory orthopedic surgery through lower pain scores and lower opioid requirements.[13] The general consensus of the literature tends to be that percutaneous PNS can be a safe, nonpharmacological treatment option for acute pain management. A 2-patient case study analyzing the use of percutaneous PNS for chronic lower back pain found there to be a decrease in average back pain intensity during the 30-day trial followed by continued relief for a few months upon removal of the leads.[14]

REFERENCES

1. Husky MM, Ferdous Farin F, Compagnone P, Fermanian C, Kovess-Masfety V. Chronic back pain and its association with quality of life in a large French population survey. *Health Qual Life Outcomes.* 2018;16(1):195. Available at: https://doi.org/10.1186/s12955-018-1018-4.
2. Choi YS, Kim DJ, Lee KY, et al. How does chronic back pain influence quality of life in Koreans: a cross-sectional study. *Asian Spine J.* 2014;8(3):346-352. Available at: doi:10.4184/asj.2014.8.3.346.
3. Dutmer AL, Preuper HRS, Soer R, et al. Personal and societal impact of low back pain: the Groningen spine cohort. *Spine.* 2019;44(24):E1443-E1451.
4. Chou R, Qaseem A, Snow V, et al. Diagnosis and treatment of low back pain: a joint clinical practice guideline from the American College of Physicians and the American Pain Society. *Ann Intern Med.* 2007;147(7):478-491.
5. Deer TR, Gilmore CA, Desai MJ, et al. Percutaneous peripheral nerve stimulation of the medial branch nerves for the treatment of chronic axial back pain in patients after radiofrequency ablation. *Pain Med.* 2021;22(3):548-560.
6. Waxenbaum JA, Reddy V, Williams C, Futterman B. Anatomy, back, lumbar vertebrae. In: StatPearls. Treasure Island (FL): *StatPearls* Publishing; August 4, 2021.
7. Deckers K, De Smedt K, van Buyten JP, et al. Chronic low back pain: restoration of dynamic stability. *Neuromodulation.* 2015; 18(6):478-486.
8. PHED301 Students. *Muscles. Advanced Anatomy.* 2nd ed. May 1, 2018. Available at: https://pressbooks.bccampus.ca/advancedanatomy1sted/chapter/muscles-6/. Accessed June 30, 2022.
9. University of Michigan. *Gross Anatomy—Muscles.* n.d. http://www.med.umich.edu/lrc/anatomy-tables/muscles_alpha.html. Accessed June 30, 2022.
10. Gilmore CA, Kapural L, McGee MJ, Boggs JW. Percutaneous peripheral nerve stimulation for chronic low back pain: prospective case series with 1 year of sustained relief following short-term implant. *Pain Pract.* 2020;20(3):310-320.
11. Gabriel RA, Ilfeld BM. Acute postoperative pain management with percutaneous peripheral nerve s.timulation: The SPRINT Neuromodulation System. *Expert Rev Med Devices.* 2021;18(2): 145-150.
12. Carayannopoulos AG. Peripheral Nerve Stimulation (PNS): Trial. In: Pope J, Deer T, eds. *Treatment of Chronic Pain Conditions.* New York: Springer; 2017. Available at: https://doi.org/10.1007/978-1-4939-6976-0_65.
13. Ilfeld BM, Plunkett A, Vijjeswarapu AM, et al. Percutaneous peripheral nerve stimulation (neuromodulation) for postoperative pain: a randomized, sham-controlled pilot study. *Anesthesiology.* 2021;135(1):95-110.
14. Kapural L, Gilmore CA, Chae J, et al. Percutaneous peripheral nerve stimulation for the treatment of chronic low back pain: two clinical case reports of sustained pain relief. *Pain Pract.* 2018;18(1):94-103.

Chapter 15

Multifidus Muscle Neurostimulator Implant

Joshua M. Martens, Kenneth J. Fiala, Alaa Abd-Elsayed, and Chris Gilligan

Chapter Outline

Introduction

Low back pain is a disabling and highly prevalent condition, with a lifetime prevalence of 23%.[1] Patients who suffer from chronic low back pain report a lower quality of life and have been shown to score higher on scales for depression, anxiety, and sleep disorders.[2] Chronic low back pain not only disables the affected patient but also presents a significant challenge to health care systems and societies, with an estimated annual productivity loss of approximately $28 billion in the United States alone.[3] Disruption of posterior stabilizing muscles allows vertebral segments to move outside of a pain-free zone, increasing patient risk for injury and pain.[4] Specifically, dysfunction of the multifidus muscle, a primary lower back stabilizer, is a common underlying mechanism of low back pain.[5] Patients with chronic low back pain have been shown to be less able than healthy patients to voluntarily contract their multifidus muscle. Improving multifidus motor control and contractility remains a primary target of therapy for refractory low back pain.

Conservative management for chronic low back pain includes exercise rehabilitation, massage, traction therapy, ultrasound, pain medications, physical therapy, and more.[4] Patients with chronic low back pain are commonly not candidates for spinal surgery, leaving them with little recourse for pain that is refractory to conservative management. The ReActiv8 system is an implantable neurostimulation system that was approved by the US Food and Drug Administration (FDA) in 2020 as an aid in the management of intractable chronic low back pain associated with multifidus muscle dysfunction.[6] It engages a restorative mechanism of action. By stimulation of the medial branch for up to 30 minutes twice a daily, it elicits strong repetitive bilateral contractions of the multifidus muscles to override the inhibition responsible for functional instability of the lumbar spine.[4] In multiple clinical trials with published outcomes for up to 4-years, the ReActiv8 system has been shown to provide statistically significant, clinically substantial and lasting improvements in pain, disability, and quality of life in patients with intractable chronic low back pain associated with multifidus dysfunction.[7–12] Providers have performed peripheral nerve stimulation (PNS) of the medial branch with systems other than the ReActiv8 system positing analgesic mechanisms of action. However, we will discuss this system specifically here as there is a wider breadth of high-quality evidence supporting its efficacy.

Procedure

The implant procedure has been described in detail[13] and peer-to-peer theoretical and surgical training and certification is mandatory for all first-time implanters. The current version of the physician manual is an easily accessible resource for the most up-to-date techniques and instructions.[14]

1. The procedure begins with the patient placed in a prone position. Padding may be used to reduce lordosis in patients as necessary. Device implantation can be conducted under general anesthesia or conscious sedation. Following the appropriate surgical preparation, an anteroposterior fluoroscopic view is used to identify the junction of the superior articular process and transverse process at the level of L3. The stimulation leads are targeted towards this junction.
2. Spinal needles (22 gauge) are placed percutaneously until bony contact is made at the junction just lateral to the accessory process. These "guide needles" should be placed as superior and medial as possible. A midline incision is made in the skin overlying the point where leads will enter the thoracolumbar fascia. This incision is typically at or above the superior aspect of the L4 spinous process and extends caudally 3 to 5 cm. Using blunt dissection, a 3-cm diameter pocket is formed above the fascia ipsilateral to the implantable pulse generator (IPG) pocket (Fig. 15.1).
3. Using the 22-gauge needles as a guide, the delivery needle is inserted through the fascia at the midline at the level of the superior aspect of the L4 spinous process and directed superiorly, toward the L3 anchor point, at a 45-degree angle with the frontal plane. The needle is further advanced superiorly and laterally toward the junction of the L3 transverse process and L3 superior articulating process until the needle has passed through the intertransversarius muscle between L2 and L3 (Figs. 15.2 and 15.3). The same procedure is repeated for needle insertion on the contralateral side.
4. Using the modified Seldinger technique, a guidewire is placed through the delivery needle which are then removed. A 7-French introducer is advanced over the guidewire such that the tip protrudes 5 mm through the intertransversarii muscles between L2 and L3 (Fig. 15.4). The contralateral introducer is placed using the same procedural steps.
5. The guidewire and dilator core are removed from the introducer to create a path for lead placement. The leads are then advanced to the end of the introducers, until the most distal electrode is just anterior to the intertransversarius muscle and held in place as introducers are withdrawn. Bilateral lead placement can be confirmed on AP and lateral fluoroscopy. (Fig. 15.5).

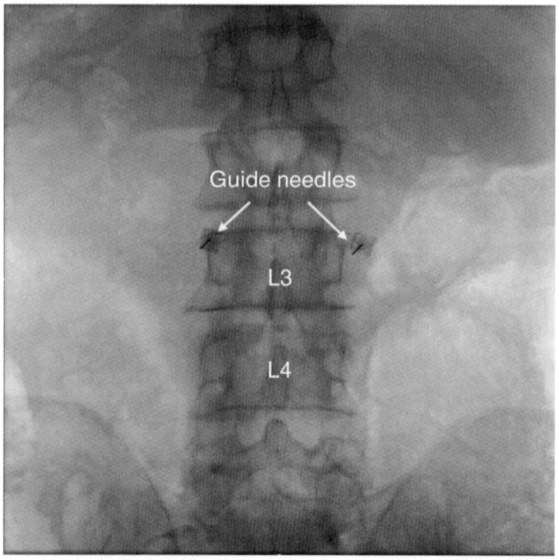

Fig. 15.1 Fluoroscopy image of guide needle placement at the L3 junction of the superior articular process and transverse process at the level of the L3 vertebra. (Courtesy Mainstay Medical Limited)

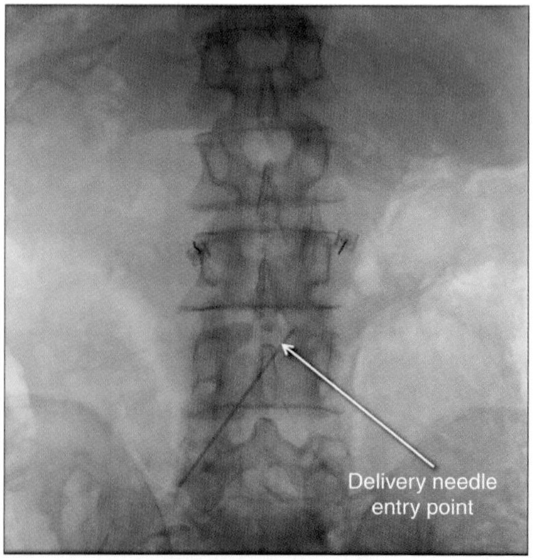

Fig. 15.2 Fluoroscopy image of delivery needle entry point approximately at the level of the superior aspect of the L4 spinous process. (Courtesy Mainstay Medical Limited)

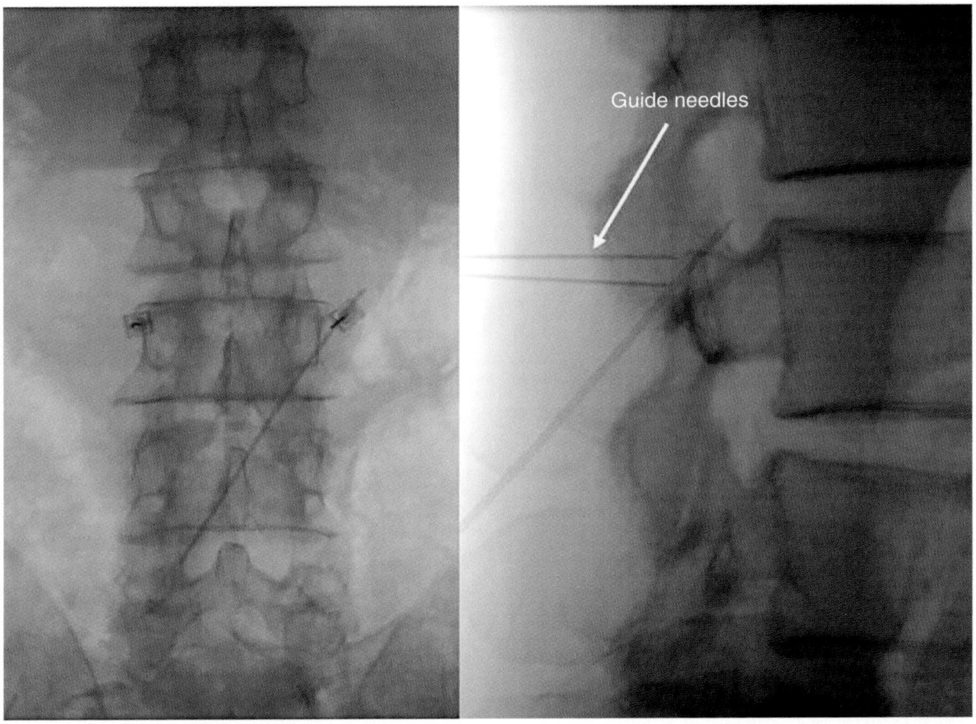

Fig. 15.3 **Fluoroscopy image of guide needles relative to delivery needle, which is positioned at a 45-degree angle with the frontal plane.** (Courtesy Mainstay Medical Limited)

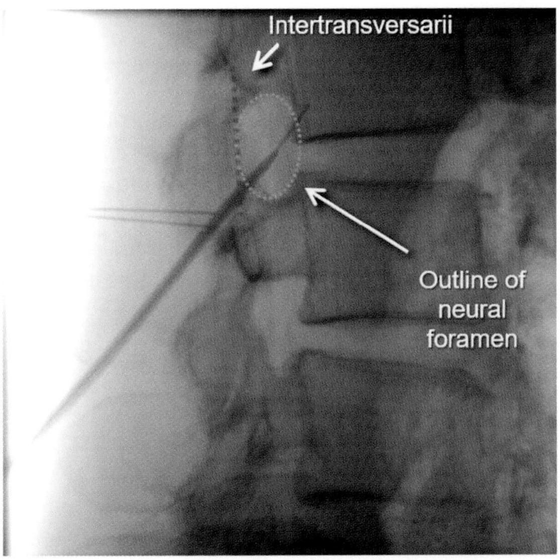

Fig. 15.4 **Fluoroscopy image of introducer positioning relative to the intertransversarii muscles and the neural foramen.** (Courtesy Mainstay Medical Limited)

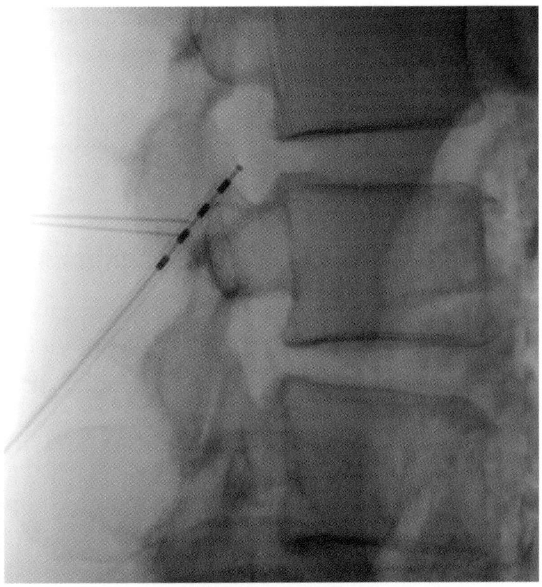

Fig. 15.5 **Fluoroscopy image of lead placement via retraction of introducer sheath.** (Courtesy Mainstay Medical Limited)

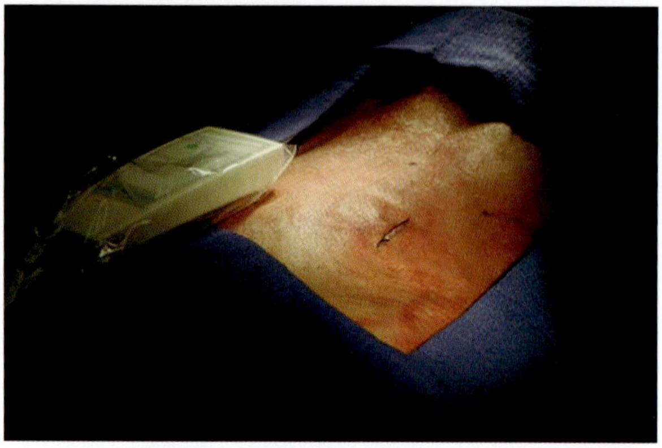

Fig. 15.6 Introduction of implantable pulse generator along with a draped programming wand for confirmatory testing. (Courtesy Mainstay Medical Limited)

6. Following lead placement, the IPG is introduced into the sterile field, along with a draped programming wand. The leads are connected to the IPG, impedances are confirmed, and bipolar stimulation is conducted with the intent to produce a palpable contraction of the multifidus. Successful contraction initiation serves as muscle confirmation of appropriate placement of the leads (Fig. 15.6).
7. A retention loop is formed, and the proximal portions of the leads are tunneled to a pocket created by blunt dissection in the subcutaneous tissue that lines the buttock. The leads are connected to the IPG which is then placed in pocket and repeat contraction testing is conducted. Following repeat testing and final fluoroscopic images, incision sites are closed (Fig. 15.7).

Intra- and Postoperative Complications

Intraoperative complications, while atypical, must be considered and planned for prior to initiation of device implant. Because lead placement is outside the spinal canal and the trajectory is directed laterally, risk of dural puncture or neurological injury is exceedingly low and has not been observed to date.

Lead migration, one of the most common complications of traditional PNS systems, has been effectively mitigated with proprietary bidirectional, flexible tines that provide distal fixation to the intertransversarii, ensuring positioning the quadripolar electrode array immediately adjacent to the medial branch. Consequently, lead migrations are exceedingly rare (<<1%) with the ReActiv8 system.

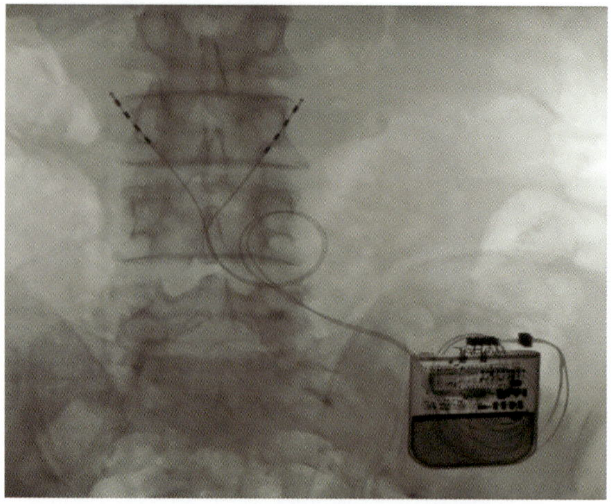

Fig. 15.7 Final fluoroscopic images to confirm implantable pulse generator and lead placement. (Courtesy Mainstay Medical Limited)

Infrequent postimplant complications include infection, seroma, pocket discomfort. Lead fracture and general hardware malfunction are rare complications which occasionally require a surgical intervention.[15,16] For cases requiring lead removal, a sheath and locking stylet are available to facilitate extraction.

General Considerations

Peer-to-peer theoretical and surgical training with certification is mandatory for all first-time implanters. In addition, it is recommended to perform the first procedures with support of an experienced proctor.

A linear trajectory of the delivery needle from the midline incision to the target location indicated by the guide needles optimizes proximity of the electrodes to the medial branch and hence stimulation efficiency. Anatomical variations and structural pathologies may require subtle adaptations of the implant procedure and trajectory. Therefore, careful preoperative review of individual patient anatomy and procedure planning should be adopted as standard for all procedures.

ReActiv8 is the only dedicated, proprietary system that has been developed, evaluated, and approved for patients with intractable chronic low back pain associated with multifidus dysfunction.

REFERENCES

1. Airaksinen O, Brox JI, Cedraschi C, et al. Chapter 4. European guidelines for the management of chronic nonspecific low back pain. *Eur Spine J*. 2006;15 Suppl 2:S192-300. doi:10.1007/s00586-006-1072-1
2. Gore M, Sadosky A, Stacey BR, Tai KS, Leslie D. The burden of chronic low back pain: clinical comorbidities, treatment patterns, and health care costs in usual care settings. *Spine*. 2012;37(11): E668-E677.
3. Rizzo JA, Abbott TA III, Berger ML. The labor productivity effects of chronic backache in the United States. *Med Care*. 1998;36(10): 1471-1488.
4. Russo M, Deckers K, Eldabe S, Kiesel K, Gilligan C, Vieceli J, Crosby P. Muscle Control and Non-specific Chronic Low Back Pain. Neuromodulation. 2018 Jan;21(1):1-9. doi: 10.1111/ner.12738.
5. Wallwork TL, Stanton WR, Freke M, Hides JA. The effect of chronic low back pain on size and contraction of the lumbar multifidus muscle. *Man Ther*. 2009;14(5):496-500.
6. US Food and Drug Administration. *Premarket Approval (PMA)*. (n.d.). Available at: https/www.accessdata.fda.gov/scripts/cdrh/cfdocs/cfpma/pma.cfm?id=P190021. Accessed June 30, 2022.
7. Gilligan C, Volschenk W, Russo M, Green M, Gilmore C, Mehta V, Deckers K, De Smedt K, Latif U, Georgius P, Gentile J, Mitchell B, Langhorst M, Huygen F, Baranidharan G, Patel V, Mironer E, Ross E, Carayannopoulos A, Hayek S, Gulve A, Van Buyten JP, Tohmeh A, Fischgrund J, Lad S, Ahadian F, Deer T, Klemme W, Rauck R, Rathmell J, Levy R, Heemels JP, Eldabe S; ReActiv8-B investigators. An implantable restorative-neurostimulator for refractory mechanical chronic low back pain: a randomized sham-controlled clinical trial. Pain. 2021 Oct 1;162(10):2486-2498. doi: 10.1097/j.pain.0000000000002258.
8. Gilligan C, Volschenk W, Russo M, Green M, Gilmore C, Mehta V, Deckers K, De Smedt K, Latif U, Georgius P, Gentile J, Mitchell B, Langhorst M, Huygen F, Baranidharan G, Patel V, Mironer E, Ross E, Carayannopoulos A, Hayek S, Gulve A, Van Buyten JP, Tohmeh A, Fischgrund J, Lad S, Ahadian F, Deer T, Klemme W, Rauck R, Rathmell J, Maislin G, Heemels JP, Eldabe S; ReActiv8-B Investigators. Long-Term Outcomes of Restorative Neurostimulation in Patients With Refractory Chronic Low Back Pain Secondary to Multifidus Dysfunction: Two-Year Results of the ReActiv8-B Pivotal Trial. Neuromodulation. 2021 Dec 18:S1094-7159(21)06386-8. doi: 10.1016/j.neurom.2021.10.011. Epub ahead of print.
9. Gilligan C, Volschenk W, Russo M, Green M, Gilmore C, Mehta V, Deckers K, De Smedt K, Latif U, Sayed D, Georgius P, Gentile J, Mitchell B, Langhorst M, Huygen F, Baranidharan G, Patel V, Mironer E, Ross E, Carayannopoulos A, Hayek S, Gulve A, Van Buyten JP, Tohmeh A, Fischgrund J, Lad S, Ahadian F, Deer T, Klemme W, Rauck R, Rathmell J, Schwab F, Maislin G, Heemels JP, Eldabe S; Three-Year Durability of Restorative Neurostimulation Effectiveness in Patients with Chronic Low Back Pain and Multifidus Muscle Dysfunction. Neuromodulation. [Accepted for publication on Aug 23, 2022].
10. Deckers K, De Smedt K, Mitchell B, Vivian D, Russo M, Georgius P, Green M, Vieceli J, Eldabe S, Gulve A, van Buyten JP, Smet I, Mehta V, Ramaswamy S, Baranidharan G, Sullivan R, Gassin R, Rathmell J, Gilligan C. New Therapy for Refractory Chronic Mechanical Low Back Pain-Restorative Neurostimulation to Activate the Lumbar Multifidus: One Year Results of a Prospective Multicenter Clinical Trial. Neuromodulation. 2018 Jan;21(1):48-55. doi: 10.1111/ner.12741.
11. Mitchell B, Deckers K, De Smedt K, Russo M, Georgius P, Green M, Gulve A, van Buyten JP, Smet I, Mehta V, Baranidharan G, Rathmell J, Gilligan C, Goss B, Eldabe S. Durability of the Therapeutic Effect of Restorative Neurostimulation for Refractory Chronic Low Back Pain. Neuromodulation. 2021 Aug;24(6):1024-1032. doi: 10.1111/ner.13477.
12. Thomson S, Chawla R, Love-Jones S, Sharma M, Vajramani G, Williams A, Eldabe S; ReActiv8 PMCF Investigators. Restorative Neurostimulation for Chronic Mechanical Low Back Pain: Results from a Prospective Multi-centre Longitudinal Cohort. Pain Ther. 2021 Dec;10(2):1451-1465. doi: 10.1007/s40122-021-00307-3.
13. Chakravarthy K, Lee D, Tram J, et al. Restorative Neurostimulation: A Clinical Guide for Therapy Adoption. 2022;(May): 1759-1774.
14. ReActiv8 Physician Manual [Add source]
15. Eldabe S, Buchser E, Duarte RV. Complications of spinal cord stimulation and peripheral nerve stimulation techniques: a review of the literature. Pain Med. 2016;17(2):325-336.
16. Woods DM, Hayek SM, Bedder M. Complications of neuro stimulation. Tech Region Anesth Pain Manage. 2007;11: 178-182.

Chapter 16

Programming

Behnum Habibi, Gustaf Van Acker, and Chong Kim

Chapter Outline

Introduction

The incidence of chronic pain in the United States is increasing[1]—50,000,000 people in the United States, or 20.4% of the population, have chronic pain.[2] Of US adults, 8% have chronic pain that limits their life or work activities on most days.[2] The annual cost of care for chronic pain in also increasing.

According to the National Academy of Medicine (formerly called the Institute of Medicine), the annual cost of care for chronic pain in the United States is estimated to be up to $635 billion annually.[3] First performed in the mid-20th century, stimulation of the spinal cord using electrical leads has emerged as a successful therapy for refractory neuropathic pain.

Stimulation of the spinal cord, typically with lead placement in the epidural space posterior to the dorsal columns, is indicated for failed back surgery syndrome (FBSS), complex regional pain syndrome (CPRS) types I and II, and intractable low back and leg pain.[4] Associated conditions and etiologies may include radicular pain, epidural fibrosis, degenerative disc disease, arachnoiditis, and multiple back surgeries. Uses of spinal cord stimulation (SCS) in clinical practice vary more broadly and include the treatment of FBSS and CPRS as well as peripheral vascular disease, visceral pain in the chest/abdomen/pelvis, and peripheral neuropathy.[5]

A major factor influencing the clinical efficacy of these devices is programming of the stimulation parameters. Programming guidelines are typically specific to an individual manufacturer's device and not as well described in the scientific literature. This chapter will serve as an introductory guide to common principles of SCS programming.

Basic Overview of Interrogation and Programming of Spinal Cord Stimulation

SCS systems contain two primary elements, electrical leads and an implantable pulse generator (IPG). The IPG controls the electrical pulses delivered by the leads. During a trial period, electrodes are inserted but the IPG remains external (and might be more accurately referred to as an external pulse generator, or EPG; Fig. 16.1). Upon implantation of the leads, either during a trial or after permanent implants, impedance checks are an essential aspect of confirming proper placement. Once verified, remaining programming adjustments all occur at the EPG. Determining successful programs during a trial period is an essential step, as it will inform programming of the fully implanted device.

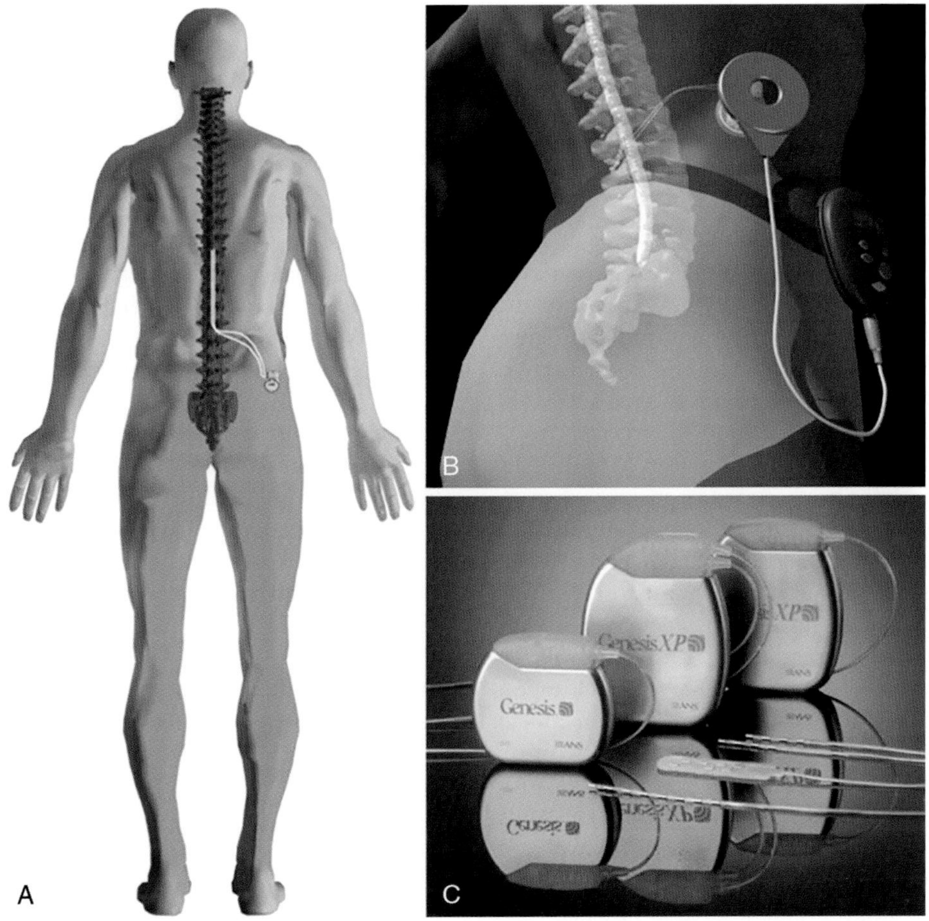

Fig. 16.1 Sample images of (A) spinal cord stimulator implanted system, (B) external pulse generator, and (C) implantable pulse generator.[6]

Interrogation is typically performed on the table in the procedure or operating room immediately after electrode placement into the dorsal epidural space at the targeted vertebral level. During a trial, the interrogation device communicates with the EPG and can provide impedance values for every contact on each lead. A contact should have a resistance below 3000 ohms. In a review of 36 patients undergoing percutaneous trial stimulation, medial impedance in the thoracolumbar stimulators was 547 ± 151 ohms.[7] Median impedance was even lower in the cervical region, 351 ± 90 ohms. This difference is likely due to the relatively smaller distance in the cervical spine between the cord and epidural space. Nonfunctional high impedance connections may be secondary to anatomy such as epidural fat or postsurgical scarring or from problems with lead placement, including trapped air from a loss-of-resistance syringe or inaccurate placement of a lead.

Upon implantation, battery life expectancy is an important variable regarding programming selection. Energy consumption (E) of an IPG is proportional to the product of the pulse width (PW), impedance at the stimulator output (R), and the square of the stimulation current (I).[7]

$$E = I^2 * R * PW$$

Different programming settings will consume different amounts of energy. IPG life will often dictate initial programming settings—that is, the lowest energy programs that offer adequate pain relief will likely be used first. Battery life of a primary cell IPG is typically 5 to 7 years. For rechargeable IPGs, the battery life span in significantly increased. However, in rechargeable devices, charging frequency is similarly influenced by the energy consumption of the program. Thus, programs with lower energy consumption will allow for longer periods between charges. This has driven research into novel energy-conserving strategies. For example, in 2019, Vesper et al. published results of "microdosed" burst waveform stimulation that was compared with standard burst SCS (i.e., 5 seconds of burst waveform stimulation alternating with 10 seconds vs. 5 seconds of no stimulation).[8] In the 25-subject randomized controlled trial, there was no significant difference between groups.

Typically, patients will choose at least 2 to 3 different programs. Major parameters to consider when reprogramming an SCS system include contact selection, amplitude, pulse width, and frequency.[9] These factors will be addressed individually in this chapter. In general, programming adjustments postoperatively should begin with a radiograph to confirm that the leads are in the appropriate location, followed by an impedance check of each contact. Traditionally, each contact is then systematically checked to find those with the best coverage of the painful areas of the body. If no contacts can be found that cover the painful areas, differing anode/cathode combinations can be explored. However, recent clinical data suggest that generating paresthesias in targeted painful area is not necessary for successful treatment.[10,11]

Initial settings can utilize traditional tonic stimulation or paresthesia-free, subperception programs. Regardless of which is used, the selected initial contacts and parameters should provide the maximum pain relief to the patient. For tonic programs, lower amplitudes correlate with milder paresthesias, while higher amplitudes will cause more intense paresthesias. In tonic programming, lower frequencies will typically cause noticeable paresthesias, while higher frequencies will cause fewer paresthesias. Finally, shorter pulse widths will typically cover small areas of the body, while longer pulse widths will cover larger areas of the body. Once the ideal first program is selected, additional programs should be sought. Often, the second program will be different from the original in terms of tonic versus paresthesia-free programming. Alternative parameters, such as duty cycle and charge per second, may also be useful ways to conceptualize the "dose" of stimulation applied to the target tissues.[12] However, this will not be discussed in detail in this chapter.

Contact Selection

Appropriate contact selection is vital for covering pain in the affected area of the body as well as for optimizing the efficacy of adjustments of other parameters. Each lead contains a number of metal contacts, each of which can be programmed as anodes or cathodes. Current flows from anodes and toward cathodes. The electrical fields generated between anodes and cathodes can be manipulated by changes in contact selection. For instance, when two adjacent leads are placed in the spinal column, selecting anodes and cathodes on different leads can allow for control of the electric field in the medial-lateral direction.

In theory, with monopolar stimulation from a point source electrode, the extracellular potentials (Ve) generated are proportional to the current and inversely proportional to the distance between electrode and tissue.[13] When represented as an equation,

$$Ve = \frac{I}{4\pi\sigma r},$$

I is the current in amperes, σ represents electrical conductivity in siemens per meter, and r is the distance in meters between the electrode and the target point in the tissue. This relationship conveys how the distance between the contact and target tissue affects neural stimulation. Thus, it should be no surprise that small distances between the selected contacts results in deeper and wider dorsal column stimulation compared with configurations with larger distances between contacts.[14] With larger distances between contacts, there may also be increased power usage.

Using a single cathode will concentrate the current delivered to a single area. Most devices can split energy between multiple cathodes, reducing the current density at an individual contact. This can reduce the intensity of paresthesias at a given site but may require additional power delivery from the IPG and, thus, shorten battery life. Clinically, stimulation of the dorsal columns is typically achieved using bipolar, not unipolar, configurations. This was, in part, a byproduct of multiple animal studies that showed preferential stimulation of the dorsal columns using short distances between electrodes in bipolar/tripolar configurations.[7] For example, with tonic stimulation, a simple bipolar program is typically trialed first with a single anode and single cathode paired together. Tripolar configurations, with a single cathode between anodes, or with two cathodes programmed between anodes, are also frequently used. These configurations may provide deeper current penetration compared with simple bipolar configurations.[15,16]

The two primary lead types, percutaneous and paddle, have different lead configurations (Fig. 16.2). The contacts may have varying length, width, shape, and number. For instance, typical leads have 8 contacts compared with some systems having up to 32 contacts. Percutaneous leads and their contacts are usually cylindrical. Paddle leads and contacts are usually rectangular or round. Both lead types are safe, effective, and have low complication rates. Paddle leads have lower dislocation rates; however, they typically require laminectomy for placement.[17]

For unilateral pain, the cathode is typically selected on the ipsilateral side (painful side). Similarly, for bilateral pain, the cathode is typically selected on the more painful side. Cathode selection in the rostrocaudal direction will depend on the painful area of the body. Classically, C2 corresponds to the face/occiput, C2 to C4 to the axial neck/shoulder, C4 to C7 to the distal upper extremity, T1 to T4 to the chest wall, T5 to T6 to the abdomen, T7 to T10 to the lower back and lower extremity, L1 to L2 to the pelvis/buttock, L5 to S1 to the distal lower extremity, and S2 to S4 to the pelvis/perineum.[18]

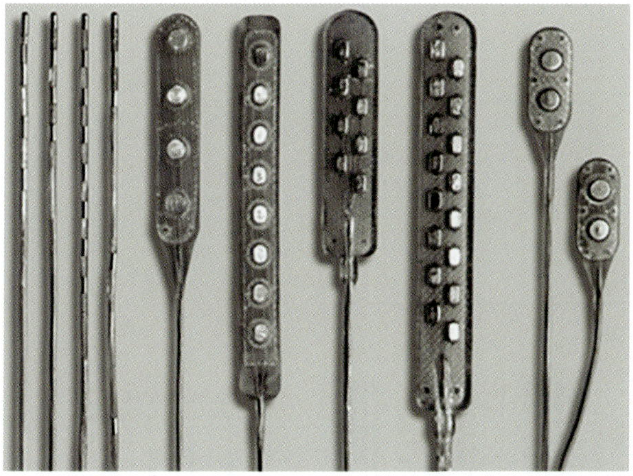

Fig. 16.2 Sample spinal cord stimulator lead configurations. Percutaneous leads are the most commonly used, followed by paddle leads. The percutaneous leads are the four leftmost electrodes; the paddle leads are the five rightmost electrodes. (Reproduced with permission of Abbott, © 2022. All rights reserved.)

Amplitude

Amplitude, in general, is defined as the maximum displacement or distance moved by a point on a vibrating body or wave measured from its equilibrium position.

The amplitude of an IPG output signal can vary in either voltage or current. Traditionally, either the current or voltage will be held constant by the IPG, whereas the other is modified by the user. In a rat model using side-by-side comparison of constant current versus constant voltage SCS, constant current SCS was more effective for treating complex pain.[19] In small clinical studies, the difference between these two approaches was less evident—one 2014 study showed a patient preference for constant current SCS, whereas another 2010 study concluded that patients were unable to detect the difference between constant current and constant voltage stimulation. Additionally, with constant voltage stimulation, paresthesia-based SCS, additional current utilizes more energy and there is a greater degree of perceived stimulation. Currently, all SCS manufacturers use constant current stimulation.

Typically, the minimum amplitude is selected that generates a perceived sensation. Maximum amplitudes are typically set at the level where paresthesias become uncomfortable or other unwanted effects are perceived. Typically, the target amplitude will be set below 1 to 5 mA (lower for cervical leads). In general, paddle leads require lower amplitudes than percutaneous leads.

Pulse Width

Pulse width is defined as a measure of the elapsed time between the leading and trailing edges of a single pulse of energy. Pulse width is typically measured in microseconds. Increasing the pulse width widens the electric field, resulting in a greater degree of stimulation and potentially wider areas of body coverage.[20] The increased body area coverage typically extends in the caudal direction, with both thoracolumbar as well as cervical dorsal column stimulation. This phenomenon is sometimes described as *caudal extension*. Increasing the pulse width is limited by unwanted anatomical recruitment, such as stimulation of the dorsal roots, which can be unpleasant. For paresthesia-free stimulation, pulse width can similarly be adjusted, though the ranges may be more limited.

The baseline pulse width for tonic stimulation is generally within 200 to 500 μs. Some devices allow pulse widths up to 1000 μs. In one small study, the median pulse width of patients upon completion of a trial and programming optimization was 400 μs.[21] Increasing the baseline pulse width is advisable when baseline stimulation does not cover all of the desired body areas. Increases in pulse width, however, must be balanced with the potential for side effects such as stimulation of unwanted body areas or unpleasant paresthesias.

In cervical stimulation, as well as dorsal root ganglion stimulation, lower pulse widths at baseline are generally advisable given the risk for increased recruitment and unpleasant paresthesias.

Frequency

Frequency of stimulation patterns, measured in pulses/second or Hz, typically start at 40 Hz, particularly for tonic/traditional dorsal column stimulation. Waveforms of varying frequencies can be either fixed, that is, there is a fixed pulse train, or variable, for example, burst stimulation (Fig. 16.3). A fixed waveform, at around 40 Hz, stimulates the dorsal columns and produces pleasant paresthesias. As the frequency increases, to about 100 Hz, paresthesias are felt more intensely, which may improve pain relief. This should be balanced against the possibility of unpleasant paresthesias at higher frequencies.

Frequency can be increased such that paresthesias are no longer perceived. High-frequency stimulation has been defined in different ways. Some texts define high-frequency stimulation as 500 Hz or greater. Others define it as 10,000 Hz or greater. Increases in frequency to achieve paresthesia-free stimulation appear to provide similar pain relief and, in some cases, particularly for low back pain, superior relief compared with traditional tonic stimulation.[10,22,23] However, increased frequency typically increases power consumption and, thus, shortens battery life.

Burst patterns of stimulation provide repeated pulse trains of varying intervals. Initial studies of burst stimulation used 40-Hz bursts of 5 spikes at 500 Hz. The pulse widths were fixed at 1 ms, with 1-ms interspike intervals and with the cumulative charge of the five 1-ms spikes balanced in the following 5 ms.[24] These bursts typically cycle, sometimes ranging from

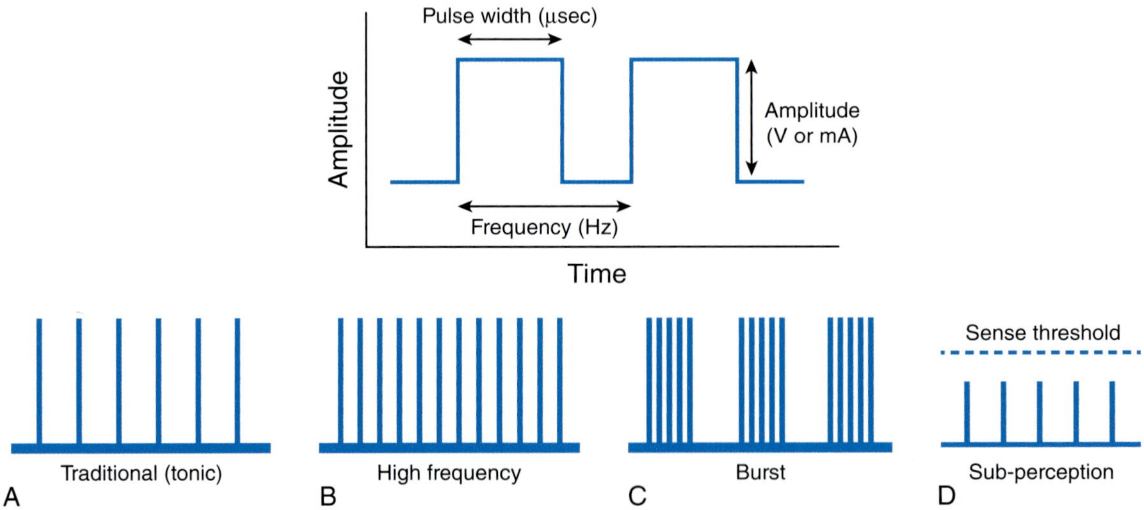

Fig. 16.3 Sample spinal cord stimulation waveform.

30 to 90 s of on time, followed by 3 to 6 minutes of off time, preserving battery life. Burst stimulation likely provides pain relief via mechanisms at the level of the spinal cord as well as the brain.[25] The latter may have implications for affective components of chronic pain. Results from a 2017 randomized controlled trial suggest that burst stimulation is safe, effective, noninferior to tonic stimulation, and possibly superior to tonic stimulation for the treatment of chronic pain.[26] BurstDR stimulation is a variant waveform with cumulative/stacking charges, whereas traditional burst waveforms use unchanging individual charges.

Open Loop Versus Closed Loop

Tonic/traditional stimulation, high-frequency stimulation, and burst stimulation are all considered open-loop stimulation devices, wherein stimulation is applied through an implanted electrode without any electrical recording of the target tissue. The stimulation settings in such systems are fixed until changed by the patient or a medical professional. Closed-loop systems can record activity in target tissues—in this case, via evoked compound action potentials (ECAPs)—and self-adjust the stimulation parameters based on this feedback.[27] ECAPs represent a summation of activity of groups of neurons in the recording electrode's vicinity. They have been shown to change in response to different SCS settings[28] as well as to normal physiological changes such as variations with respiration. In a trial of 51 patients who underwent a trial procedure with a closed-loop SCS system, 36 progressed to permanent implants.[29] The proportion of those 36 patients with $>$ 50% pain relief was 93% for those with back pain and 91% for those with leg pain at 3 months post implantation. Most patients still had pain relief 6 months postoperatively. Results from a randomized, double-blind, controlled trial of 134 patients using an intention-to-treat analysis to compare closed-loop systems with open-loop systems was published in 2020.[30] At 3 months postimplantation, the closed-loop system provided a greater number of patients with a reduction of 50% or more of overall back and leg pain. There were no differences in safety profiles between the two groups. These two studies suggest that closed-loop systems may provide superior relief for patients with chronic, intractable pain of the back and legs. Further studies will likely elucidate the validity of these findings, expand on the current proposed mechanisms of action, and perhaps improve the analgesic effect of closed-loop systems. For example, there have been recent publications on time-dynamic pulses, whereby stimulation parameters continuously change based on a modulation signal. In at least one animal trial, SCS using time-dynamic pulses improved analgesia more than fixed SCS stimulation settings.[31]

Conclusion

The basic parameters of SCS programming of contact selection, amplitude, pulse width, and frequency have significant clinical implications. High-frequency, burst, and closed-loop stimulation may offer advantages over tonic stimulation, as some data suggest that these types of stimulation are better tolerated and may provide pain relief to patients who fail traditional tonic stimulation.[32]

REFERENCES

1. Dagenais S, Caro J, Haldeman S. A systematic review of low back pain cost of illness studies in the United States and internationally. *Spine J*. 2008;8(1):8-20. Available at: https://doi.org/10.1016/j.spinee.2007.10.005.
2. Dahlhamer J, Lucas J, Zelaya C, et al. Prevalence of chronic pain and high-impact chronic pain among adults—United States, 2016. *MMWR Morb Mortal Wkly Rep*. 2018;67(36):1001-1006. Available at: https://doi.org/10.15585/mmwr.mm6736a2.
3. Pizzo PA, Clark NM. Alleviating suffering 101—pain relief in the United States. *N Engl J Med*. 2012;366(3):197-199. Available at: https://doi.org/10.1056/NEJMp1109084.
4. U.S. Food and Drug Administration. Premarket Approval Application P030017-S275: *Summary of Safety and Effectiveness Data (SSED)*. Available at: https://www.accessdata.fda.gov/cdrh_docs/pdf3/P030017S275B.pdf. Accessed July 1, 2022.
5. Mekhail NA, Mathews M, Nageeb F, Guirguis M, Mekhail MN, Cheng J. Retrospective review of 707 cases of spinal cord stimulation: indications and complications. *Pain Pract*. 2011;11(2):148-153.
6. Durbhakula S, Malik K. Spinal cord stimulation. In: Benzon H, ed, et al. *Essentials of Pain Medicine*. Philadelphia, PA: Elsevier; 2018:663-676.
7. Alo K, Varga C, Krames E, et al. Factors affecting impedance of percutaneous leads in spinal cord stimulation. *Neuromodulation*. 2006;9(2):128-135. Available at: https://doi.org/10.1111/j.1525-1403.2006.00050.x.
8. Vesper J, Slotty P, Schu S, et al. Burst SCS microdosing is as efficacious as standard burst SCS in treating chronic back and leg pain: results from a randomized controlled trial. *Neuromodulation*. 2019;22(2):190-193. doi:10.1111/ner.12883.
9. Sheldon B, Staudt MD, Williams L, et al. Spinal cord stimulation programming: a crash course. *Neurosurg Rev*. 2021;44:709-720. Available at: https://doi.org/10.1007/s10143-020-01299-y.

10. Kapural L, Yu C, Doust MW, et al. Novel 10-kHz high-frequency therapy (HF10 therapy) is superior to traditional low-frequency spinal cord stimulation for the treatment of chronic back and leg pain: The SENZA-RCT randomized controlled trial. *Anesthesiology*. 2015;123(4):851-860. doi:10.1097/ALN.0000000000000774.
11. Al-Kaisy A, Baranidharan G, Palmisani S, et al. Comparison of paresthesia mapping to anatomical placement in burst spinal cord stimulation: initial trial results of the prospective, multicenter, randomized, double-blinded, crossover, CRISP study. *Neuromodulation*. 2020;23(5):613-619. doi:10.1111/ner.13104.
12. Miller JP, Eldabe S, Buchser E, Johanek LM, Guan Y, Linderoth B. Parameters of spinal cord stimulation and their role in electrical charge delivery: a review. *Neuromodulation*. 2016;19(4):373-384. Available at: https://doi.org/10.1111/ner.12438.
13. Molnar G, Barolat G. Principles of cord activation during spinal cord stimulation. *Neuromodulation*. 2014;17(suppl 1):S12-S21. Available at: https://doi.org/10.1111/ner.12171.
14. Sankarasubramanian V, Buitenweg JR, Holsheimer J, Veltink P. Triple leads programmed to perform as longitudinal guarded cathodes in spinal cord stimulation: a modeling study. *Neuromodulation*. 2011;14(5):401-410; discussion 411. Available at: https://doi.org/10.1111/j.1525-1403.2011.00383.x.
15. Holsheimer J, Wesselink WA. Effect of anode-cathode configuration on paresthesia coverage in spinal cord stimulation. *Neurosurgery*. 1997;41:654-659; discussion 659-660. doi:10.1097/00006123-199709000-00030.
16. North RB, Ewend MG, Lawton MT, Piantadosi S. Spinal cord stimulation for chronic, intractable pain: superiority of "multichannel" devices. *Pain*. 1991;44(2):119-130. Available at: https://doi.org/10.1016/0304-3959(91)90125-h.
17. Kinfe TM, Quack F, Wille C, Schu S, Vesper J. Paddle versus cylindrical leads for percutaneous implantation in spinal cord stimulation for failed back surgery syndrome: a single-center trial. *J Neurol Surg A Cent Eur Neurosurg*. 2014;75(06):467-473. Available at: https://doi.org/10.1055/s-0034-1371517.
18. Deer TR. Programming spinal cord stimulation systems. In: Deer TR, Pope JE, eds. *Atlas of Implantable Therapies for Pain Management*. New York, NY: 2nd ed. Springer-Verlag; 2016;49-56.
19. Qin C, Martinez M, Tang R, et al. Is constant current or constant voltage spinal cord stimulation superior for the suppression of nociceptive visceral and somatic stimuli? A rat model. *Neuromodulation*. 2012;15(2):132-142; discussion 143. Available at: https://doi.org/10.1111/j.1525-1403.2012.00431.x.
20. Holsheimer J, Buitenweg JR, Das J, de Sutter P, Manola L, Nuttin B. The effect of pulse width and contact configuration on paresthesia coverage in spinal cord stimulation. *Neurosurgery*. 2011;68(5):1452-1461. Available at: https://doi.org/10.1227/NEU.0b013e31820b4f47.
21. Hershey B, Valencia CA, Yearwood TL. Pulse width programming in spinal cord stimulation: a clinical study. *Pain Physician*. 2010;13:321-335.
22. Crapanzano JT, Harrison-Bernard LM, Jones MR, Kaye AD, Richter EO, Potash MN. High frequency spinal cord stimulation for complex regional pain syndrome: a case report. *Pain Physician*. 2017;20:e177-e182.
23. Tiede J, Brown L, Gekht G, Vallejo R, Yearwood T, Morgan D. Novel spinal cord stimulation parameters in patients with predominant back pain. *Neuromodulation*. 2013;16(4):370-375. Available at: https://doi.org/10.1111/ner.12032.
24. De Ridder D, Vanneste S, Plazier M, van der Loo E, Menovsky T. Burst spinal cord stimulation: toward paresthesia-free pain suppression. *Neurosurgery*. 2010;66(5):986-990. Available at: https://doi.org/10.1227/01.NEU.0000368153.44883.B3.
25. Chakravarthy K, Fishman MA, Zuidema X, Hunter CW, Levy R. Mechanism of action in burst spinal cord stimulation: review and recent advances. *Pain Med*. 2019;20(suppl 1):S13-S22. Available at: https://doi.org/10.1093/pm/pnz073.
26. Deer T, Slavin KV, Amirdelfan K, et al. Success using neuromodulation with BURST (SUNBURST) study: results from a prospective, randomized controlled trial using a novel burst waveform. *Neuromodulation*. 2018;21(1):56-66. Available at: https://doi.org/10.1111/ner.12698.
27. Anaya CJ, Zander HJ, Graham RD, Sankarasubramanian V, Lempka SF. Evoked potentials recorded from the spinal cord during neurostimulation for pain: a computational modeling study. *Neuromodulation*. 2020;23(1):64-73. Available at: https://doi.org/10.1111/ner.12965.
28. Parker JL, Karantonis DM, Single PS, Obradovic M, Cousins MJ. Compound action potentials recorded in the human spinal cord during neurostimulation for pain relief. *Pain*. 2012;153(3):593-601. Available at: https://doi.org/10.1016/j.pain.2011.11.023.
29. Russo M, Cousins MJ, Brooker C, et al. Effective relief of pain and associated symptoms with closed-loop spinal cord stimulation system: preliminary results of the Avalon Study. *Neuromodulation*. 2018;21(1):38-47. Available at: https://doi.org/10.1111/ner.12684.
30. Mekhail N, Levy RM, Deer TR, et al. Long-term safety and efficacy of closed-loop spinal cord stimulation to treat chronic back and leg pain (Evoke): a double-blind, randomised, controlled trial. *Lancet Neurol*. 2020;19(2):123-134. doi:10.1016/S1474-4422(19)30414-4.
31. Edhi MM, Heijmans L, Vanent KN, et al. Time-dynamic pulse modulation of spinal cord stimulation reduces mechanical hypersensitivity and spontaneous pain in rats. *Sci Rep*. 2020;10:20358. Available at: https://doi.org/10.1038/s41598-020-77212-w.
32. Pope JE, Falowski S, Deer TR. Advanced waveforms and frequency with spinal cord stimulation: burst and high-frequency energy delivery. *Expert Rev Med Devices*. 2015;12(4):431-437. Available at: https://doi.org/10.1586/17434440.2015.1026805.

Chapter 17

Sacral Neuromodulation

Steven Zhou, Lakshmi Akhila Nerusu, Nasir Hussain, and Alaa Abd-Elsayed

Chapter Outline

Introduction

Sacral neuromodulation (SNM) refers to a minimally invasive technique to modulate spinal nerves that innervate the bladder, bowel, sphincter, and pelvic floor muscles to restore micturition and defecation irregularities.[1] The idea of electrical stimulation for the treatment of bladder stimulation was first proposed by Danish surgeon, Dr. M.H. Saxtorph in 1878.[2] Later, Tanagho and Schmidt found that stimulation of ventral sacral nerve roots was effective in initiation of micturition.[3] While SNM was initially approved by the US Food and Drug Administration (FDA) in 1997,[4] its use has gained in popularity secondary to technological advancements, including a reduction in device size and improvement in leads to decrease migration.[5] In recent years, SNM research has transitioned to tackle a challenging diagnosis: chronic pelvic pain. Defined as persistent noncyclic pain in the pelvic area that lasts greater than 6 months, treatment is often difficult and often eludes traditional therapies.[6] In conjunction with SNM, spinal cord stimulation (SCS) and dorsal root ganglion stimulation (DRGS) have also emerged as experimental interventions for this puzzling disease. Due to the emerging challenges of chronic pelvic pain, it remains critical to review the current literature pertaining to its treatment options. In this chapter, we will briefly detail these three commonly used neuromodulation interventions, including their indications, procedural technique, and evidence.

General Indications

The primary indications of SNM continue to be those initially approved by the FDA: urinary urgency, incontinence, and nonobstructive urinary retention.[7] The American Urological Association (AUA) and the

European Association of Urology have also recommended SNM as a treatment option for patients with severe refractory overactive bladder with or without urinary incontinence. Nonobstructive chronic underactive bladder defined as nonpainful bladder with chronic high postvoid residual is another FDA-approved indication for SNM since 1999. Over time, these have evolved to now include patients with fecal incontinence due to idiopathic sphincter degeneration or iatrogenic internal sphincter damage.[4,8] SNM has also been proven to be effective in patients with micturition center abnormalities in neurological diseases, such as Parkinson disease, Alzheimer disease, and fecal incontinence.[9] Although not approved by the FDA, preliminary data suggest that SNM may be beneficial in patients with interstitial cystitis or painful bladder syndrome.[8] Furthermore, a number of case reports have been published regarding the off-label use of SNM for chronic pelvic pain.

Sacral Neuromodulation

MECHANISM OF ACTION

While the exact mechanism of action of SNM is not well understood, several theories have been postulated. As S2 to S4 nerve roots provide autonomic and somatic innervation to the bladder, urethra, and pelvic floor, neuromodulation has been thought to help with dysfunctional bladder and rectal symptoms by stimulation or inhibition.[10] It is hypothesized that SNM inhibits the guarding reflex that lowers the sphincter tone and intravesical pressure, thereby facilitating bladder emptying.[11] This has been primarily thought to be mediated by modulation of afferent nerve endings that mediated spinal activity and brain reflexes. Specifically, the sensory cortical area may be involved, including areas of sensorimotor learning.[12-14]

PATIENT SELECTION

As with all pain procedures, appropriate patient selection remains the key to positive outcomes. Although no factors guarantee success, it is known that certain comorbidities play an important role in the success of therapy, especially in older adults.[15] In a recent systematic review, Jairam et al. found that a successful diagnostic test stimulation was the only reliable predictor of treatment success after SNM implantation.[16] In another study by Amundsen et al., age more than 55 years and the presence of three or more comorbidities were associated with lower likelihood of remission of symptoms following SNM.[17] Comorbid conditions identified as being associated with a lower likelihood of success include hypertension, diabetes mellitus, arthritis, history of back surgery, stroke, and multiple sclerosis.[16] In addition, patients with partial urinary obstruction may be more likely to respond to SNM as compared with those with complete urinary obstruction. Males have also been found to have lower success rates when compared with females owing to the complex voiding dysfunction in males related to prostatic obstruction. Some patient-specific factors should also be considered prior to implantation. Since the ability to use complex therapeutic equipment is crucial prior to implantation of a sacral nerve stimulator, older patients with advanced dementia may not be ideal candidates. Finally, all patients who are being considered for SNM should have a complete history and physical examination, with an emphasis on genitourinary and neurological systems. Additional information, including voiding diaries and urodynamic studies, should be thoroughly evaluated.

Patient selection for the use of SNM (or SCS and DRGS) in the treatment of chronic pelvic pain remains nebulous. At a minimum, as the devices are used off label, patients should have exhausted all available FDA-approved therapies before attempting placement. They must also be carefully counseled regarding the possible benefits and risks, with explicit repeat back regarding the experimental nature of the procedure. Another challenging aspect for patients is that without FDA approval, insurance companies are often hesitant to approve or pay for associated costs, further burdening those most in need.

TECHNIQUE

All techniques for neuromodulation rely on the same general steps: initial temporary stimulation followed by permanent pacemaker implantation.

Test Procedure

The test procedure is performed as a short-term trial of 3 to 7 days to determine whether the patient would benefit from permanent implantation of a neurostimulator device.[18] The test procedure is usually performed

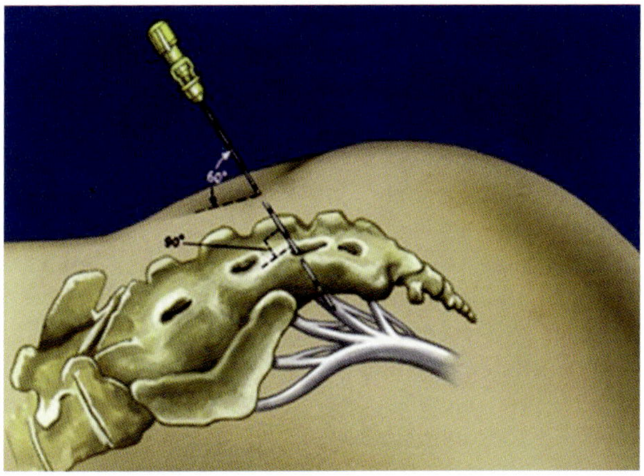

Fig. 17.1 Optimal positioning of needle in S3 foramen. (From Noblett KL, Cadish LA. Sacral nerve stimulation for the treatment of refractory voiding and bowel dysfunction. *Am J Obstet Gynecol.* Feb 2014;210[2]:99–106.)

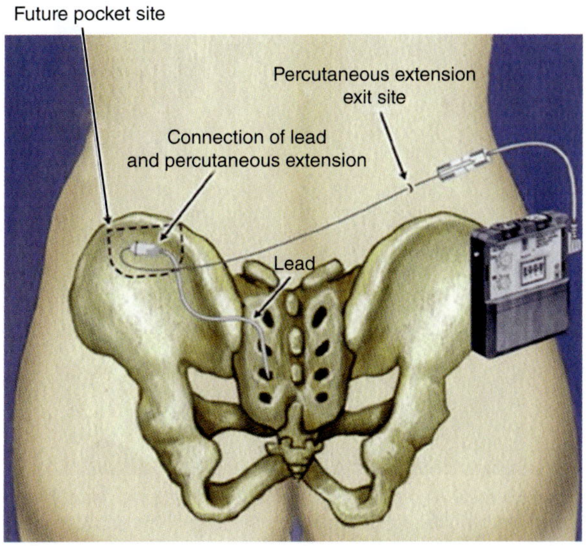

Fig. 17.2 Components of sacral neuromodulation during trial period. (From Noblett KL, Cadish LA. Sacral nerve stimulation for the treatment of refractory voiding and bowel dysfunction. *Am J Obstet Gynecol.* Feb 2014; 210[2]:99–106.)

in the outpatient setting under local anesthesia. After preparing the sacral area with povidone-iodine, appropriate landmarks are identified by palpation and 1% lidocaine is used to achieve local anesthesia. An insulated needle is then passed through the S3 or S4 foramen at a 60-degree angle and motor and sensory nerve root responses are identified (Fig. 17.1). Motor responses include tightening of the levators or plantar flexion of the great toe. Sensory responses include a vibratory response or a pulling sensation in the rectum or vagina. A guidewire is then inserted into the insulated needle, and the needle is subsequently removed. This wire is securely taped and connected to the external neurostimulator (Fig. 17.2). The position is confirmed with sacral radiographs. The patient is discharged home and instructed to maintain the void diary for 3 to 7 days. The stimulator and the wire are removed during follow-up at 3 to 7 days and the voiding diary is repeated. The diaries are compared and patients with a significant improvement in subjective and objective parameters (> 50% change) are considered for permanent device implantation.

Implant Procedure

Patients who have responded to SNM in the test procedure are considered candidates for the implantation of a permanent device, such as InterStim. It is prudent to inform the patients upfront about the benefits and risks of the planned procedure, including battery life, which is known to range from 6 months to 10 years depending on device settings and frequency of use.

Although the type of anesthesia is again on a case-by-case basis, general anesthesia is favored. Broad-spectrum antibiotic prophylaxis is usually preferred prior to initiation of the procedure. For prosthetic devices, the AUA recommends prophylactic coverage of skin flora for procedures such as SNM that do not involve direct entry into the urinary tract. There is also no evidence to support prolonged antibiotic use during the trial period.[19] The patient is placed in the prone position and the sacral area is prepped with multiple layers of povidone-iodine. A midline sacral incision is made and carried down to the level of lumbodorsal fascia, which is at least 1.5 cm from the midline. The paravertebral muscles are separated and the sacral foramen identified by palpation. An insulated needle is then placed into the foramen and motor responses are elicited until the appropriate foramen is identified (Fig. 17.3). A quadripolar lead is placed in the foramen and the collar is sutured to the periosteum to prevent migration of the lead. The lead is tested again to confirm that there is excellent motor response on at least three of the four lead contacts. A

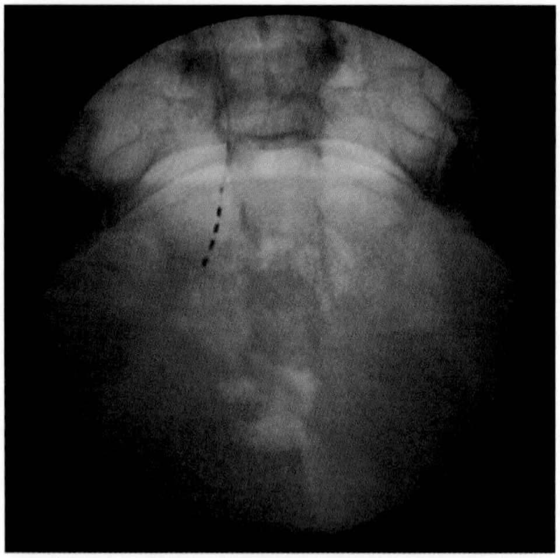

Fig. 17.3 Ideal lead position, anteroposterior view. An ideally positioned lead originates close to the medial edge of the sacral foramen and the lead curves out laterally, with the appearance of the proximal contacts more close together and the distal contacts further apart, due to positioning in space along the nerve. (From Liberman K, Ehlert MJ, Siegel SW. Sacral neuromodulation in urological practice. *Urology.* 2017; 99:14–22.)

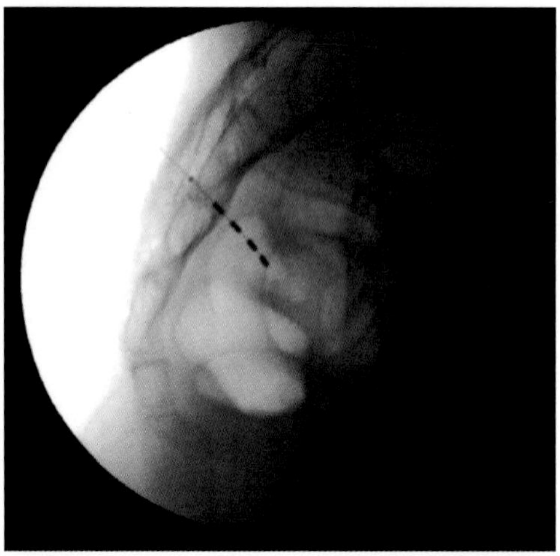

Fig. 17.4 Ideal lead position, lateral view. The lead course parallels the fusion plane of the sacral foramen and exits about 1 cm above the bony protrusion or hillock at the S3 level. (From Liberman K, Ehlert MJ, Siegel SW. Sacral neuromodulation in urological practice. *Urology.* 2017;99:14–22.)

new incision is then made about 3 to 5 cm below the superior posterior iliac crest for the implant generator/battery (Fig. 17.4). A tunnel is created such that the free end of the quadripolar lead is transferred to the buttock incision through a 10-cm-long connecting lead that is ultimately connected with the InterStim neurostimulator device. The incisions are finally closed in layers. Alternatively, the generator/battery can be placed subcutaneously in the anterior abdomen. The device settings can be adjusted through an external programmer.

In patients who have only partially responded to the test stimulation, a variation of the implant procedure—in which the connecting lead is tunneled subcutaneously and brought through the skin—has been dscribed.[20] The lead is then attached to the temporary neurostimulator, which is placed externally on the skin. If the trial is successful, a permanent InterStim device is then implanted as described earlier.

Ideal Lead Position

An ideal lead is positioned in the most superior and medial position within the foramen. It should yield similar motor responses at both the levator and greater toe at a threshold less than or equal to 2 volts with each contact. Ideal lead placement will result in longer battery life, less frequent reprograming, and lower risk of complications.

COMPLICATIONS

Some of the commonly reported complications with SNM include infection, pain at generator site, and lead migration.[18] In the initial years after its introduction, at least one-third of implants required surgical revision, including temporary or permanent device explantation during the first 6 months.[21] However, this risk seems to have been reduced over the years, likely secondary to operator experience. Moreover, many current devices are magnetic resonance imaging (MRI) incompatible.

EVIDENCE FOR USE

Chronic Pelvic Pain

Notoriously difficult to treat, chronic pelvic pain afflicts both males and females, with numerous etiologies. A number of neuromodulation techniques have been evaluated, including SNM, SCS, and DRGS.

Although broad, SNM has been trialed on a number of chronic pelvic pain syndromes, with the strongest evidence for bladder pain syndrome/interstitial cystitis (Table 17.1).[22] In 2017, Wang et al. conducted a systemic review and meta-analysis, finding that SNM may be effective and safe for patients refractory to conventional therapies with minimal adverse events.[22]

TABLE 17.1 Characteristics of Studies Evaluating SMN for Chronic Pelvic Pain

Study	Type	Year	Patient Population (n)	Results
Wang J et al.,[22]	Meta-analysis	2018	Bladder pain syndrome/ interstitial cystitis	• 17 studies with 583 patients • Pooled analyses demonstrated that SNM was associated with great reduction in pelvic pain (weighted mean difference –3.99; 95% confidence interval [CI], –5.22 to –2.76; $P < 0.00001$) • The pooled treatment success rate was 84% (95% CI, 76% to 91%). SNM-related adverse events were minimal
Martellucci J et al.,[23]	Prospective observational	2012	Chronic pelvic pain (17)	• Eight (47%) patients fulfilled the criteria for definitive implantation and were followed for a mean of 39 months • VAS pain levels fell from 8.2 preoperatively to 1.9, 2.1, 2.0 and 1.8 at 6, 12, 24 and 36 months • Age < 60 years and duration of symptoms of < 24 months were good predictors and stapling was a poor predictor of success
Kim J et al.,[24]	Case series	2010	Cauda equina syndrome/ chronic pelvic pain	• Case 1 had pain score reduction from 9/10 to 3 post implantation. At 18-month follow-up, VAS maintained at 4 without medications • Case 2 had pain score reduction from 10/10 to 5 post implantation. At 20-month follow-up, VAS maintained at 5 with intermittent medications
Valovska A et al.,[25]	Case report	2014	Pudendal neuralgia	• VAS 10/10 preoperatively with significant limits in daily function • > 75% pain reduction with trial, pain 2/10 on NRS at subsequent pain management visits with significant decrease in medication use and OMEs

NRS, Numeric rating scale; *OMEs*, oral morphine equivalents; *SNM*, sacral neuromodulation; *VAS,* visual analog scale.

Furthermore, they found not only improvements in pain but also in symptom scoring. In addition, Martellucci et al. found in a case series of 27 patients that SNM proved effective for chronic pelvic pain, with a mean visual analog scale (VAS) score decrease of 8.1 preoperatively to 2.1 at 6 months.[23] Isolated case reports have also been cited for the successful treatment of pudendal neuralgia and cauda equina syndrome (among others). However, the overall evidence is weak and further randomized controlled trials (RCTs) need to be completed.[24,25]

Sacroiliac Joint Dysfunction

Sacroiliac joint (SIJ) dysfunction (or pain) is often difficult to treat, with typical treatments involving a combination of pharmaceuticals, intra-articular injections, or radiofrequency ablation.[26] To date, the use of neuromodulation on this disease has been limited to case reports or small studies. Recently, Guentchev et al. has demonstrated successful long-term treatment of SIJ pain using peripheral nerve field stimulation (PNFS).[27] Evidence for sacral nerve stimulation is even more weak, limited to individual case studies.[28]

Urinary Incontinence

SNM has robust evidence for the treatment of refractory urinary incontinence (Table 17.2). Hassouna et al. evaluated 51 patients across 12 centers worldwide and found that SNM improved number of voids daily (16.9 to 9.3), volume per void (118 to 126 mL) and degree of urgency (2.2 to 1.6) at 6 months.[29] Further, an RCT by Schmidt et al. found that SNM was associated with a significant reduction in daily incontinent episodes, severity of episodes, and absorbent pads used compared with standard therapy.[21] In an RCT by Weil et al., 44 patients with refractory incontinence were

TABLE 17.2 Characteristics of Studies Comparing SNM vs Control Therapy in Urinary Incontinence

Study	Type	Year	Patient Population (n)	Results
Schmidt RA et al.,[21]	RCT	1999	SNM (30) vs Conservative therapy (42)	• Reduction in mean ± SD of incontinent episodes per day with SNM, 9.7 ± 6.3 at baseline compared with 2.6 ± 5.1 at 6 months; while in control group there was an increase, 9.3 ± 4.8 at baseline compared with 11.3 ± 5.9 at 6 months. • Mean ± SD absorbent pads used per day was decreased with SNM at 6 months, 6.2 ± 5 at baseline, compared with 1.1 ± 2 at 6 months, while the usage increased in the control group, 5.0 ± 3.7 at baseline, 6.3 ± 3.6 at 6 months.
Hassouna MM et al.,[29]	Prospective observational	2000	SNM (25) vs Conservative therapy (26)	• Mean ± SD volume (mL) voided per void increased with SNM, 118 ± 74 at baseline, compared with 226 ± 124 at 6 months; while it remained similar in control group, 124 ± 66 at baseline compared with 123 ± 75 at 6 months. • At 6 months, degree of urgency was reduced with SNM, while it remained the same in control group.
Weil EHJ et al.,[30]	RCT	2000	SNM (21) vs conservative therapy (23)	• Mean incontinence episodes/day was also reduced with SNM with 13.5 (95% CI: 10.3 – 16.7) at baseline and 1.4 (95% CI: 0 – 3.2) at 6 months; while there was an increase in control group, 10 (95% CI: 7.5 – 12.5) at baseline and 11.2 (95%CI: 8.9 – 13.5) at 6 months.
Siegel S et al., (InSite)[31]	RCT	2014	SNM (70) vs Conservative therapy (77)	• Therapeutic success rate at 6 months was higher for SNM compared with conservative therapy (61% vs 42%, $p= 0.02$). • Complete continence at 6 months was higher for SNM compared with conservative therapy (39% vs 21%, $p= 0.06$).
Wallace PA et al.,[32]	Case series	2006	Underlying neurological disease ex MS and Parkinsons (33)	• 68% reduction in daily incontinence with a 72% reduction in daily pad use, and nearly a 43% reduction in daily voiding frequency

RCT: Randomized controlled trial; *SNM:* Sacral neuromodulation; *SD:* Standard deviation; *CI:* confidence interval; *mL:* milliliters; *SNM:* sacral neuromodulation; *n:* sample size.

randomized to either conservative treatment (23 patients) or SNM. At 6 months, mean number of incontinence episodes, leakage severity, and mean pad usage was significantly lower with SNM compared with conservative therapy.[30] In the InSite RCT that randomized patients who failed at least one anticholinergic drug, SNM was associated with improved quality of life as measured on the International Consultation on Incontinence Modular Questionnaire–Overactive Bladder Quality of Life (ICIQ-OABqol) instrument compared with standard therapy.[31] In a study by Wallace et al., patients with underlying neurological disease, such as multiple sclerosis and Parkinson disease, had a 68% reduction in daily incontinence with a 72% reduction in daily pad use and nearly a 43% reduction in daily voiding frequency with SNM.[32]

Fecal Incontinence

In contrast to urinary incontinence, there is a lack of high-quality evidence on the efficacy of SNM for the treatment of fecal incontinence (Table 17.3). A systematic review of all available case series by the National Institute for Clinical Excellence (NICE) concluded that SNM significantly improved fecal

TABLE 17.3 Characteristics of Studies Evaluating SNM for Fecal Incontinence

Study	Type	Year	Patient Population (n)	Results
Fraser C et al.,[33]	Meta-analysis	2003	Urinary incontinence (266)	• 41-75% of patients achieved complete fecal continence and 75-100% experienced an improvement of 50% or more in the number of fecal incontinence episodes • All studies reported a decrease in the number of episodes of incontinence per week, with statistical significance achieved in four studies • Five studies employing the American Society of Colon and Rectal Surgery (ASCRS) fecal incontinence quality of life instrument reported improvements in all categories
Melenhorst J et al.,[34]	Prospective observational	2007	Fecal incontinence (100)	• The mean number of incontinence episodes decreased significantly during the test stimulation (baseline, 31.3; test, 4.4; $P < 0.0001$) and at follow-up (36 months postoperatively, 4.8; $P < 0.0001$) • The squeeze pressures were significantly higher at 6 months (109.8 mmHg; $P = 0.03$), 12 months (114.1 mmHg; $P = 0.02$) and 24 months postoperatively (113.5 mmHg; $P = 0.007$).

TABLE 17.4 Characteristics of Studies Comparing SNM vs Control Therapy in Urinary Retention

Study	Type	Year	Patient Population (n)	Results
Jonas U et al.,[35]	RCT	2001	SNM (29) vs Control (22)	• Catheterization volume per catheterization (mL) at 6 months was lower with SNM (median: 49; IQR: 0-155) compared with control group (median: 319; IQR: 124-514) • Total catheter volume per day (mL) at 6 months was lower with SNM (median: 237; IQR: 0-801) compared with control group (median: 1305; IQR: 415-2195) • Total volume voided per day (mL) at 6 months was lower with SNM (median: 1808; IQR: 929-2687) compared with control group (median: 488; IQR: 0-1218)
Dasgupta R et al.,[36]	Case series	2004	SNM (26)	• Spontaneous voiding in 20 patients (77%) at 6 months with SNM use
Gross C et al.,[37]	Meta-analysis	2010	SNM vs Conservative therapy	• Median difference in PVR decrease was 236 mL (IQR: 219-253) with SMN in comparison to conservative therapy ($p < 0.00001$). • Median difference in voided volume increase was 299 mL (IQR: 280-318) with SMN in comparison to conservative therapy ($p < 0.00001$)

SNM: Sacral neuromodulation; *IQR:* Interquartile range; *PVR:* Post void residual; mL: milliliters; *IQR:* interquartile range; *n:* sample size

incontinence among patients who were refractory to medical or conservative treatment.[33] Melenhorst et al. found that patients with bowel incontinence with an SNM device had a reduction in mean number of incontinent episodes from 31.3 to 4.8.[34]

Urinary Retention

There is only one RCT that evaluated the role of SNM in urinary retention (Table 17.4). Jonas et al. initially recruited 177 patients with urinary retention who underwent SNM test stimulation.[35] Among them, only 68 patients had procedural success and were randomized to receive SNM (37 patients) or conservative therapy (31 patients). However, 17 patients were missing at the time of final reporting. SNM was found to significantly reduce the number of catheterizations as well as catheter volume from 613 mL to 72 mL. In a retrospective study by Dasgupta et al., among 26 women who underwent SNM, 20 patients (77%) were able to void spontaneously during a median follow-up of 37 months.[36] Finally, in a meta-analysis by Gross et al., including one RCT and 13 observational studies, SNM was found to decrease postvoid residual volume by 236 mL and increase voiding volume by 299 mL.[37]

Constipation

Although not currently approved in the United States, SNM is being used internationally for refractory constipation (Table 17.5). The European SNM Bowel Study Group currently recommends SNM for patients who have refractory symptoms for more than a year after failed conservative therapy in the absence of mechanically correctable etiology.[1] Ganio et al. revealed that SNM increased squeeze pressure and reduced the volume needed for urge sensation.[38] Further, in the largest multicenter prospective study evaluating the utility of SNM for fecal constipation, Kamm et al. found that SNM was associated with an increase in bowel frequency from 3.5 to 7.1 episodes per week.[39] Additionally, there was a decrease in straining, incomplete evacuation, and abdominal pain with SNM.[39]

Spinal Cord Stimulation

MECHANISM OF ACTION

The exact mechanism of action is largely unknown, but is believed to be based on Melzack and Wall's gate control theory of pain.[40] It is postulated that stimulation of non-nociceptive fibers of peripheral nerves can inhibit the activity of small nociceptive projections in the dorsal horn of the spinal cord. This activity can also activate GABA and adenosine receptors that lead to pain activity, another proposed mechanism.

INDICATIONS

Traditionally, SCS has enjoyed success in treating a variety of chronic pain syndromes. Overall, the strongest evidence for SCS remains for complex regional pain syndrome (CRPS), failed back surgery syndrome (FBSS), and ischemic lower extremity pain.[41] Experimentally, there is growing support for a number of off-label uses, including refractory angina pectoris and peripheral ischemic limb pain, among others.[40] However, owing to the complexity in anatomy and contributing innervations from both the lumbar and sacral regions, evidence for chronic pelvic pain remains relatively weak.[42]

TECHNIQUE

Spinal cord stimulator implantation technique is similar to that for SNM stimulator placement, as discussed previously. Placement can be completed under local anesthesia, spinal, or even general anesthesia if needed. A small cut is made on the patient's back to

TABLE 17.5 Characteristics of Studies Evaluating SMN for Constipation

Study	Type	Year	Patient Population (n)	Results
Giano E et al.,[38]	Prospective observational	2001	SNM (40)	• At 9.9 days, there was an increase in maximum rest pressure (39.4 +/- 7.3 vs. 54.3 +/- 8.5 mmHg; $P = 0.014$), maximum squeeze pressure (84.7 +/- 8.8 vs. 99.5 +/- 1.1 mmHg; $P = 0.047$) and urge sensation (123.8 +/- 0.6 vs. 78.3 +/- 8.9 ml; $P = 0.05$)
Kamm M et al.,[39]	Prospective observational	2010	SNM (62)	• At 28 month follow up, defecation frequency/week increased from 2.3 to 6.6 ($p < 0.001$), straining frequency decreased from 75% to 46% ($p < 0.001$), sensation of incomplete evacuations decreased from 71.5% to 46% ($p < 0.001$)

SNM: Sacral neuromodulation.

insert the epidural needle and leads.[43] Placement is usually in the T12 to L1 region near, but can be advanced closer to the desired area of pain control. After careful insertion with fluoroscopy, the leads are anchored and a tunnel track created for the generator.

COMPLICATIONS

Overall, complications are similar to those of SNM, mostly leading to infection or lead migration. These are more commonly seen with permanent implants, with limited risk for SCS trials.[40] More serious risks—such as epidural hematoma, dural puncture, and nerve or spinal cord injury—may be possible but the incidence is low.

EVIDENCE FOR USE

Chronic Pelvic Pain

In 2015, Buffenoir et al. evaluated 27 patients for permanent implantation of a conus medullaris spinal cord stimulator in patients with refractory pudendal neuralgia (Table 17.6).[44] Out of the 27 patients, 20 were deemed responders (> 50% reduction in pain or > 50% increase in sitting time), with a 55% estimated improvement with long-term evaluation. In addition, Kapural et al. placed SCS in six female patients with long-standing pelvic pain after trials of both hypogastric and neurolytic hypogastric blocks.[45] Overall, patients reported a mean VAS score decrease from 8 to 3, alongside significant decreases in pain disability index (57 to 19.5) and opiate use (average of 22.5 to 6.6 mg morphine equivalents per day). Abd-Elsayed et al. and Romero-Serano et al. also published case reports showing > 80% pain improvement after SCS placement for previously intractable pain.[46,47]

Dorsal Root Ganglion Stimulation

MECHANISM OF ACTION

The dorsal root ganglion (DRG) is located bilaterally from the spinal cord and houses the cell bodies of sensory neurons. As such, it is often implicated in the development of chronic pain.[48] Research done first by Koopmeiners et al. helped establish the idea that low-frequency stimulation can increase calcium in the DRG neurons, thus decreasing action potential frequency and conduction velocity.[48,49] Other hypothesized mechanisms of action include reduced cytokine release, downregulation of ion channels, and decreased DRG hyperexcitability.[48,50]

TABLE 17.6 Characteristics of Studies Evaluating SCS for Chronic Pelvic Pain

Study	Type	Year	Patient Population (n)	Results
Buffenoir K et al.,[44]	Prospective observational	2015	Refractory pudendal neuralgia (27)	• Twenty of the 27 patients were considered to be responders to spinal cord stimulation and 100% of implanted patients remained long-term responders (mean tripling of sitting time, and mean estimated percent improvement (EPI) of 55.5%)
Kapural L et al.,[45]	Case series	2006	Chronic visceral pelvic pain (6)	• Median visual analog scale pain score decreased from 8 to 3 • All patients had more than 50% of the pain relief. Pain Disability Index changed from an average of 57.7 +/- 12 to 19.5 +/- 7 • Opiate use decreased from an average 22.5 mg to 6.6 mg of morphine sulfate milligram equivalents per day
Abd-Elsayed A.et al.,[46]	Case report	2017	Chronic pelvic pain (1)	• >80% improvement in trial week with continued relief at 1-year follow-up
Romer-Serrano E et al.,[47]	Case report	2021	Chronic pelvic pain (1)	• 80% pain reduction at 2 weeks with cessation of opioids • Improvement in EuroQOL-5D and VAS

VAS, visual analog scale.

INDICATIONS

Dorsal root ganglion stimulation (DRGS) has been used to treat chronic pain, and recently has been approved by the FDA for the treatment of lower extremity CRPS. Contrary to SCS, DRGS can theoretically deliver targeted stimulation to focal areas and does not rely on paresthesias, making it an emerging area of research for chronic pelvic pain.[51] In addition, as the CSF layer surrounding the DRG is lower in volume than the spinal cord, lower stimulation amplitudes can be used with less postural variation.[48]

TECHNIQUE

The technique for DRGS implantation is very similar to that of SCS, except that the dorsal root ganglion is stimulated instead of the spinal cord. As such, the leads are directed under fluoroscopy via a percutaneous incision through the epidural space, exiting through the foramen, and to rest near the target DRG (Fig. 17.5).[52] A generator is then placed and a tunnel created. Recent techniques describe placement near the L1 to S1 or S2 DRG for treatment of chronic pelvic pain.[51,53]

COMPLICATIONS

Complications for DRGS are similar to that of SNM and SCS. As it is a newer technique, data are limited. Thus, more research is needed to further ascertain complication rates.

EVIDENCE FOR USE

Chronic Pelvic Pain

Hunter and Yang reported 7 patients successfully treated with DRGS who failed a variety of pharmaceutical and interventional therapies (Table 17.7).[51] All patients in the case series reported significant pain relief as well as reduction in opioid consumption. Of the 7 patients, 4 were implanted and continued to experience pain relief with high satisfaction and functional improvement at long-term follow-up. Patel reported a case series of 15 patients with permanent implantation of DRG stimulation leads, with significant improvement in disability and a 70% to 90% pain score decrease at 3-month follow-up.[53] At long-term follow-up, 13 of 15 patients were even able to stop taking opioids.

Future Directions

SNM remains an exciting avenue for future research. Strong evidence currently exists for the use of SNM for a variety of urogenital conditions, including urinary/fecal incontinence, urinary retention, and constipation.

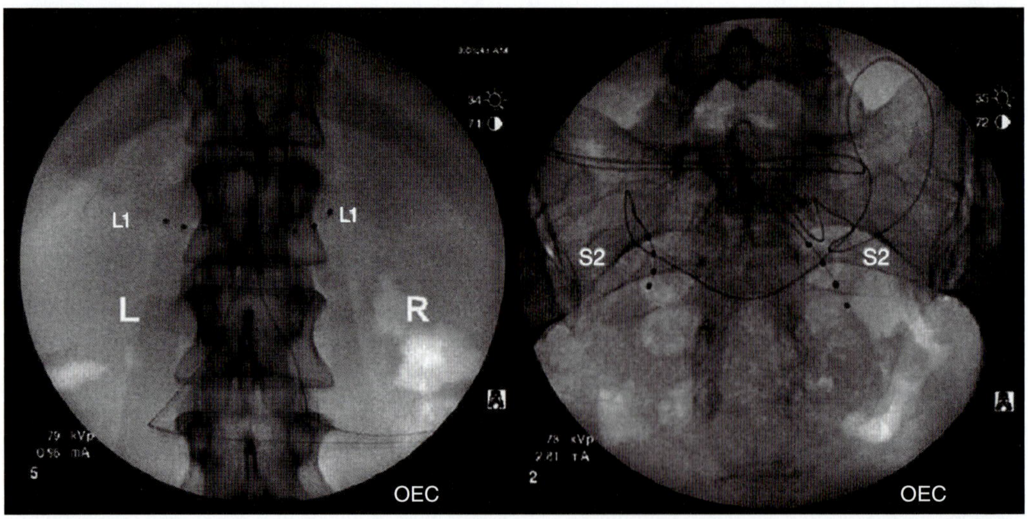

Fig. 17.5 Dorsal root ganglion stimulation (DRGS) lead placement. Left: bilateral L1 DRGS lead placement. Right: bilateral S2 DRGS lead placement. (From Hunter CW, Yang A. Dorsal root ganglion stimulation for chronic pelvic pain: a case series and technical report on a novel lead configuration. *Neuromodulation.* 2019;22[1]:87–95.)

TABLE 17.7 Characteristics of Studies Evaluating DRGS for Chronic Pelvic Pain

Study	Type	Year	Patient Population (n)	Results
Hunter CW et al.,[51]	Case series	2019	Chronic pelvic pain (7)	• All seven patients experienced significant pain relief as well as reduction in opioid consumption and some cases improvement with sexual function and urination • Four of these patients have been implanted and continue to self-report sustained pain relief with high-satisfaction and functional improvement • To date no explants or instances of loss of efficacy have occurred (>1 year since implant)
Patel KV[53]	Case series	2019	Chronic pelvic pain (15)	• At 3 months post implant, all 15 patients reported an improvement from crippled to minimal disability and a 70-90% decrease in NRS • All patients reported improving symptoms and less interference of pain with activities of daily living. • Long term follow-up showed ODI and NRS remained consistent or displayed further improvement • 13 out of 15 patients, were able to stop taking opioid medication following the initiation of DRG therapy

DRGS, Dorsal root ganglion stimulation; *NRS,* Numeric Rating Scale; *ODI,* Oswestry Disability Index.

However, the field of neuromodulation is still relatively new, with boundless opportunities for future growth. Even now, research continues regarding its expanded use in patients with chronic pelvic pain, a costly and debilitating condition with no clearly established efficacious treatments. Looking to the future, much work remains to increase adoption of this exciting field.

Conclusions

In a relatively short period of time, SNM has evolved from an experimental technique to an essential tool providing symptomatic relief in patients with refractory bowel and bladder dysfunction. With the proven successes in the field, SNM, along with SCS and DRGS, are increasingly being studied as potential therapies for chronic pelvic pain. While current evidence remains limited in the form of mostly case reports, cautious optimism remains in their ability to deliver efficacious yet safe neuromodulatory care. Although still in its early stages, future research should focus on exploring mechanisms of action and facilitating its rapid uptake in clinical practice.

REFERENCES

1. Maeda Y, O'Connell PR, Lehur PA, Matzel KE, Laurberg S, European SNS Bowel Study Group. Sacral nerve stimulation for faecal incontinence and constipation: a European consensus statement. *Colorectal Dis*. 2015;17(4):O74-O87. doi:10.1111/codi.12905.
2. Saxtorph MH. *Strictura urethrae—Fistula perinei—Retentio urinae*. Copenhagen: Clinisk Chirurgi, Gyldendalske Forlag; 1878: 265-280.
3. Tanagho EA, Schmidt RA. Bladder pacemaker: scientific basis and clinical future. *Urology*. 1982;20(6):614-619. doi:10.1016/0090-4295(82)90312-0.
4. Felony MP, Strauss K, Leslie SW. *Sacral Neuromodulation*. Treasure Island, FL: StatPearls; 2022. doi:NBK567751.
5. De Wachter S, Knowles CH, Elterman DS, et al. New technologies and applications in sacral neuromodulation: an update. *Adv Ther*. 2020;37(2):637-643. doi:10.1007/s12325-019-01205-z.
6. Speer LM, Mushkbar S, Erbele T. Chronic pelvic pain in women. *Am Fam Physician*. 2016;93(5):380-387.
7. Steele SS. Sacral nerve stimulation: 50 years in the making. *Can Urol Assoc J*. 2012;6(4):231-232. doi:10.5489/cuaj.12194.
8. Noblett KL, Cadish LA. Sacral nerve stimulation for the treatment of refractory voiding and bowel dysfunction. *Am J Obstet Gynecol*. 2014;210(2):99-106. doi:10.1016/j.ajog.2013.07.025.
9. Bosch JL, Groen J. Sacral nerve neuromodulation in the treatment of patients with refractory motor urge incontinence: long-term results of a prospective longitudinal study. *J Urol*. 2000; 163(4):1219-1222.
10. De Wachter S, Vaganee D, Kessler TM. Sacral neuromodulation: mechanism of action. *Eur Urol Focus*. 2020;6(5):823-825. doi:10.1016/j.euf.2019.11.018.

11. Lavelle JP, Teahan S, Kim DY, Chancellor MB. Medical and minimally invasive treatment of urinary incontinence. *Rev Urol*. 1999;1(2):111-119.
12. Wenzler DL, Burks FN, Cooney M, Peters KM. Proof of concept trial on changes in current perception threshold after sacral neuromodulation. *Neuromodulation*. 2015;18(3):228-231; discussion 232. doi:10.1111/ner.12213.
13. Blok BF, Groen J, Bosch JL, Veltman DJ, Lammertsma AA. Different brain effects during chronic and acute sacral neuromodulation in urge incontinent patients with implanted neurostimulators. *BJU Int*. 2006;98(6):1238-1243. doi:10.1111/j.1464-410X.2006.06521.x.
14. Braun PM, Baezner H, Seif C, et al. Alterations of cortical electrical activity in patients with sacral neuromodulator. *Eur Urol*. 2002;41(5):562-566; discussion 566-567. doi:10.1016/s0302-2838(02)00029-5.
15. Secretariat MA. Sacral nerve stimulation for urinary urge incontinence, urgency-frequency, urinary retention, and fecal incontinence: an evidence-based analysis. *Ont Health Technol Assess Ser*. 2005;5(3):1-64.
16. Jairam R, Drossaerts J, Marcelissen T, van Koeveringe G, Vrijens D, van Kerrebroeck P. Predictive factors in sacral neuromodulation: a systematic review. *Urol Int*. 2022;106(4):323-343. doi:10.1159/000513937.
17. Amundsen CL, Webster GD. Sacral neuromodulation in an older, urge-incontinent population. *Am J Obstet Gynecol*. 2002;187(6):1462-1465; discussion 1465. doi:10.1067/mob.2002.130004.
18. Das AK, White MD, Longhurst PA. Sacral nerve stimulation for the management of voiding dysfunction. *Rev Urol*. Winter 2000;2(1):43-60.
19. Lightner DJ, Wymer K, Sanchez J, Kavoussi L. Best Practice Statement on Urologic Procedures and Antimicrobial Prophylaxis. *J Urol*. 2020 Feb;203(2):351-356. doi: 10.1097/JU.0000000000000509.]
20. Janknegt RA, Weil EH, Eerdmans PH. Improving neuromodulation technique for refractory voiding dysfunctions: two-stage implant. *Urology*. 1997;49(3):358-362. doi:10.1016/S0090-4295(96)00506-7.
21. Schmidt RA, Jonas U, Oleson KA, et al. Sacral nerve stimulation for treatment of refractory urinary urge incontinence. Sacral Nerve Stimulation Study Group. *J Urol*. 1999;162(2):352-357.
22. Wang J, Chen Y, Chen J, Zhang G, Wu P. Sacral neuromodulation for refractory bladder pain syndrome/interstitial cystitis: a global systematic review and meta-analysis. *Sci Rep*. 2017;7(1):11031. doi:10.1038/s41598-017-11062-x.
23. Martellucci J, Naldini G, Carriero A. Sacral nerve modulation in the treatment of chronic pelvic pain. *Int J Colorectal Dis*. 2012;27(7):921-926. doi:10.1007/s00384-011-1394-2.
24. Kim JH, Hong JC, Kim MS, Kim SH. Sacral nerve stimulation for treatment of intractable pain associated with cauda equina syndrome. *J Korean Neurosurg Soc*. 2010;47(6):473-476. doi:10.3340/jkns.2010.47.6.473.
25. Valovska A, Peccora CD, Philip CN, Kaye AD, Urman RD. Sacral neuromodulation as a treatment for pudendal neuralgia. *Pain Physician*. 2014;17(5):E645-E650.
26. Chakrabortty S, Kumar S, Gupta D, Rudraraju S. Intractable sacroiliac joint pain treated with peripheral nerve field stimulation. *J Anaesthesiol Clin Pharmacol*. 2016;32(3):392-394. doi:10.4103/0970-9185.173336.
27. Guentchev M, Preuss C, Rink R, Peter L, Sailer MHM, Tuettenberg J. Long-term reduction of sacroiliac joint pain with peripheral nerve stimulation. *Oper Neurosurg*. 2017;13(5):634-639. doi:10.1093/ons/opx017.
28. Kim YH, Moon DE. Sacral nerve stimulation for the treatment of sacroiliac joint dysfunction: a case report. *Neuromodulation*. 2010;13(4):306-310. doi:10.1111/j.1525-1403.2009.00270.x.
29. Hassouna MM, Siegel SW, Nÿeholt AA, et al. Sacral neuromodulation in the treatment of urgency-frequency symptoms: a multicenter study on efficacy and safety. *J Urol*. 2000;163(6):1849-1854.
30. Weil EH, Ruiz-Cerdá JL, Eerdmans PH, Janknegt RA, Bemelmans BL, van Kerrebroeck PE. Sacral root neuromodulation in the treatment of refractory urinary urge incontinence: a prospective randomized clinical trial. *Eur Urol*. 2000;37(2):161-171. doi:10.1159/000020134.
31. Siegel S, Noblett K, Mangel J, et al. Results of a prospective, randomized, multicenter study evaluating sacral neuromodulation with InterStim therapy compared to standard medical therapy at 6-months in subjects with mild symptoms of overactive bladder. *Neurourol Urodyn*. 2015;34(3):224-230. doi:10.1002/nau.22544.
32. Wallace PA, Lane FL, Noblett KL. Sacral nerve neuromodulation in patients with underlying neurologic disease. *Am J Obstet Gynecol*. 2007;197(1):96.e1-e5. doi:10.1016/j.ajog.2007.04.016.
33. Fraser CGC, Grant G, Mowatt G. *Systematic Review of the Efficacy and Safety of Sacral Nerve Stimulation for Faecal Incontinence*. Available at: https://www.nice.org.uk/guidance/ipg99/evidence/systematic-review-of-the-efficacy-and-safety-of-sacral-nerve-stimulation-for-faecal-incontinence-pdf-302617261. Accessed July 2, 2022.
34. Melenhorst J, Koch SM, Uludag O, van Gemert WG, Baeten CG. Sacral neuromodulation in patients with faecal incontinence: results of the first 100 permanent implantations. *Colorectal Dis*. 2007;9(8):725-730. doi:10.1111/j.1463-1318.2007.01241.x.
35. Jonas U, Fowler CJ, Chancellor MB, et al. Efficacy of sacral nerve stimulation for urinary retention: results 18 months after implantation. *J Urol*. 2001;165(1):15-19. doi:10.1097/00005392-200101000-00004.
36. Dasgupta R, Wiseman OJ, Kitchen N, Fowler CJ. Long-term results of sacral neuromodulation for women with urinary retention. *BJU Int*. 2004;94(3):335-337. doi:10.1111/j.1464-410X.2004.04979.x.
37. Gross C, Habli M, Lindsell C, South M. Sacral neuromodulation for nonobstructive urinary retention: a meta-analysis. *Female Pelvic Med Reconstr Surg*. 2010;16(4):249-253. doi:10.1097/SPV.0b013e3181df9b3f.
38. Ganio E, Masin A, Ratto C, et al. Short-term sacral nerve stimulation for functional anorectal and urinary disturbances: results in 40 patients: evaluation of a new option for anorectal functional disorders. *Dis Colon Rectum*. 2001;44(9):1261-1267. doi:10.1007/BF02234782.
39. Kamm MA, Dudding TC, Melenhorst J, et al. Sacral nerve stimulation for intractable constipation. *Gut*. 2010;59(3):333-340. doi:10.1136/gut.2009.187989.
40. Jeon YH. Spinal cord stimulation in pain management: a review. *Korean J Pain*. 2012;25(3):143-150. doi:10.3344/kjp.2012.25.3.143.
41. Christelis N, Simpson B, Russo M, et al. Persistent spinal pain syndrome: a proposal for failed back surgery syndrome and ICD-11. *Pain Med*. 2021;22(4):807-818. doi:10.1093/pm/pnab015.
42. Hunter CW, Stovall B, Chen G, Carlson J, Levy R. Anatomy, pathophysiology and interventional therapies for chronic pelvic pain: a review. *Pain Physician*. 2018;21(2):147-167.

43. Dydyk AM, Tadi P. *Spinal Cord Stimulator Implant*. Treasure Island (FL): StatPearls Publishing; 2021 Sep 29. Available at: https://www.ncbi.nlm.nih.gov/books/NBK555994/.
44. Buffenoir K, Rioult B, Hamel O, Labat JJ, Riant T, Robert R. Spinal cord stimulation of the conus medullaris for refractory pudendal neuralgia: a prospective study of 27 consecutive cases. *Neurourol Urodyn*. 2015;34(2):177-182. doi:10.1002/nau.22525.
45. Kapural L, Narouze SN, Janicki TI, Mekhail N. Spinal cord stimulation is an effective treatment for the chronic intractable visceral pelvic pain. *Pain Med*. 2006;7(5):440-443. doi:10.1111/j.1526-4637.2006.00165.x.
46. Abd-Elsayed A, Lee S, King C. Retrograde placement of spinal cord stimulator leads for treating resistant pelvic pain. *Saudi J Anaesth*. 2017;11(3):366-367. doi:10.4103/sja.SJA_129_17.
47. Romero-Serrano E, Esparza-Miñana JM. Spinal cord stimulation in the approach to chronic pelvic pain: a case report and literature review. *Medicine (Baltimore)*. 2021;100(52):e28379. doi:10.1097/md.0000000000028379.
48. Huygen F, Kallewaard JW, Nijhuis H, et al. Effectiveness and safety of dorsal root ganglion stimulation for the treatment of chronic pain: a pooled analysis. *Neuromodulation*. 2020;23(2):213-221. doi:10.1111/ner.13074.
49. Koopmeiners AS, Mueller S, Kramer J, Hogan QH. Effect of electrical field stimulation on dorsal root ganglion neuronal function. *Neuromodulation*. 2013;16(4):304-311; discussion 310-311. doi:10.1111/ner.12028.
50. Krames ES. The dorsal root ganglion in chronic pain and as a target for neuromodulation: a review. *Neuromodulation*. 2015;18(1):24-32; discussion 32. doi:10.1111/ner.12247.
51. Hunter CW, Yang A. Dorsal root ganglion stimulation for chronic pelvic pain: a case series and technical report on a novel lead configuration. *Neuromodulation*. 2019;22(1):87-95. Available at: https://doi.org/10.1111/ner.12801.
52. Deer TR, Levy RM, Kramer J, et al. Dorsal root ganglion stimulation yielded higher treatment success rate for complex regional pain syndrome and causalgia at 3 and 12 months: a randomized comparative trial. *Pain*. 2017;158(4):669-681. doi:10.1097/j.pain.0000000000000814.
53. Patel KV. Dorsal Root Ganglion stimulation for chronic pelvic pain [39T]. *Obstet Gynecol*. 2019;133:223S. doi:10.1097/01.AOG.0000559141.59342.5f.

Chapter 18

Spinal Cord Stimulation: Controversial Topics

R. Scott Stayner and David M. Schultz

Chapter Outline

Introduction

Spinal cord stimulation (SCS) was first used to treat a human patient by Dr. Norman Shealy at Gunderson Lutheran Hospital in 1967. The patient had metastatic cancer and a prognosis of 1 to 2 months' life expectancy, with pain in the chest, abdomen, and legs. By today's standards, the device was crude. It required laminectomy for placement and was sutured to the dura and subcutaneous jacks for the external plug-in to power the electrode and modulate the stimulation delivered to the dorsal columns. However, the patient reported near complete pain relief when the device was turned on and the pain relief was maintained by changing pulse frequency.[1] Unfortunately, the patient died 2 days after implantation due to a thromboembolic event precipitated by undiagnosed endocarditis. This complication was not attributed to the implant. The widespread use of SCS and its variants, such as dorsal root ganglion stimulation (DRGS), to treat chronic intractable pain has led to efforts to reduce the risk of complications. The recommendations outlined are taken from published guidelines, when available, as well as practical experience when no published research or guidelines are available.

Obesity

Obesity is usually defined as a body mass index (BMI) of 30 to 39.9 kg/m^2 and morbidly obese as greater than 40 kg/m^2.[2] Obesity is associated with inherent risk for surgical procedures. For elective spine procedures, morbidly obese patients are at significantly higher risk for increased operative time, higher blood loss, increased postsurgical medical complications, increased risk for surgical site infection (SSI) and poorer surgical outcomes.[3] However, one retrospective study of orthopedic spine surgeries found that obese patients had an odds ratio of 3.5 for SSI though morbidly obese patients had an odds ratio of 2.6.[4] Two studies that examined risk factors for SCS infection rates concluded that there was no significant increase in infection rates for obese patients compared with nonobese patients.[5,6] The difference in infection risk for SCS implantation versus spinal surgery may be attributed to the relatively minimal invasive ness of this procedure compared with open spine surgery. Additionally, though the number of obese SCS patients has increased, health care utilization as measured by total hospital cost is not significantly different than with patients who are not obese.[7] However, another study reviewed the efficacy of SCS for obese patients and found a negative correlation between increasing BMI and spinal cord stimulator efficacy measured by reduction in the visual analog scale (VAS) score.[2]

RECOMMENDATIONS FOR OBESE PATIENTS

1. Advise patients that increased weight adds risk to any surgery, especially from an anesthetic perspective.
2. Consider hospital setting for morbidly obese SCS implantation due to potential airway issues with anesthesia.
3. Utilize weight-based dosing of antibiotics.[5]
4. Consider post-surgery antibiotic for 7 to 10 days after surgery.[5]

Diabetes

SCS is considered a definitive treatment for diabetic peripheral neuropathy.[8-10] However, diabetes has been associated with postoperative complications, especially an increase in SSIs. In a retrospective study of patients undergoing spine surgery, the odds ratio of developing an SSI was 8.4 for patients with a diagnosis of diabetes compared with patients without diabetes.[4] A study in 2010 found SSI after SCS implantation in 9% of diabetic patients compared with 4% of the patients without diabetes.[11] However, two more recent studies showed no increased risk of SSI after SCS implantation for diabetic patients.[5,6] The researchers did not track preoperative attempts at glycemic control, but it was assumed that the diabetic patients in the studies had well-controlled blood glucose prior to surgery and in the postoperative period.

RECOMMENDATIONS FOR DIABETIC PATIENTS

1. Good glycemic control perioperatively.
2. Check for and treat any open sores or ulcers.
3. Consider postoperative antibiotics for 7 to 10 days postsurgery.

Intraoperative Dural Puncture

Dural puncture can occur during percutaneous placement of spinal cord stimulator leads. Potential sequelae of dural puncture include postdural puncture headache (PDPH), neck pain, photophobia, cerebrospinal fluid collection in the midline pocket site, and, potentially, intracranial hemorrhage and neurological injury.[12,13] The incidence of dural puncture with SCS and subsequent PDPH is estimated to be between 0.2% to 3%.[12,14,15] Factors that are thought to increase risk of dural puncture with percutaneous spinal cord stimulator lead placement include spinal deformities, obesity, previous surgery at needle entry site, and spinal stenosis at the needle entry site.[12,16,17] Although the risk of serious neurological injury is extremely low, development of a PDPH can interfere with interpretation of relief of chronic pain during the SCS trial and add to postsurgical pain after an implant.

The risk of dural puncture during epidural access for SCS lead placement can be reduced by optimal patient positioning to reduce the lordosis in the spine at the epidural access site. If possible, avoid stenotic levels and previous surgical sites for epidural access. We also find that bending the 14-gauge introducer needle can be very helpful in navigating the needle around osteophytes that may interfere with the needle path. It is necessary to lubricate the stylette prior to bending the needle or the stylette will be difficult to remove (Fig. 18.1).

Another technique to reduce the risk of inadvertent dural puncture is to use the contralateral oblique fluoroscopic view to visualize the needle tip as it enters the epidural space. We have found this technique

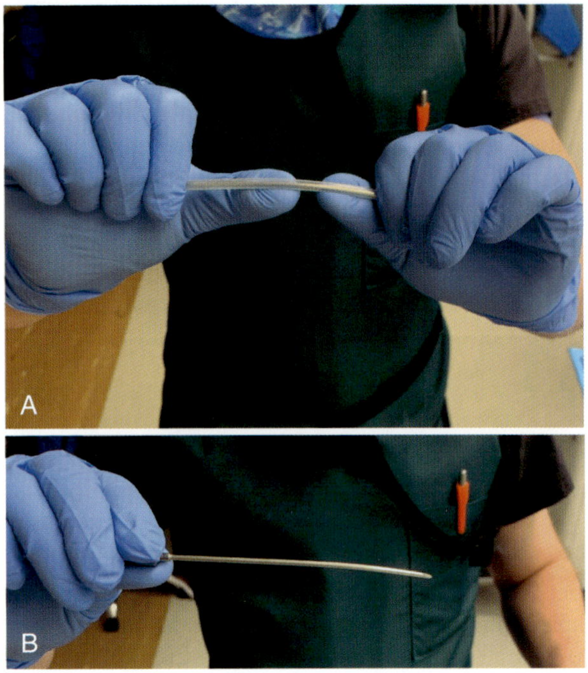

Fig. 18.1 Demonstration of bending the Tuohy introducer needle to enable easier navigation of osteophytes and other anatomic barriers when accessing the epidural space for spinal cord stimulator lead placement.

especially useful if loss of resistance has been achieved but advancement of the SCS lead into the epidural space is blocked by the superior lamina. In such cases, switching the fluoroscope to the contralateral oblique view (45–50 degrees) to visualize the introducer needle tip is helpful. In this view, rotating the bevel caudal and then advancing the needle a few millimeters will often allow the needle to advance slightly further into the epidural space beyond any osteophytes on the lamina without dural puncture. The SCS lead will then advance easily into the epidural space.

If an inadvertent dural puncture does occur, there is no consensus regarding next steps. A conservative strategy is to abort the procedure and try it again on a different day. However, this can be very unsatisfactory for patients who are anticipating pain relief from the SCS lead placement and have often made special arrangements to have the procedure. In such rare cases, we attempt to access the epidural space at a more cephalad level and then place the SCS lead. It is prudent to check the stimulator lead contact impedances before anchoring the lead to help confirm that the lead is indeed in the epidural space.

As some patients, especially older ones, do not develop PDPH after a dural puncture, we do not routinely perform a prophylactic blood patch at the time of lead placement. We recommend keeping the patient flat in the recovery room for 30 minutes and infusing 500 to 1000 mL of intravenous (IV) fluids prior to discharge. It is best to advise the patient of the possibility of developing a positional headache. If that does occur, we recommend that the patient return to have a blood patch performed under aseptic conditions and leave the device intact. If postoperative antibiotics were not prescribed, it would be prudent to prescribe antibiotics as a precaution.

RECOMMENDATIONS FOR MANAGEMENT OF DURAL PUNCTURE

1. Avoid attempts to access the epidural space at levels previously treated with spine surgery and/or significant spinal stenosis.
2. If dural puncture occurs, immediately retract the needle until cerebrospinal fluid flow subsides. Consider the following strategies.
   a. Abandon the procedure and reschedule. However, this may be very inconvenient for the patient.
   b. Attempt epidural access at adjacent level, cephalad to the dural puncture level if possible. Once leads are placed, check impedances in addition to checking a lateral view before anchoring the leads. This can help determine whether a lead has been placed in the intrathecal space.
   c. Educate the patient in strategies to manage a spinal headache, such as resting in the recumbent position the remainder of the day, drinking plenty of fluids and caffeine.
   d. Inform the patient to observe for signs of a spinal headache, including headache that is less severe when in the recumbent position, photosensitivity, and nausea.
   e. If a spinal headache develops, offer the patient a blood patch under aseptic conditions at or near the level of the presumed dural puncture.

Anticoagulant Use

Concomitant anticoagulation use when placing percutaneous spinal cord stimulator leads is contraindicated by all published pain society guidelines. These guidelines also strongly recommend holding anticoagulation medications for the duration of a percutaneous spinal cord stimulator trial.[18,19] However, some patients may not be able to safely do without anticoagulant medication for the usual 5- to 7-day spinal cord stimulator trial period. In such cases, the stimulator trial can be shortened to 48 to 72 hours.

In exceptional circumstances when holding anticoagulation for even 2 days is contraindicated, a staged spinal cord stimulator trial can be performed. The patient is usually transitioned to low-molecular-weight (LMW) heparin, which is held 24 hours prior to placement of the spinal cord stimulator leads. The leads are placed percutaneously but anchored to the fascia underneath the skin at the midline spine, as would be done for a permanent spinal cord stimulator implant. However, instead of attaching the distal lead contacts to an internal pulse generator battery, the leads are attached to lead extensions. Our practice is to tunnel these leads to the flank opposite the side that a permanent implantable pulse generator (IPG) battery would be placed, where the extensions would exit the skin. The midline pocket is then closed in the usual fashion and an external battery is attached to the externalized lead extensions. Anticoagulation medication, usually LMW heparin, can be restarted 12 to 24 hours, as recommended by the guidelines. The trial can then proceed for a typical duration of 5 to 10 days.

If the trial is deemed successful, the midline incision is re-incised using the usual sterile operating room protocol. However, the extension lead exit site is not prepared in the sterile field. The lead extensions are cut at the midline incision and an operating room nurse or other personnel gently pulls the contaminated lead extensions through the flank side exit site. The sterile leads are then tunneled to a pocket on the side contralateral to the extension exit wound. The leads are then attached to the IPG, tested, and the battery implanted per the usual protocol for permanent SCS system implantation. If the trial is deemed unsuccessful, the midline leads are surgically removed after the extension leads have been cut and removed via the flank exit wound. In either case, anticoagulation medication can be resumed in 12 to 24 hours per the usual guideline recommendations.

RECOMMENDATIONS FOR PATIENTS ON ANTICOAGULANT MEDICATIONS

1. All patients should hold anticoagulant medications for 5 half-lives prior to placement of percutaneous spinal cord stimulator leads for trial or permanent implantation. Consult specific guidelines for duration that various anticoagulants must be held prior to surgery.[16,18,20]
2. Patients should hold anticoagulation medications throughout the duration of the spinal cord stimulator trial if the leads are anchored at the skin. Anticoagulation medication can be restarted within 12 to 24 hours after trial lead removal as recommended by specific guidelines.[18,20]
3. If a patient cannot hold anticoagulation medication for the duration of a spinal cord stimulator trial period, there are two potential options:
   a. Shorten the trial duration (i.e., 3 days instead of 5 to 7, as is often considered standard practice).
   b. If the patient cannot hold anticoagulation for even 72 hours after trial lead placement, a staged trial can be performed as described earlier.

Choice of Anesthesia and Neuromonitoring

Percutaneous placement of SCS leads with 14-gauge introducer needles can result in transient pain for the patient but also poses risk of injury to the spinal cord and the spinal nerve roots. The reported frequency of spinal cord injury has been reported to be as high as 2.35%,[21] but other large studies have found no injuries.[22,23] There is no standard anesthetic modality agreed upon for percutaneous SCS or DRGS lead placement. Some authors speculate that use of deep sedation likely increases the risk of spinal cord injury.[12] However, other experts note that SCS and especially DRGS lead placement can be very uncomfortable for the patient. Most patients undergoing these procedures are hypersensitive to pain. Thus, the added pain of needle placement and lead navigation through the epidural space, especially near the DRG, can be intolerable with local anesthetic and light intravenous anesthesia with fentanyl and versed. Additionally, sudden movement by the patient can potentially result in unanticipated needle movement and result in neural injury.[24] Many centers have used deeper sedation, in which the patient is not responsive to painful response with no major adverse outcomes reported.[25] Neuromonitoring has been used to optimize SCS lead placement for patients under general anesthesia; specific protocols for this have been published.[26] However, neuromonitoring for percutaneous SCS lead placement is not widely used and large-scale studies have not yet been performed to determine whether variation in anesthetic practice and the use of adjunct neuromonitoring has a clinically significant effect on outcomes.[12,25]

In our practice, we offer patients a choice of anesthesia for percutaneous SCS and DRGS trials. Some patients tolerate these procedures with local anesthetic and a small amount of IV fentanyl and versed. Others require monitored anesthesia care (MAC) sedation for these procedures without neuromonitoring. Most of our permanent implantation of SCS and DRGS systems are performed with MAC anesthesia in an ambulatory surgery center. Permanent system placement for morbidly obese patients (BMI $>$ 50) is performed in a hospital operating room under general anesthesia with a secure airway. Our experience reflects that of published studies in that we do not observe incidence of permanent neurological damage regardless of anesthetic technique. We have observed that if the patient is uncomfortable during the placement of the trial system, the patient seems more likely to report that the system does not help with chronic pain.

RECOMMENDATIONS FOR ANESTHESIA AND NEUROMONITORING

1. At this writing, there is no consensus on the mode of anesthesia and use of neuromonitoring for SCS and DRGS trials and permanent system implants. Practices vary from minimal sedation to deeper sedation, including general anesthesia. Neuromonitoring during lead placement is not currently widely performed. However, documented risk for permanent neurological injury secondary to SCS lead placement is estimated to be 0% to 2.35%.[11,21,22]
2. Use the least amount of anesthesia tolerated by the patient for SCS and DRGS trials and implant procedures. This is often a combination of local anesthetic and IV fentanyl and versed.
3. If deeper anesthesia is used, consider neuromonitoring to reduce the risk of spinal cord or spinal nerve root injury.

Surgical Site Infection: Risk Factors, Diagnosis, and Management

SSI after SCS device implantation is one of the most dreaded complications associated with this therapy. Recent studies indicate device infection rates to be 2.4% to 3.1%,[5,6] though older studies reported infection rates of 3% to 6%.[11,17] Although mortality from SSI after SCS device implantation is rare, treatment involves weeks of antibiotic therapy, occasional hospitalization, and usually requires removal of the device. This, in turn, prevents patients from receiving adequate pain management.

The pathogenesis for SSI is mainly from the patient's skin flora contaminating the IPG pocket or midline lumbar pocket and the corresponding device hardware. This is consistent with the finding that the most frequently isolated bacteria from wound cultures is *Staphylococcus aureus*.[27-29] Bacteria readily adhere to foreign body surfaces to form a biofilm; thus, the body can isolate only growing bacteria rather than neutralizing the infection by phagocytizing and regenerating affected tissue, as occurs in soft-tissue infections. Antibiotics administered prior to infection can neutralize bacteria before the biofilm has formed but are ineffective at halting foreign body bacteria growth.[30,31]

RISK FACTORS AND MITIGATION FOR SURGICAL SITE INFECTION AFTER SPINAL CORD STIMULATOR IMPLANTATION

Patient comorbidity risk factors for SSI after SCS permanent implantation were often thought to be similar to other surgical procedures. However, two recent studies found that obesity, diabetes, smoking, revision surgery, underlying malignancy, ongoing chemotherapy, and radiation were not associated with higher rates of infection in permanent SCS device implantation.[5,32] However, history of previous surgical infection and younger age[5,6] were associated with increased risk of SSI.[5,6]

Perioperative and intraoperative factors affect rates of infection up to 12 months after implantation, the timeline outlined by guidelines for which SSI can occur.[16] Factors associated with increased risk of SSI include prolonged surgical time in one study (215 ± 93 minutes for SSI vs. 123 ± 52 minutes for no SSI)[32] and longer trial duration (> 5 days).[5] Perioperative and intraoperative factors that were associated with decreased SSI rates include staged trial (i.e., permanent trial), administration of IV antibiotics prior to skin incision, postoperative antibiotics for an average of 7.6 days after surgery, and application of an occlusive dressing in the operating room that is kept intact for at least 24 hours after surgery.[5] Perioperative and intraoperative factors that do not appear to affect rate of SSI include choice of lead (paddle vs. cylindrical), length of time between trial and permanent implant, and choice of intraoperative antibiotic.[5]

Some perioperative and intraoperative factors that cannot yet be evaluated due to inadequate data for SCS device implantation include skin closure technique and volume or type of wound irrigation. Additionally, methicillin-resistant *Staphylococcus aureus* (MRSA) screening and decolonization has not been adequately studied for SCS device implantation. However, several studies document that wound infections that progress to SCS device explantation had cultures positive for MRSA.[27,32] If patients have a history of MRSA, it would be prudent to choose an intraoperative and postoperative antibiotic to which MRSA is likely to be sensitive, such as vancomycin or clindamycin.

RECOMMENDATIONS TO REDUCE RISK OF SURGICAL SITE INFECTION

1. Administer IV antibiotics prior to surgical incision.
2. If the patient has a history of MRSA, consider nasal decolonization and select an appropriate antibiotic (i.e., vancomycin or clindamycin).
3. Although diabetes has not been associated with increased wound infection rates, communicate with the patient's primary care provider to ensure appropriate perioperative and postoperative glycemic control.
4. Prescribe postoperative antibiotics for up to 10 days, as this has been associated with decreased wound infections.
5. Apply an occlusive wound dressing in the operating room immediately after wound closure and instruct the patient to leave this dressing intact for at least 24 hours after the surgery.
6. Follow up within 7 days to monitor wound healing progress.

Surgical Site Infection: Diagnosis and Management after Spinal Cord Stimulator Implantation

Surgical site infections tend to present on average within 1 to 2 months after implantation. Most infections occur at the generator pocket site and secondarily at the midline lead pocket site.[5,6,16,33] Superficial infections present with pain, erythema, and edema at the surgical incision. Deep infections have additional symptoms of dehiscence, fluctuance, purulent drainage, and, potentially, erosion through the skin. Systemic symptoms are always a risk, but uncommon.[29] Epidural abscess may present as back pain, fever, and neurological deficits. If untreated, the infection can potentially progress to meningitis. However, incidence of meningitis after SCS device implantation is exceedingly rare.[27]

In our practice, the first sign of a potential SSI is usually fluctuance with erythema around the incision site. We initially aspirate any fluid from the affected sites and send a sample to the laboratory for culture and antibiotic sensitivity testing. We also obtain blood work, including complete blood cell count with differential, C-reactive protein, and sedimentation rate. Although nonspecific, the results of these tests can assist in determining whether the fluid in the surgical pocket is a noninfectious seroma or deep wound infection. We often start the patient on empiric antibiotic medication, such as trimethoprim/sulfamethoxazole unless the patient has a sulfa allergy. Other choices include cephalexin or clindamycin depending on the patient's individual antibiotic medication allergy profile. If the patient has no signs of systemic infection and the aspirate is nonpurulent, sanguinous, or serosanguinous, we wait for blood lab results and wound culture aspirates before proceeding to device explantation.

If the patient has any signs of systemic infection or deep wound infection with device contamination, such as purulent drainage from the wound, purulent aspirate, or wound dehiscence and/or visualization of the underlying device through a skin erosion, we quickly proceed to surgical explantation. It is our practice to remove the entire system as partial removal of SCS systems has been associated with higher rates of recurrence of infection or failure to heal.[34] Intraoperatively, fluid samples are taken from both the IPG pocket and the midline lumbar pocket and sent for culture. We debride the wound and excise any devitalized or necrotic skin tissue surrounding the incision site prior to wound closure.

Closure with nonresorbable nylon suture with a vertical mattress stitch is the most conservative choice for significantly compromised wounds. However, this can leave an undesirable scar. In the case of an infection identified in early stages, we have found that closure with resorbable suture is adequate. The addition of a surgical drain can be considered, but we often find this unnecessary.

After device explantation, we refer the patient to infectious disease experts to help with postoperative antibiotic therapy based on culture sensitivities. Once the wound has healed completely and the patient has been off antibiotics for several weeks, we consider reimplantation of the device according to the patient's wishes.

RECOMMENDATIONS FOR SURGICAL SITE INFECTION DIAGNOSIS AND MANAGEMENT AFTER SPINAL CORD STIMULATOR IMPLANTATION

1. Consider image-guided needle aspiration under aseptic conditions of any fluctuant fluid in a wound that is tender and/or has signs of erythema or drainage. Send a sample of the aspirated fluid to the lab for culture. Obtain blood work, including complete blood count with differential, C-reactive protein, and sedimentation rate to help establish the presence of infection. Consider starting empiric antibiotics with trimethoprim/sulfamethoxazole or another antibiotic if the patient has a sulfa allergy.
2. If there is evidence of systemic infection or signs of hardware contamination, such as purulent fluid in the pocket, significant dehiscence, or visualization of the underlying hardware, consider urgent surgical removal of all associated SCS hardware.
3. If the decision is made to remove the SCS hardware, obtain fluid cultures from both the IPG and lumbar midline pockets.
4. Adequately debride all infected or necrotic wound tissue and consider an elliptical incision around the original surgical incision to excise any devitalized skin.
5. Copiously irrigate all wounds and consider application of vancomycin powder in the infected wound sites.
6. Consider closing using a vertical mattress stitch with a nonresorbable suture (i.e., braided nylon) for significantly infected wounds. Otherwise, consider closure with resorbable sutures. If the patient is to be hospitalized after the explantation, consider the use of a Jackson-Pratt drain that can be pulled once drainage from the site has subsided and the patient is ready to discharge.
7. Refer the patient to infectious disease experts for management of infection as guided by culture sensitivities.
8. Consider reimplantation of the SCS system, per the patient's wishes, once the wounds have completely healed and the patient has finished the course of antibiotic regimen recommended by the infectious disease team.

REFERENCES

1. Shealy CN, Mortimer JT, Reswick JB. Electrical inhibition of pain by stimulation of the dorsal columns: preliminary clinical report. *Anesth Analg.* 1967;46(4):489-491. doi:10.1213/00000539-196707000-00025.
2. Mekhail N, Mehanny D, Armanyous S, Saweris Y, Costandi S. The impact of obesity on the effectiveness of spinal cord stimulation in chronic spine-related pain patients. *Spine J.* 2019;19(3):476-486. doi:10.1016/j.spinee.2018.08.006.
3. Epstein N. More risks and complications for elective spine surgery in morbidly obese patients. *Surg Neurol Int.* 2017;8(1):66. doi:10.4103/sni.sni_49_17.
4. Olsen MA, Nepple JJ, Riew KD, et al. Risk factors for surgical site infection following orthopaedic spinal operations. *J Bone Joint Surg Am.* 2008;90(1):62-69. doi:10.2106/JBJS.F.01515.
5. Hoelzer BC, Bendel MA, Deer TR, et al. Spinal cord stimulator implant infection rates and risk factors: a multicenter retrospective study. *Neuromodulation.* 2017;20(6):558-562. doi:10.1111/ner.12609.
6. Falowski SM, Provenzano DA, Xia Y, Doth AH. Spinal cord stimulation infection rate and risk factors: results from a United States payer database. *Neuromodulation.* 2019;22(2):179-189. doi:10.1111/ner.12843.

7. Orhurhu V, Khan F, Salisu Orhurhu M, et al. Obesity trends amongst hospitalized patients with spinal cord stimulator implants. *Adv Ther*. 2020;37(11):4614-4626. doi:10.1007/s12325-020-01487-8.
8. Koetsier E, Franken G, Debets J, et al. Effectiveness of dorsal root ganglion stimulation and dorsal column spinal cord stimulation in a model of experimental painful diabetic polyneuropathy. *CNS Neurosci Ther*. 2019;25(3):367-374. doi:10.1111/cns.13065.
9. Pluijms WA, Slangen R, Joosten EA, et al. Electrical spinal cord stimulation in painful diabetic polyneuropathy, a systematic review on treatment efficacy and safety. *Eur J Pain*. 2011;15(8):783-788. doi:10.1016/j.ejpain.2011.01.010.
10. Duarte RV, Andronis L, Lenders MWPM, de Vos CC. Quality of life increases in patients with painful diabetic neuropathy following treatment with spinal cord stimulation. *Qual Life Res*. 2016;25(7):1771-1777. doi:10.1007/s11136-015-1211-4.
11. Mekhail NA, Mathews M, Nageeb F, Guirguis M, Mekhail MN, Cheng J. Retrospective review of 707 cases of spinal cord stimulation: indications and complications. *Pain Pract*. 2011;11(2):148-153. doi:10.1111/j.1533-2500.2010.00407.x.
12. Deer TR, Lamer TJ, Pope JE, et al. The Neurostimulation Appropriateness Consensus Committee (NACC) safety guidelines for the reduction of severe neurological injury. *Neuromodulation*. 2017;20(1):15-30. doi:10.1111/ner.12564.
13. Eldabe S, Buchser E, Duarte RV. Complications of spinal cord stimulation and peripheral nerve stimulation techniques: a review of the literature. *Pain Med*. 2016;17:325-336. doi:10.1093/pm/pnv025.
14. Deer TR, Stewart CD. Complications of spinal cord stimulation: identification, treatment, and prevention. *Pain Med*. 2008;9(suppl 1):S93-S101. doi:10.1111/j.1526-4637.2008.00444.x.
15. Bendersky D, Yampolsky C. Is spinal cord stimulation safe? A review of its complications. *World Neurosurg*. 2014;82(6):1359-1368. doi:10.1016/j.wneu.2013.06.012.
16. Deer TR, Provenzano DA, Hanes M, et al. The Neurostimulation Appropriateness Consensus Committee (NACC) recommendations for infection prevention and management. *Neuromodulation*. 2017;20(1):31-50. doi:10.1111/ner.12565.
17. Deer TR, Mekhail N, Provenzano D, et al. The appropriate use of neurostimulation: avoidance and treatment of complications of neurostimulation therapies for the treatment of chronic pain. Neurostimulation Appropriateness Consensus Committee. *Neuromodulation*. 2014;17(6):571-597; discussion 598. doi:10.1111/ner.12206.
18. Narouze S, Benzon HT, Provenzano D, et al. Interventional Spine and Pain Procedures in Patients on Antiplatelet and Anticoagulant Medications (Second Edition): Guidelines from the American Society of Regional Anesthesia and Pain Medicine, the European Society of Regional Anaesthesia and Pain Therapy, the American Academy of Pain Medicine, the International Neuromodulation Society, the North American Neuromodulation Society, and the World Institute of Pain. *Reg Anesth Pain Med*. 2018;43(3):225-262. doi:10.1097/AAP.0000000000000700.
19. Manchikanti L. Responsible, safe, and effective use of Antithrombotics and Anticoagulants in patients undergoing interventional techniques: American Society of Interventional Pain Physicians (ASIPP) guidelines. *Pain Phys*. 2019;22(1S):S75-S128. doi:10.36076/ppj/2019.22.s75.
20. Deer TR, Narouze S, Provenzano DA, et al. The Neurostimulation Appropriateness Consensus Committee (NACC): recommendations on bleeding and coagulation management in neurostimulation devices. *Neuromodulation*. 2017;20(1):51-62. doi:10.1111/ner.12542.
21. Petraglia FW, Farber SH, Gramer R, et al. The incidence of spinal cord injury in implantation of percutaneous and paddle electrodes for spinal cord stimulation. *Neuromodulation*. 2016;19(1):85-90. doi:10.1111/ner.12370.
22. Cameron T. Safety and efficacy of spinal cord stimulation for the treatment of chronic pain: a 20-year literature review. *J Neurosurg*. 2004;100(3 Suppl Spine):254-267. doi:10.3171/spi.2004.100.3.0254.
23. Kumar K, Wilson JR, Taylor RS, Gupta S. Complications of spinal cord stimulation, suggestions to improve outcome, and financial impact. *J Neurosurg Spine*. 2006;5(3):191-203. doi:10.3171/spi.2006.5.3.191.
24. Falowski SM, Celii A, Sestokas AK, Schwartz DM, Matsumoto C, Sharan A. Awake vs. asleep placement of spinal cord stimulators: a cohort analysis of complications associated with placement. *Neuromodulation*. 2011;14(2):130-135. doi:10.1111/j.1525-1403.2010.00319.x.
25. Deer TR, Pope JE, Lamer TJ, et al. The Neuromodulation Appropriateness Consensus Committee on best practices for dorsal root ganglion stimulation. *Neuromodulation*. 2019;22(1):1-35. doi:10.1111/ner.12845.
26. Shils JL, Arle JE. Neuromonitoring for spinal cord stimulation lead placement under general anesthesia. *J Clin Neurol*. 2018;14(4):444-453. doi:10.3988/jcn.2018.14.4.444.
27. Bendel MA, O'Brien T, Hoelzer BC, et al. Spinal cord stimulator related infections: findings from a multicenter retrospective analysis of 2737 implants. *Neuromodulation*. 2017;20(6):553-557. doi:10.1111/ner.12636.
28. Yusuf E, Bamps S, Ursi JP, et al. Characteristics of infections associated with a spinal cord stimulator system. *J Infect*. 2016;73(5):515-517. doi:10.1016/j.jinf.2016.08.012.
29. Esquer Garrigos Z, Farid S, Bendel MA, Sohail MR. Spinal cord stimulator infection: approach to diagnosis, management, and prevention. *Clin Infect Dis*. 2020;70(12):2727-2735. doi:10.1093/cid/ciz994.
30. Vuong C, Otto M. *Staphylococcus epidermidis* infections. *Microbes Infect*. 2002;4(4):481-489. doi:10.1016/s1286-4579(02)01563-0.
31. Fey PD, Olson ME. Current concepts in biofilm formation of *Staphylococcus epidermidis*. *Future Microbiol*. 2010;5(6):917-933. doi:10.2217/fmb.10.56.
32. Engle MP, Vinh BO, Harun N, Koyyalagunta D. Infectious complications related to intrathecal drug delivery system and spinal cord stimulator system implantations at a comprehensive cancer pain center. *Pain Phys*. 2013;16(3):251-257.
33. Hayek SM, Veizi E, Hanes M. Treatment-limiting complications of percutaneous spinal cord stimulator implants: a review of eight years of experience from an academic center database. *Neuromodulation*. 2015;18(7):603-609. doi:10.1111/ner.12312.
34. Follett KA, Boortz-Marx RL, Drake JM, et al. Prevention and management of intrathecal drug delivery and spinal cord stimulation system infections. *Anesthesiology*. 2004;100(6):1582-1594. doi:10.1097/00000542-200406000-00034.

Chapter 19

Patient Selection for Intrathecal Drug Delivery Systems

Alyson M. Engle

Chapter Outline

Introduction

Intrathecal drug delivery systems are devices often referred to as intrathecal pumps (ITPs) or targeted drug delivery systems (TDDSs). The system functions to effectively administer an infusion of a medication into the intrathecal (IT) space by means of a strategically placed catheter in the cerebrospinal fluid of the neuroaxis. TDDSs are often used as a last resort for pain control when conservative therapies fail. Delivering drugs into the fluid that surrounds the spinal cord near areas of pain sensation allows for concentrated dosing at the spinal cord. This method allows for less medication to be used, thereby reducing systemic side effects experienced with oral medications. This is one benefit for the use of TDDSs in patients with intractable chronic pain states.

Patient Selection

Determining the right therapy for the right patient is essential for delivering appropriate medical care. TDDS candidates include patients with refractory pain due to malignant cancer pain, spasticity refractory to oral medications, end-of-life care, and some types of chronic intractable nonmalignant pain. Nonmalignant pain that is intractable comprises facial pain syndromes, pelvic pain syndromes, abdominal pain syndromes, painful diabetic neuropathy, failed back surgery syndrome, plexopathies, complex regional pain syndrome types I and II, compression fractures, spondylosis, spondylolisthesis, and spinal stenosis. Malignant pain includes painful neoplastic disorders, bone tumors, gastrointestinal malignancies, and pathological spine fractures with myelomalacia.

Absolute contraindications to ITP placement include patient refusal or inability to provide informed consent, allergy to implantable materials or drugs, uncorrected coagulopathy, infection that is systemic or localized to the site of implantation, psychosis, dementia, and active substance abuse. Patients with a history of psychosis or another organic brain cognitive disorder are absolute contraindications to ziconotide. A patient with a bleeding diathesis is a contraindication to surgical placement since implantation requires accessing the neuraxial space. Relative contraindications include impaired wound healing states, such as uncontrolled diabetes, immunosuppressed states, and active tobacco use.

Anatomical Considerations

Patient body habitus is important in periprocedural planning for positioning and equipment selection.

Spinal deformities and prior back surgery also need to be evaluated to determine location of needle entry and potential obstruction to needle placement. Spinal hardware, prior back fusions, scar tissue, and deformities such as scoliosis have implications in procedural technique. If there is any concern for cancer, bony metastasis needs to be evaluated before performing the procedure. Needle entry below L1 to L2 is preferred to avoid direct contact with the conus medullaris. A paramedian approach is also preferred to midline because a paramedian approach will decrease the risk of the catheter becoming compressed between the spinous processes, which may lead to catheter maceration.

Complications Associated With Patient Selection

There is an increased risk of complications in certain patient populations, such as those with psychosocial implications. See Table 19.1 for an outline of patient-related complications. For example, personality disorders, conversion disorder, poor coping mechanisms, and addiction may contribute to complications when TDDSs are implanted. In addition, patients with coagulopathy and those taking anticoagulant medications or herbal supplements may have an increased risk of bleeding. Uncontrolled bleeding may lead to a soft tissue seroma, poor wound healing, or a more serious complication such as an epidural hematoma. Metastatic disease with ongoing chemotherapy, radiation, and surgery needs to be given special consideration based on multidisciplinary team meetings.

TABLE 19.1 Patient-Related Complications Associated with Intrathecal Drug Delivery System Implantation

Patient-specific comorbidities
- Psychiatric comorbidities
- Cancer metastasis
- Smoking
- Diabetes
- Immunosuppression
- Obstructive sleep apnea

Pharmacological complications
- Allergic reactions
- Withdrawal
- Overdose
- Medication-specific side effects
    - Endocrinopathies (e.g., hypogonadism)
    - Low bone mineral density

Other patient-related factors that may increase the risk of complications include active infections, active smoking, diabetic states, and immunosuppression. Obstructive sleep apnea is an important consideration for the use of sedatives in the intrathecal space and plays a role in medication selection. Ziconotide is an absolute contraindication for patients with a history of psychosis. Guidelines and best practice recommendations released by the Centers for Disease Control and Prevention (CDC), the Polyanalgesic Consensus Committee (PACC), and the American Society of Regional Anesthesia and Pain Medicine (ASRA) help to guide the clinician to reduce patient-related complications and provide the safest therapy.[1-3]

General Considerations

PHARMACOLOGY COMPLICATIONS

In addition to complications secondary to patient comorbidities, there are also medication-related complications that can occur in the setting of a TDDS. Adverse drug reactions are the most common complications of a TDDS.[4] Severe adverse reactions include anaphylaxis, respiratory depression, and infection secondary to contaminated medication use.

The drug ziconotide is most efficacious if used as a first-line stand-alone agent in a pump. It must be trialed very slowly with only small dose changes due to its narrow therapeutic window. Side effects of ziconotide include psychosis, cognitive dysfunction, balance issues, uncontrolled eye movements, and elevated creatinine kinase (CK) serum levels, among others. CK levels should be checked at baseline and during initiation of ziconotide therapy as they may increase twofold.

Intrathecal administration of clonidine has side effects of light-headedness, dizziness, hypotension, withdrawal, and increased fall risk. The clinical presentation of withdrawal from clonidine is usually rebound hypertension. Prevention includes careful calculation of dosing and timing of follow-up for refills.

Baclofen's adverse effect profile includes oversedation and weakness. Weakness and sedation place the patient at an increased risk of falls. Therefore, baclofen should be carefully titrated, especially in the elderly or those with underlying comorbidities. When stopping baclofen, there is the potential for life-threatening withdrawal, which could present clinically with high fevers, rigidity, myoclonus, seizures, rhabdomyolysis, and possibly death. Therefore, baclofen treatment should incorporate education and shared decision-making with patients regarding the complications and when to seek emergency medical care.[5] Prevention includes careful calculation of dosing and ensuring that patients follow up on time for refills to avoid withdrawal.

Intrathecal bupivacaine has the potential to result in hypotension, numbness, motor block, seizures, cardiotoxicity, and local anesthetic systemic toxicity (LAST) if accidentally administered intravascularly. Prevention of LAST includes always aspirating before injection, as in the case of refill.

Certain medications are higher risk for specific complications than others. For example, there is a higher risk of respiratory depression with the administration of IT opioids. Patient-related factors that increase the risk of respiratory depression involve being in the elderly age bracket, concomitant sedative use, obstructive sleep apnea, chronic obstructive lung disease, and neurological disease states. In addition, the use of higher opioid doses and the selection of lipophilic opiates will increase the chances of respiratory depression. When a patient presents with a decline in respiratory status requiring naloxone administration, the provider should be vigilant with dosing to avoid also precipitating withdrawal symptoms. For example, when reversing an opioid with a half-life longer than naloxone, a low-dose naloxone infusion can be useful.

Other complications include granuloma formation and endocrinopathies. The use of morphine and hydromorphone are more commonly associated with granuloma formation at the catheter tip.[4] Hormone shifts can also be seen with the use of TDDS.[6-10] Low bone mineral density has been seen with intrathecal opioid use.[8] Opioids directly affect bone turnover through opioid receptors present on osteoblasts. Opioids also inhibit the hypothalamic-pituitary-adrenal axis, which also decreases bone mineral density. Surveillance of patients on long-term IT opioid therapy may decrease the clinical risk of alterations in the endocrine system resulting in osteoporosis and potential fractures.

A secondary clinical effect of opioid inhibition of the hypothalamic-pituitary-adrenal axis is hypogonadotropic hypogonadism, also referred to as *opioid-induced androgen deficiency* (OPIAD).[7,10,11] Lower testosterone concentrations have been observed in patients with IT opioid administration.[8,9,12] There are no criteria for monitoring and managing opioid-induced hypoadrenalism or hypogonadism. Screening of symptomatic patients should include hormone and lipid panels. Low testosterone levels may present with symptoms of fatigue, erectile dysfunction, decreased libido, depression, and sexual dysfunction. Treatment may include weaning opioids, switching to another medication, and hormone replacement therapy. In OPIAD treatment, 7.5 mg per day of transdermal testosterone has improved symptoms.[13]

Opioids administered intrathecally are less likely to result in systemic side effects, such as constipation, nausea, and urinary retention. However, patients with intrathecal opioid pumps may still experience systemic issues. Opioid-induced nausea and vomiting happens because of cephalad migration of intrathecal opioids, which results in activity in the chemoreceptor trigger zone (CTZ) area postrema.[14] Pruritis may also result from cephalad migration of opioids when in contact with the trigeminal nucleus in the superficial medulla.[15] Symptomatic relief of these side effects can be achieved with a low-dose naloxone infusion. Nalbuphine provides an alternative pruritic treatment. Gastrointestinal side effects, such as constipation, are due to the affinity for opioid receptors in the spinal cord, which leads to decreased gastrointestinal motility.[16] Treatment options include adequate hydration, stool softeners, and prokinetic agents. Urinary retention may be encountered with IT opioid administration. The mechanism is thought to be due to the decreased sacral parasympathetic outflow to the detrusor muscle.[17]

Avoiding pharmacological adverse effect profiles can be achieved by following the manufacturers' refill protocols; double checking medication names, doses, location of injections, and programs; starting at low doses with slow titration; and close monitoring of the patient and patient education. Early recognition and action will help decrease the risk of experiencing patient decline. The PACC guidelines as outlined in Table 19.2 can aid the clinician on best practices for preventing side effects.

TABLE 19.2 Summary of the Polyanalgesic Consensus Conference Recommendations on Intrathecal Drug Infusion Systems, 2017[1]

Psychology

- Psychological assessment, counseling, and after care are recommended in appropriate candidates. The use of an assessment is critical in all noncancer patients receiving an IDDS.
- Psychological screening is not required for end-of-life patients, but psychological counseling should be considered.

Pharmacology

- First-line, FDA-approved medications to be used in the IT space:
  - Morphine
  - Ziconotide
- Off-label drug monotherapy or combination therapy is not recommended until FDA-approved drugs are tried and failed or are contraindicated. In cancer pain, the on-label drugs can be used during the trial phase. If the results are not acceptable due to lack of efficacy or side effects, an admixture with bupivacaine of the primary use of fentanyl is supported by our consensus guidelines.
- The PACC algorithms are based on improving safety and efficacy in clinical practice, which includes the use of off-label drugs.
- Ziconotide has strong clinical evidence for efficacy.
- There are no cases of death from ziconotide overdose and no granuloma formation has been reported.
- Unless contraindicated, ziconotide should be the first drug selected in the population of noncancer patients.
- The initiating dose of IT opioids and ziconotide should be as low as reasonably expected to provide analgesia.
- The initiating dose of IT opioids and ziconotide delivered continuously should be 50% or less of the dose used during bolus trialing.
- The PACC recommends that the primary medication be weaned and discontinued when converting medications from one single medication to a different single medication in the algorithm.
- The use of ziconotide and bupivacaine do not have the risk of withdrawal; thus, weaning is not needed. The abrupt stopping of an opioid is not recommended.
- The PACC recommends careful attention to side effects when adding any adjuvant drug to a primary drug.
- Medications with significant withdrawal syndromes, including clonidine and baclofen, require rescue strategies in the event of abrupt cessation or interruption in IT delivery.
- Before proceeding with aggressive dose titration above 1000 μg per day of IT fentanyl, clinicians should closely monitor the outcome of each dose increase and, if efficacy is not being established, consider dose reduction with taking into account IT tolerance and hyperalgesia.

Patient-related factors

- Patients with comorbidities that negatively affect cardiopulmonary function need increased vigilance when instituting opioid therapy.
- Localized, diffuse, and global pain can be adequately treated with IT therapy. The evidence for global pain treatment is less well defined and should be approached cautiously.
- The algorithms are based on evidence and consensus on safety. The patient's physician and good clinical judgment should guide individual patient care.
- The disease process should be considered when making decisions on algorithms for patient care.
- IT therapies should be used at an appropriate time in the algorithm and not as a salvage treatment.
- The stage of cancer and survival time should be considered when performing drug titration.
- IT therapy should be considered within the same line as neurostimulation.
- IT therapy should be considered after neurostimulation if the pain is isolated and unlikely to spread.
- IT therapy should be considered before neurostimulation for active cancer-related pain that is mechanical and likely to spread.

FDA, US Food and Drug Administration; *IDDS,* intrathecal drug delivery system; *IT,* intrathecal; *PACC,* Polyanalgesic Consensus Conference.

REFERENCES

1. Deer TR, Pope JE, Hayek SM, et al. The Polyanalgesic Consensus Conference (PACC): recommendations on intrathecal drug infusion systems best practices and guidelines. *Neuromodulation*. 2017;20(2):96-132. doi:10.1111/ner.12538.
2. Narouze S, Benzon HT, Provenzano D, et al. Interventional Spine and Pain Procedures in Patients on Antiplatelet and Anticoagulant Medications (Second Edition): Guidelines from the American Society of Regional Anesthesia and Pain Therapy, the American Academy of Pain Medicine, the International Neuromodulation Society, the North American Neuromodulation Society, and the World Institute of Pain. *Reg Anesth Pain Med*. 2018;43(3):225-262. doi:10.1097/AAP.0000000000000700.
3. Berriós-Torres SI, Umscheid CA, Bratzler DW, et al. Centers for Disease Control and Prevention Guideline for the prevention of surgical site infection, 2017. *JAMA Surg*. 2017;152(8):784-791. doi:10.1001/jamasurg.2017.0904.
4. Bhatia G, Lau ME, Koury KM, Gulur P. Intrathecal Drug Delivery (ITDD) systems for cancer pain. F1000Res. 2013; Mar 28;2:96. doi: 10.12688/f1000research.2-96.v4.
5. Coffey RJ, Edgar TS, Francisco GE, et al. Abrupt withdrawal from intrathecal baclofen: recognition and management of a potentially life-threatening syndrome. *Arch Phys Med Rehabil*. 2002;83(6):735-741. doi:10.1053/apmr.2002.32820.
6. Acurcio FA, Moura CS, Bernatsky S, Bessette L, Rahme E. Opioid use and risk of nonvertebral fractures in adults with rheumatoid arthritis: a nested case-control study using administrative databases. *Arthritis Rheumatol*. 2016;68(1):83-91. doi:10.1002/art.39422.
7. Coluzzi F, Pergolizzi J, Raffa RB, Mattia C. The unsolved case of "bone-impairing analgesics": the endocrine effects of opioids on bone metabolism. *Ther Clin Risk Manag*. 2015;11:515-523. doi:10.2147/TCRM.S79409.
8. Duarte RV, Raphael JH, Southall JL, Labib MH, Whallett AJ, Ashford RL. Hypogonadism and low bone mineral density in patients on long-term intrathecal opioid delivery therapy. *BMJ Open*. 2013;3(6):e002856. doi:10.1136/bmjopen-2013-002856.
9. Kim CH, Garcia R, Stover J, Ritchie K, Whealton T, Ata MA. Androgen deficiency in long-term intrathecal opioid administration. *Pain Physician*. 2014;17(4):543-548.
10. Smith HS, Elliott JA. Opioid-induced androgen deficiency. *Pain Physician*. 2012;15(suppl 3):SE145-SE156.
11. Daniell HW. An opioid contribution to low bone mineral density in cannabis smokers. *Am J Med*. 2017;130(10):e453. doi:10.1016/j.amjmed.2017.03.048.
12. Rubinstein A, Carpenter D, Minkoff J. Hypogonadism in men with chronic pain linked to the use of long-acting rather than short-acting opioids. *Clin J Pain*. 2013;29(10):840-845.
13. Daniell HW, Lentz R, Mazer NA. Open-label pilot study of testosterone patch therapy in men with opioid-induced androgen deficiency. *J Pain*. 2006;7(3):200-210.
14. Wang SC, Borison HL. The vomiting center. *Arch Neurol Psychiatry*. 1950;63(6):928-941.
15. Ballantyne J, Loach A, Carr D. Itching after epidural and spinal opiates. *Pain*. 1988;33:149-160.
16. Porreca F, Filla A, Burks T. Spinal cord mediated opiate effects on gastrointestinal transit in mice. *Eur J Pharmacol*. 1983;86: 135-136.
17. Kari M, Jaycox M, Lubenow TR. Complications associated with intrathecal drug delivery systems. In: Diwan S, Buvanendran, Deer T, eds. *Intrathecal Drug Delivery for Pain and Spasticity*. Volume 2 in *Interventional and Neuromodulatory Techniques for Pain Management*. Elsevier Inc.; 2012:102-110. doi:10.1016/b978-1-4377-2217-8.00014-3.

Chapter 20

Perioperative Care with Intrathecal Drug Delivery Systems

Alyson M. Engle

Chapter Outline

Introduction

Intrathecal drug delivery system (IDDS) devices provide continuous infusion of a drug into the intrathecal (IT) space via a sialastic catheter placed within the cerebrospinal fluid (CSF). An IDDS device is inserted after conservative therapies fail to achieve pain relief or generate intolerable side effects. The IDDS device is composed of a pump and catheter. The IDDS pump can be programmed as a constant flow device, with complex programming or with an ability to administer "dosing on demand." IDDS devices offer a tool for physicians to provide personalized precision medicine by effectively delivering therapeutic drug levels for extended periods of time at a specified target. The delivery of medication into the intrathecal space allows for targeted dosing at the spinal cord and reduces systemic side effects. The option to deliver personalized therapy with precision is one key advantage of IDDSs in the pain care algorithm. The Polyanalgesic Consensus Conference (PACC) best practices and guidelines in conjunction with the SAFE principles help guide clinicians in the decision-making process of when to consider using the IDDS.[1,2]

Anatomical Considerations

Patient body habitus is important in periprocedural planning for positioning and equipment selection. Spinal deformities and prior back surgery also need to be evaluated to determine location of needle entry and potential obstruction to needle placement. The history of back fusions, presence of spinal hardware, scar tissue and deformities, such as scoliosis, have implications in procedural technique. If there is any concern for cancer, bony metastasis needs to be evaluated before performing the procedure. Needle entry below L1 to L2 is preferred to avoid direct contact with the conus medullaris. A paramedian approach is also preferred to the midline since a paramedian approach will decrease the risk of the catheter becoming compressed between the spinous processes, which may lead to catheter maceration.

Procedural Technique

Either general anesthesia or monitored anesthesia care are acceptable anesthetic modalities for IDDS implantation. In both cases, the patient is placed in the lateral decubitus position and the patient's pressure points are positioned and padded appropriately. The lower spine and abdomen are sterile prepped. Fluoroscopic guidance is used to identify the appropriate landmarks for skin and dural insertion—the inferior aspect of the right L5 lamina and entry site of L3 to L4 interspace. Next, local anesthetic consisting of 7 to 10 mL of 0.25% bupivacaine with 1:100,000 epinephrine for areas of skin incision is administered. A skin incision is made with a 10-blade scalpel. Dissection is then performed with Bovie cautery and blunt dissection down into the supraspinous ligament. A Tuohy needle is advanced under fluoroscopic guidance until CSF is obtained. The stylet is then removed. The catheter is inserted through the Tuohy needle. The catheter is then advanced under fluoroscopic guidance until reaching the appropriate level. Once there is confirmation of CSF from the catheter, the physician can be confident of intrathecal placement. Verification methods, such as flushing the catheter with preservative-free saline and performing a myelogram, may prove to be valuable as well.

The needle is left in place while a "0" nonabsorbable suture is used to place a purse string suture, secured around the needle. The purse string suture can be used as an anchoring suture if it is to exit the ligament in close approximation to the catheter exit. If the purse string suture is not used for the anchor stitch, then after the needle is removed, the stay suture for the anchor can be placed through the supraspinous ligament while the anchor is positioned over the IT catheter. The anchor is then advanced down to the supraspinous ligament, at which a free stay suture is placed around the wings of the anchor and sutured. The anchor is then carried down to the supraspinous ligament suture that was already in place and secured.

Following catheter placement, the pump pocket is made. The pocket can be made in the abdominal wall or in the paravertebral region. A skin incision and blunt dissection is used to create the appropriately sized pocket for the pump implant. Four sutures are positioned evenly to secure the pump, which minimizes risk of pump torsion or flipping in the pocket.

Next, a tunneling tool is used to the pass the catheter from the spinal incision to the pocket. The tunneler should traverse the subcutaneous tissue only. After advancing the tunneler from the spinal incision to the pocket incision, the tunneler's stylet or handle is removed. The catheter is then threaded through the tunneler into the pocket. The tunneler is then removed while holding onto the catheter to avoid manipulation. At that point, the catheter is attached to the pump and the pump is secured into the pocket using the four nonabsorbable sutures placed earlier. It should be noted that some providers trim the catheter length. If catheter length is altered, it should be noted by the provider for programming purposes. Catheter length accuracy is important to accurately determine the catheter volume for priming purposes.

A catheter dye study should be performed on the patient to ensure catheter placement and system integrity. Medication should be placed in the pump prior to implantation. Both pockets must then be thoroughly irrigated with warm normal saline with or without antibiotics. After confirming hemostasis, deep basal sutures are placed in both pockets using 3-0 Monocryl. Hemostasis, fascial closure, and subcuticular closure of each surgical pocket are essential for wound healing. After skin closure, the wound should be covered with a sterile dressing and the patient observed in the recovery room.

Intraoperative Complications and Management

There are several procedure-related complications as well as equipment and refill-related considerations to keep in mind with IDDS devices. Table 20.1 outlines complications associated with IDDS implantation. Table 20.2 contains the PACC recommendations for IDDSs, and Table 20.3 provides updated recommendations for prevention and management of complications as published by the Centers for Disease Control and Prevention (CDC) and the Neuromodulation Appropriateness Consensus Committee (NACC).

TABLE 20.1 Procedural and Equipment Complications Associated with Intrathecal Drug Delivery System Implantation

Procedural complications
- Bleeding
- Cerebrospinal fluid leakage
- Postdural puncture headache
- Seroma formation
- Neurological injury
- Wound dehiscence
- Skin erosion
- Seroma
- Neuroma
- Infection
  - Surgical site
  - Deep infection
  - Discitis
  - Epidural abscess
  - Meningitis

Equipment complications
- Catheter malfunction
  - Dislodgement
  - Malposition
  - Migration
  - Kinking
  - Shearing
  - Puncture
  - Fracture
  - Leakage
  - Granuloma formation
- Pump malfunction
  - Pump failure
  - Battery failure
  - Pump rotation or flipping in the pocket
  - Overfilling

Refill-related complications
- Subcutaneous pocket
- Medication error
- Pump programming error

PROCEDURAL COMPLICATIONS

General procedure-related complications include bleeding, infection, wound dehiscence, and neurological injury. Complications specific to IDDS implantation include CSF leakage, postdural puncture headache, pump malposition, implant pocket seroma, meningitis, epidural abscess, epidural hematoma, spinal cord injury, and death. The conus medullaris could be damaged—its location should be evaluated on preprocedural imaging before placement.

TABLE 20.2 Polyanalgesic Consensus Conference Recommendations on Intrathecal Drug Infusion Systems, Training and Techniques Summary, 2017[1]

Training and Techniques
- Limited data exist as to appropriate and best catheter tip placement. The catheter should ideally be centered in the spinal dermatome associated with the pain generator. The consensus recommendation is that the doctor use clinical judgement based on the clinical setting.
- Each accredited facility should have the ability to evaluate an indwelling implanted device, including pump and catheter system.
- All patients admitted to a medical facility should have their IDDS documented as part of the medical record to include: IDDS type, manufacturer, medication(s), respective concentrations, daily dose, delivery modes, and if applicable electronic pump interrogation.
- Documentation of IDDS type and manufacturer of pump identification for drug delivery should be considered the standard of care prior to performing an MRI or pursuing elective surgery and is imperative for all patients admitted to a hospital.
- The training of all personnel for device evaluation and refilling is an important part of patient care. This training should be device specific and supervised carefully. The PACC recommends that 20 refills be supervised before independent practice is approved. Two or more trained individuals should check all reprogramming.
- In order to offer IT therapies regardless of primary specialty, the physician should be supervised in a minimum of 10 implant and/or explant cases.
- In order to maintain skills, the implanter should be involved in five cases over the course of two years or should undergo additional hands-on certified educational training to refresh skills.
- The training to manage an IT device is critical to the long-term success of the therapy. All pump management physicians should have ongoing educational training that includes knowledge of all current and FDA-approved devices and future devices approved by regulatory bodies for research and found to be clinically relevant.
- Managing physicians who are not implanting physicians are expected to be trained at the same level as those who both implant and manage devices.

FDA, US Food and Drug Administration; *IDDS,* intrathecal drug delivery system; *IT,* intrathecal; *MRI,* magnetic resonance imaging; *PACC,* Polyanalgesic Consensus Conference.

TABLE 20.3 Summary of Infection Management Practices from the Neurostimulation Appropriateness Consensus Committee and the Centers for Disease Control and Prevention Guidelines for the Prevention of Surgical Site Infections, 2017[3,4] (CDC Evidence Rank, NACC Consensus Strength)

Perioperative measures

- Optimize glucose control before implantation of device (IB, strong).
- Discontinue tobacco use before implantation of device (IB, strong).
- Decolonize MSSA and MSRA carriers through the application of mupirocin nasal ointment and chlorhexidine baths (strong).
- Antibiotics
  - Prophylactic antibiotics should be used for both trials and implants (IA, strong).
  - Weight-based antibiotic dosing is strongly recommended (IA, strong).
  - Use appropriate timing of prophylactic antimicrobial such that the bactericidal concentration is established in the serum and tissues at incision (IB, strong).
  - Vancomycin should not be used routinely (IB).
  - In clean and clean-contaminated procedures, do not administer additional prophylactic antimicrobial agent doses after the surgical incision is closed in the operating room, even in the presence of a drain (IA, strong).
- If hair is to be removed, use electric clippers immediately before surgery (IA).
- Keep nails short and do not wear artificial nails for both trials and implants (IB, strong).
- Do not wear hand or arm jewelry for trials or implants (IB, strong).

Intraoperative measures

- Utilize chlorhexidine gluconate for preoperative skin antiseptic agent (IB, strong).
- Perform preoperative surgical scrub for a minimum of 2–5 min with an appropriate antiseptic prior to neuromodulation trials and implants (IB, strong).
- Limit operating room (OR) traffic (II, strong).
- Maintain positive pressure ventilation and HEPA filters in the OR for implants (IB, strong).
- Keep the operating room doors closed during the procedure (IB, strong).
- Wear a surgical mask and fully cover hair for both trials and implants (IB, strong).
- Wear sterile gown and gloves for both trials and implants (IB, strong).
- Double glove (II, strong).
- If an incise drape is used, then iodophor-impregnated drape for implants is recommended (strong).
- Handle tissue gently, eradicate dead space, maintain hemostasis and avoid electrocautery at tissue surface (IB).
- Irrigate with saline through bulb syringe prior to closure of surgical wound (strong).
- Employ implant strategies to limit operative time (strong).

Postoperative measures

- Apply an occlusive sterile dressing following trials and implants for 24–48 h postoperatively (IB, strong).
- Do not routinely use topical antimicrobial agents for surgical wounds that are healing by primary intention (strong).
- If a dressing change is required, use hand washing (IB, strong) and sterile technique (II, moderate).
- Do not continue antimicrobial agents beyond 24 hours (strong).
- Understand maximum time criterion for defining a deep surgical site infection (SSI) of an implanted device: 1 year postimplant (strong).
- Educate patient and family on proper incision care, signs of infection, and reporting symptoms (II, strong).
- When SSI is suspected, prescribe an antibiotic that covers the likely causative organisms. Consider local resistance patterns and culture results in choosing an antibiotic (strong).

CDC Evidence Rankings. IA: Strongly recommended for implementation and supported by well-designed experimental, clinical, or epidemiological studies. IB: Strongly recommended for implementation and supported by some experimental, clinical, or epidemiological studies and strong theoretical rationale. II: Suggested for implementation and supported by suggestive clinical or epidemiological studies or theoretical rationale.

HEPA, High-efficiency particulate air; *MRSA,* methicillin-resistant *Staphylococcus aureus*; *MSSA,* methicillin-sensitive *S. aureus*.

Bleeding

Bleeding into the epidural space is rare with a pump placement performed by skilled clinicians. More commonly, bleeding of the surrounding tissue can result in seroma formation or bruising. This results from coagulopathy, ineffective intraoperative hemostasis, and trauma during epidural access. An epidural hematoma is a serious complication that every interventional pain physician should be able to recognize and appropriately work up in a timely manner. Acute epidural hematoma signs and symptoms include severe back pain, new leg weakness or spasms, new loss of distal extremity reflexes, and acute loss of bowel or bladder control. Suspicion of an epidural hematoma is considered a neurosurgical emergency, which requires urgent neurosurgical evaluation and immediate imaging. Acceptable imaging modalities include magnetic resonance imaging (MRI) or non–contrast computed tomography (CT) if MRI is unavailable or contraindicated.

Prevention of bleeding complications starts with the preoperative assessment and identification of coagulopathy based on comorbidities, anticoagulants, antiplatelet agents, nonsteroidal antiinflammatory medications, and the use of herbal supplements (e.g., ginkgo, garlic, ginseng, turmeric). Patient-related factors that may increase bleeding risk include quantitative or qualitative platelet abnormalities, abnormalities in clotting factors, and hepatic disease states. Medication decisions that affect clotting function should follow the 2017 guidelines from the NACC and the American Society of Regional Anesthesia and Pain Medicine for interventional spine and pain procedures in patients on antiplatelet and anticoagulant medications.[5,6]

Neurological Injury

Neurological injury is a serious complication that may result from trauma to the spinal cord during catheter placement into the IT space. This complication is rare, especially when performed by properly trained clinicians. Following the NACC guidelines helps reduce the risk of severe neurological injury.[7] Every patient should have a detailed baseline neurological examination preoperatively. Planning implantation should include reviewing the patient's imaging, such as X-rays, CT myelograms, and MRIs. Pathologies identified on imaging that may increase the risk of neurological injury comprise spinal metastasis, spinal stenosis, scoliosis, and areas of concern for compression fractures. In particular, patient positioning should be checked to avoid nerve compression since it is common to place the patient in the lateral position. Placement of the catheter in the lateral position may present challenges such as steering or resistance to advancing the catheter. Procedural skill is essential for prevention of intraoperative neurological trauma and equipment-related complications. For example, when encountering the challenge of inability to advance the catheter due to high resistance, then the needle and catheter together should be withdrawn. This technique is used to avoid sheering of the catheter. A conversive patient is important to ensure safety and is helpful in monitored anesthesia cases. In cases in which the physician chooses general anesthesia, neuromonitoring can help improve patient safety and reduce overall procedural risks. Postoperatively, a neurological examination should be well documented. New symptoms or physical examination signs warrant immediate evaluation with the indicated imaging, labs, and consideration of surgical exploration.

Cerebrospinal Fluid Leak

CSF leakage may result from intended dural puncture at the entry site or unintended dural puncture from catheter fracture, dislodgement, and migration. The reported incidence of IDDS procedure-related CSF leaks is about 20%.[8] The purse string method is used with the intended goal to reduce the number of dural punctures. During insertion, the catheter is threaded through a large-bore Touhy needle. Once the catheter is in the correct position, the Touhy needle is removed, leaving behind a dural puncture that is larger than the catheter. A CSF leak could occur around the catheter as a result but usually is self-limited. CSF leaking may persist, leading to symptoms of a postdural puncture headache. Postdural puncture headaches present as positional headaches, with exacerbation in the upright position and alleviation in the supine position. First-line management of postdural puncture headaches is conservative therapy, which consists of hydration, abdominal binder, positioning, caffeine, sumatriptan, and theophylline. If conservative therapies fail to effectively manage the symptoms, an epidural blood patch may be considered. An epidural blood patch is performed by taking 15 to 20 cc of autologous blood and readministering it at the puncture site. The epidural blood patch should be performed with aseptic technique under fluoroscopic guidance to avoid infection or catheter damage. Upon injection of whole blood, the dural puncture seals off, thereby resolving symptoms immediately. CSF leakage is rare when the clinician carefully plans preoperatively, takes intraoperative steps to minimize the number of spinal punctures, uses appropriate purse string placement, performs careful wound closure, and provides postoperative management.

Another consideration of CSF leakage is when the CSF leak occurs along the catheter, at the pump connection site, or through the incision. CSF leakage through the incision requires surgical revision to resuture the surgical wound.[9] When CSF leaks along the catheter or at the pump connection site, it may form a sterile collection of CSF in the subcutaneous tissue, termed a *CSF hygroma*. CSF hygromas present as a subcutaneous fluid collection on physical examination. CSF hygromas are usually small and self-resolve without clinical consequence. Management includes observation and avoiding aspiration due to concern for introduction of microorganisms that may lead to infection. If CSF hygromas are large and require aspiration, then strict aseptic technique should be followed and care taken to avoid damage to the implanted device.[9] If there is concern for infection, then hospitalization, explantation, and systemic antibiotics are warranted.

Measures that prevent the incidence of CSF leaks include consideration of preoperative risk factors and intraoperative procedural technique. Such techniques that may decrease the incidence of persistent CSF leakage include inserting the Tuohy needle with a steep paramedian approach to the spinal canal and suturing the catheter to the fascia.[9]

Seroma Formation

Occasionally, pockets develop a serosanguinous fluid collection that may last from a few days up to 2 months postimplantation (Fig. 20.1). These are more common with poor surgical technique, including poor management of hemostasis and rough handling of tissue. These seroma formations are usually self-limiting, with no clinical consequence. Management includes observation and patient reassurance. Similar to management of CSF hygromas, aspiration is avoided unless the fluid collection is excessive, persistent, and uncomfortable. Strict aseptic technique should be followed if aspiration is required.

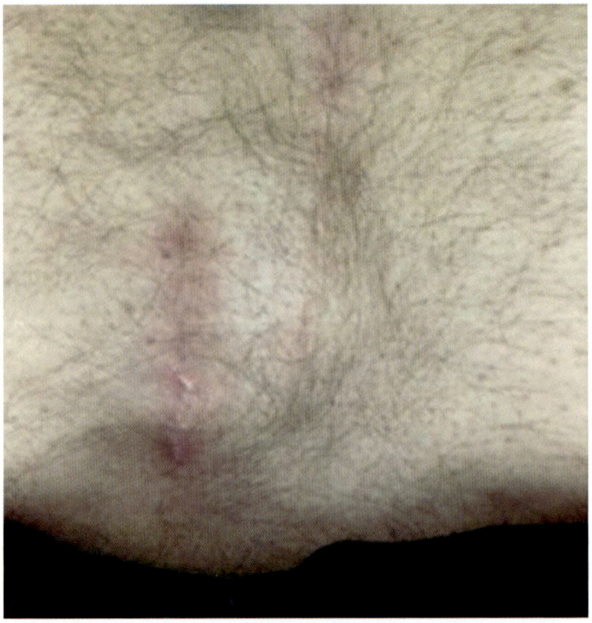

Fig. 20.1 Seroma formation along midline incision following implantation of an intrathecal drug delivery system. The patient denies positional headaches and placement of an abdominal binder has significantly reduced the size of the seroma. (From *Anesthesia Key*. Seroma or hygroma formation after implantation of an intrathecal drug delivery system or a spinal cord stimulator. Fig. 30.2. https://aneskey.com/seroma-or-hygroma-formation-after-implantation-of-an-intrathecal-drug-delivery-system-or-a-spinal-cord-stimulator)

Wound Dehiscence

Poor suture technique may result in wound breakdown and dehiscence (Fig. 20.2). In addition, patient factors may contribute to the risk of wound breakdown, such as uncontrolled diabetes, poor nutrition, chronic illness, obesity, high opioid intake, immunosuppression, smoking, direct compression due to being bed bound or wheelchair dependent, and from untreated seroma or hematoma. Other factors include significant weight loss after implantation, improper pump size to pocket ratio, improper pump positioning

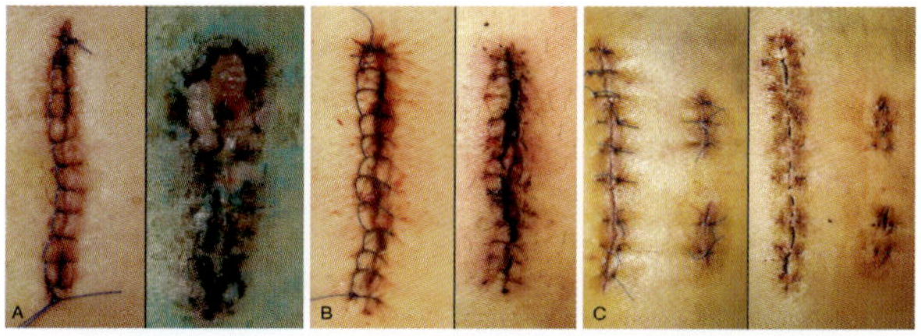

Fig. 20.2 Postoperative wound dehiscence. (Used with permission from Barrow Neurological Institute, Phoenix, Arizona)

and infection. Risk factors that could lead to wound breakdown should be considered in the preoperative evaluation to avoid dehiscence. For example, preexisting scars, ostomy sites, belt preference styles, and lifestyle concerns (e.g., wheelchair needs) should be contemplated when deciding on the surgical site since these factors could lead to excessive pressure over the wound, causing dehiscence or device malposition.

Infection

Infection of an implanted device is a serious complication. The incidence of device infection ranges from 0.7% to 5.2% and usually presents itself in the first 3 months postimplantation.[10,11] The clinical presentation of a surgical site infection may be pain at the surgical site, fever, chills, erythema, edema, fluctuant pocket, wound exudate, foul smell, induration at the incision or pump site, poor wound healing, or skin erosion. Most reported infections are superficial. However, the provider must rule out deeper infections, such as an epidural abscess (Fig. 20.3) because the catheter provides a direct path to the central nervous system. Working up a suspected infection should involve assessment of vital signs; in-office examination; and ordering white blood cell count, erythrocyte sedimentation rate (ESR), C-reactive protein, and aspiration of pocket fluid for cultures. A CT scan or MRI is essential if there is a suspicion for epidural abscess. Neurosurgical consultation is also recommended in the case of epidural abscess concern. Device removal is not required for most superficial infections. Immediate device removal is required when the patient presents with deep infections (e.g., epidural abscess or meningitis). If deep infection is present, then hospital

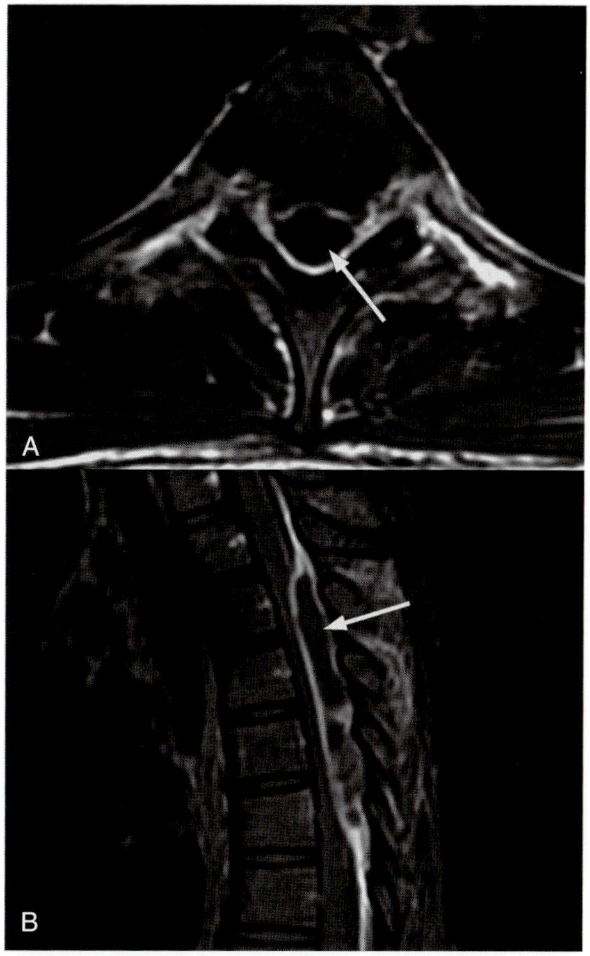

Fig. 20.3 T1-weighted, fat-suppressed, gadolinium-enhanced magnetic resonance images of the thoracic spine in a 26-year-old woman. Axial (A) and sagittal (B) images show posterior spinal epidural abscess at the T3 to T6 segments (*arrows*). Maximum measured thickness of the abscess was 8.0 mm at the level of T3/T4 vertebral bodies, whereas the spine in the narrowest region was 2.0 mm thick.[13] (Rosc-Bereza K, Arkuszewski M, Ciach-Wysocka E, Boczarska-Jedynak M. Spinal Epidural Abscess: Common Symptoms of an Emergency Condition. Neuroradiol J. 2013;26(4):464-468. doi:10.1177/197140091302600411)

admission and intravenous antibiotics based on culture sensitivities are needed as well.[10] Postoperative discitis is a serious complication, albeit rare, which is often misdiagnosed. Early diagnosis and treatment is critical to success. Management of discitis starts with antibiotics, analgesics, bed rest, and, if needed, surgical re-exploration with debridement of the disc space granulation tissue.[12] Preventing an infection begins with the preoperative evaluation. Preoperative evaluation of patient risk factors includes obesity, malnutrition, poor hygiene, decubitus ulcers, incontinence, debilitated status, insulin-dependent diabetes, chronic steroid use, autoimmune dysfunction, preexisting infection, and extremely thin body habitus. Implanting a drug delivery system should incorporate the guidelines for reducing surgical site infections, as updated by the CDC, NACC, and PACC best practice recommendations (see Table 20.2 and Table 20.3).[1,3,4]

General Considerations

EQUIPMENT-RELATED COMPLICATIONS

Equipment-related complications of IDDS include catheter and pump malfunction. Catheter-related complications comprise the majority of equipment-related complications. The reported annual incidence of such complications that require surgical revision ranges from 10.5% to 49.4%.[11]

Catheter-Related Complications

Catheter migration is the most common reported catheter-related complication.[14] Catheter migration may occur due to dislodgement at the dural entry site or from the origin of the pump. Catheter fractures often occur in areas where high stress is placed on the catheter. High stress areas include the reservoir and the anchoring site.[10] Catheter migration, fracture, kink, occlusion or dislodgement each can present with symptoms of withdrawal, new pain or increase in baseline pain levels, symptoms of a CSF leak, or spinal cord trauma. A kinked catheter may present with underdosing or motor stall. Imaging modalities employed should include plain radiography to facilitate detection of catheter tip migration, fractures, or dislodgement. A catheter contrast agent study, often referred to as a *pump-o-gram* (Fig. 20.4), can detect an occlusion, minor kink, leak, and fractures.[15] A catheter dye study employs nonionic radiocontrast dye to visualize the flow dynamics under direct fluoroscopy. Intrathecal gadolinium should be avoided because there have been case reports of fatalities and neurotoxicity with its use.[16,17] Gadolinium is not approved for IT use by the United States Food and Drug Administration. Before

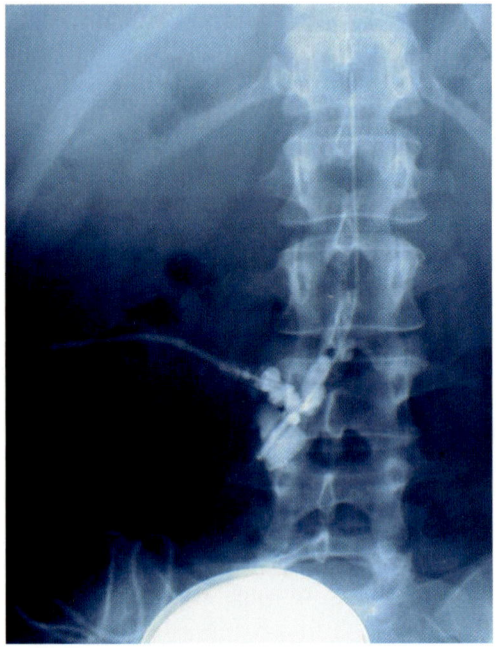

Fig. 20.4 Catheter-o-gram in a 49-year-old female patient with hereditary spastic paraparesis and implantation of a Medtronic pump for intrathecal baclofen therapy. Discontinuity/fracture of the catheter adjacent to the body of L3 on the right.[20] (Vaidyanathan, S., Soni, B.M., Oo, T. et al. Bladder stones – red herring for resurgence of spasticity in a spinal cord injury patient with implantation of Medtronic Synchromed pump for intrathecal delivery of baclofen – a case report. BMC Urol 3, 3 (2003). https://doi.org/10.1186/1471-2490-3-3)

performing a catheter contrast agent study, the side port should be accessed in a sterile fashion and aspiration attempted. If more than 0.3 mL of CSF is aspirated, then the catheter system is considered to be continuous. Contrast may then be injected into the side port. However, if CSF is not aspirated, then the clinician needs to consider the associated safety concerns of the study. Injecting the IT catheter with contrast could increase patient exposure to medications in the IDDS, leading to overdose. Before injecting dye, the clinician should assess the patient's clinical status and consider the type of medication in the pump and catheter, with attention to the catheter's dead space to understand the amount of medication that may be present in the catheter. Based on that information, the provider needs to be prepared to provide supportive care and possibly coordinate admission for observance or supportive care in the hospital depending on clinical judgment. Management of CSF leak due to IDDS catheter malfunction may include surgical revision to replace catheters that have been occluded, kinked, dislodged, or fractured.[18] In some cases, a kink may be released through simple manipulation if easily freed from scar tissue. Preventing IDDS catheter malfunction should include inserting the catheter under direct fluoroscopy, avoiding placing the catheter in spaces of high mobility and stress, and withdrawing the needle and catheter together to avoid sheering of the catheter.[19] Suturing the catheter to the underlying fascia may prevent migration. However, this does not preclude the catheter from coiling inside the IT space.

Granuloma Formation

A serious IDDS complication is granuloma formation, which happens at the catheter tip. This is a noninfectious collection of inflammatory cells. The reported incidence of granuloma formation at year 1 postimplant is 0.04%; at 6 years, it is 1.2%.[21] Intrathecal opioids at high doses or concentrations can increase the risk for granuloma development. For example, IT morphine shows a dose-dependent and concentration-dependent correlation with granuloma formation.[21] Clinical signs of granuloma development may involve poorly controlled pain and neurological signs (e.g., focal neurological deficits, numbness, bladder or bowel dysfunction, and weakness). Some devices are designed to curtail granuloma formation. These designs focus on incorporating multiple side holes at the most distal catheter tip. The design effectively achieves a larger CSF distribution of the drug.[14] It is thought that this design functions to reduce the local concentration of drug in the intrathecal space, thereby reducing the incidence of granuloma formation.

Pump Malfunction

The battery-powered IDDS pump may inadvertently rotate or flip in the pocket. The battery may also fail, and the pump may be overfilled.[9,10,18] When the pump is not correctly sutured down or if the pump pocket is larger than the pump itself, then the risk for pump torsion and flipping is increased. Pocket revision needs to be performed if the central port of the pump cannot be accessed or if torsion of the pump generates stress on the catheter, resulting in malfunction. Steps that may be taken to prevent pump malfunction include decreasing risk factors that lead to torsion. Making an appropriately sized pump pocket and appropriately anchoring the pump with four nonabsorbable sutures is beneficial.

Battery-powered pumps are programmable. Battery failure most often occurs when the battery reaches the end of its life span. At this point, battery replacement is needed. Battery life span depends on the brand and programming. Mechanical pump failure can occur when there is overpressurization (e.g., overfilling the reservoir) or filling of the pump with an incompatible medication.[9,18] Incompatible medications can damage the catheter and could force the telemetric receiver to new settings. Pump failure management requires battery replacement to continue therapy. Overfilling the pump can lead to failure because of the increased pressure placed on the IDDS. Overdose may be the presenting feature. Prevention includes using the appropriate refill kit provided by the manufacturer, following the manufacturer's protocol for pump refills, and the use of manometry.

REFILL-RELATED COMPLICATIONS

IT pump refill complications include pump programming errors, medication errors, and inadvertent drug administration into the subcutaneous tissue—a subcutaneous pocket. A subcutaneous pocket can occur when medication is inadvertently administered into the tissue space outside the pump reservoir. Incorrect drug selection and incorrect concentration are both examples of medication errors. Preventing these complications begins with following standard operation protocol for IT pump refills, which employ double checking all medications, dosing, concentrations, and documentation of pump interrogation before and after the pump refill. Inaccurate pump reprogramming, such as incorrect flow rate or incorrect medication concentration, can lead to under- or overdosing of medication, resulting in withdrawal or overdose, respectively. In the case of overdose, the pump should be aspirated for all medications and replaced with preservative-free saline followed by pump interrogation. The provider needs to be prepared to provide supportive care and arrange for possible intensive care unit transportation in the event of seizures, hemodynamic instability, respiratory depression, or cardiovascular collapse. In the case of difficult port access, the provider may choose to use direct fluoroscopy or ultrasonography to aid in locating the central refill port. Only trained providers who are comfortable with the refill technique should conduct pump refills. According to the PACC guidelines, 20 or more supervised pump refills should be undertaken before someone practices independently.[1]

REFERENCES

1. Deer TR, Pope JE, Hayek SM, et al. The Polyanalgesic Consensus Conference (PACC): recommendations on intrathecal drug infusion systems best practices and guidelines. *Neuromodulation*. 2017;20(2):96-132. doi:10.1111/ner.12538.
2. Krames E, Poree L, Deer T, Levy R. Implementing the SAFE principles for the development of pain medicine therapeutic algorithms that include neuromodulation techniques. *Neuromodulation*. 2009;12(2):104-113. doi:10.1111/j.1525-1403.2009.00197.x.
3. Berriós-Torres SI, Umscheid CA, Bratzler DW, et al. Centers for Disease Control and Prevention Guideline for the prevention of surgical site infection, 2017. *JAMA Surg*. 2017;152(8):784-791. doi:10.1001/jamasurg.2017.0904.
4. Deer TR, Provenzano DA, Hanes M, et al. The Neurostimulation Appropriateness Consensus Committee (NACC) recommendations for infection prevention and management. *Neuromodulation*. 2017;20(1):31-50. doi:10.1111/ner.12565.
5. Narouze S, Benzon HT, Provenzano D, et al. Interventional Spine and Pain Procedures in Patients on Antiplatelet and Anticoagulant Medications (Second Edition): Guidelines from the American Society of Regional Anesthesia and Pain Therapy, the American Academy of Pain Medicine, the International Neuromodulation Society, the North American Neuromodulation Society, and the World Institute of Pain. *Reg Anesth Pain Med*. 2018;43(3):225-262. doi:10.1097/AAP.0000000000000700.
6. Deer TR, Narouze S, Provenzano DA, et al. The Neurostimulation Appropriateness Consensus Committee (NACC): recommendations on bleeding and coagulation management in neurostimulation devices. *Neuromodulation*. 2017;20(1):51-62. doi:10.1111/ner.12542.
7. Deer TR, Lamer TJ, Pope JE, et al. The Neurostimulation Appropriateness Consensus Committee (NACC) safety guidelines for the reduction of severe neurological injury. *Neuromodulation*. 2017;20(1):15-30. doi:10.1111/ner.12564.
8. Knight KH, Brand FM, Mchaourab AS, Veneziano G. Implantable intrathecal pumps for chronic pain: highlights and updates. *Croat Med J*. 2007;48(1):22-34.
9. Krames ES. Intrathecal infusional therapies for intractable pain: patient management guidelines. *J Pain Symptom Manage*. 1993;8(1):36-46. doi:10.1016/0885-3924(93)90118-F.
10. Malinowski MN, Bremer N, Kim CH, Deer TR. Intrathecal drug delivery: indications, risks, and complications. In: Khelemsky Y, Malhotra A, Gritsenko K, eds. Acedemic Pain Medicine. Springer; 2019:139–142. doi:10.1007/978-3-030-18005-8.
11. Flückiger B, Knecht H, Grossmann S, Felleiter P. Device-related complications of long-term intrathecal drug therapy via implanted pumps. *Spinal Cord*. 2008;46(9):639-643. doi:10.1038/sc.2008.24.
12. Luzzati R, Giacomazzi D, Danzi MC, Tacconi L, Concia E, Vento S. Diagnosis, management and outcome of clinically-suspected spinal infection. *J Infect*. 2009;58(4):259-265.
13. Rosc-Bereza K, Arkuszewski M, Ciach-Wysocka E, Boczarska-Jedynak M. Spinal epidural abscess: common symptoms of an emergency condition. *Neuroradiol J*. 2013;26(4):464-468. doi:10.1177/197140091302600411.
14. Follett KA, Naumann CP. A prospective study of catheter-related complications of intrathecal drug delivery systems. *J Pain Symptom Manage*. 2000;19(3):209-215. doi:10.1016/S0885-3924(99)00153-0.
15. Dvorak EM, McGuire JR, Nelson ME. Incidence and identification of intrathecal baclofen catheter malfunction. *PM R*. 2010;2(8):751-756.
16. Hagedorn JM, Bendel MA, Moeschler SM, Lamer TJ, Pope JE, Deer TR. Intrathecal gadolinium use for the chronic pain physician. *Neuromodulation*. 2019;22(7):769-774. doi:10.1111/ner.13043.
17. Provenzano DA, Pellis Z, Deriggi L. Fatal gadolinium-induced encephalopathy following accidental intrathecal administration: a case report and a comprehensive evidence-based review. *Reg Anesth Pain Med*. 2019;44(7):721-729. doi:10.1136/rapm-2019-100422.
18. Krames E. Intraspinal opioid therapy for chronic nonmalignant pain: current practice and clinical guidelines. *J Pain Symptom Manage*. 1996;11(6):333-352.
19. Kari M, Jaycox M, Lubenow TR. Complications associated with intrathecal drug delivery systems. In: Deer T, ed. Intrathecal Drug Delivery for Pain and Spasticity: A Volume in the Interventional and Neuromodulatory Techniques for Pain Management Series. Philadelphia: Elsevier Inc.; 2012:102–108. doi:10.1016/b978-1-4377-2217-8.00014-3.
20. Vaidyanathan S, Soni BM, Oo T, et al. Bladder stones—red herring for resurgence of spasticity in a spinal cord injury patient with implantation of Medtronic Synchromed pump for intrathecal delivery of baclofen—a case report. *BMC Urol*. 2003;3(1):3. doi:10.1186/1471-2490-3-3.
21. Yaksh TL, Hassenbusch S, Burchiel K, Hildebrand KR, Page LM, Coffey RJ. Inflammatory masses associated with intrathecal drug infusion: a review of preclinical evidence and human data. *Pain Med*. 2002;3(4):300-312. doi:10.1046/j.1526-4637.2002.02048.x.

Chapter 21

Medications Used in Pain Pumps

David M. Schultz, Caitlin Bakke, and Amy Commers

Chapter Outline

Introduction

The first use of intrathecal opioid in humans occurred in 1979 at the Mayo Clinic in Rochester, Minnesota. In that year, Mayo anesthesiologist Josef Wang, MD injected morphine into the lumbar intrathecal spaces of eight patients with intractable cancer pain involving the low back and legs. Of the eight patients, six experienced dramatic pain relief. Dr. Wang published a three-page case report that ushered in a new era of targeted spinal drug delivery.[1] The first intrathecal (IT) drug delivery pump and catheter system was introduced in 1981. Over the past 40 years, technological and pharmacological advances have combined to make targeted spinal drug delivery a mainstay of 21st century pain management and a treatment of choice for the most difficult and refractory pain problems (Fig. 21.1).

In the early 1980s, shortly after its first IT use in humans, the US Food and Drug Administration (FDA) approved preservative-free morphine (Duramorph, Infumorph) for use in continuous IT infusion pumps.[2] Since that time, the only other IT pain pump medication to be approved by the FDA is ziconotide (Prialt), a neurotoxin derived from marine snail venom, which was approved in 2004.[3]

Many experienced pain specialist physicians who manage IT pain pumps believe that IT drugs other than morphine and ziconotide are safer and more effective at relieving pain and/or that IT drug admixtures provide overall better pain relief at lower medication dosages. In addition, some patients find monotherapy morphine or Prialt to be ineffective at relieving pain or patients experience debilitating side effects, leaving the managing physician to switch to off-label IT medications or to abandon IT therapy entirely. Morphine and ziconotide are FDA approved only as monotherapies because all admixtures of IT medications are unapproved, as are all compounded medications, and any approved medication that is altered in any way from the commercially available product—for example, Prialt—that has been diluted for IT use is off-label (Table 21.1).

Manufacturer registry data from Medtronic's Product Surveillance Registry (PSR)—formerly called the Implantable Systems Performance Registry (ISPR)—for Medtronic's targeted drug delivery (TDD) products reveal that over 80% of pain pump patients treated for chronic pain of noncancer origin receive IT medications that are not currently FDA approved in the United States for chronic IT use. Additionally, the percentage for off-label use escalates to greater than 90% in the patient population treated for cancer pain syndromes. In the United States therefore, most IT medications used in pain pumps are not FDA approved for this purpose.[4]

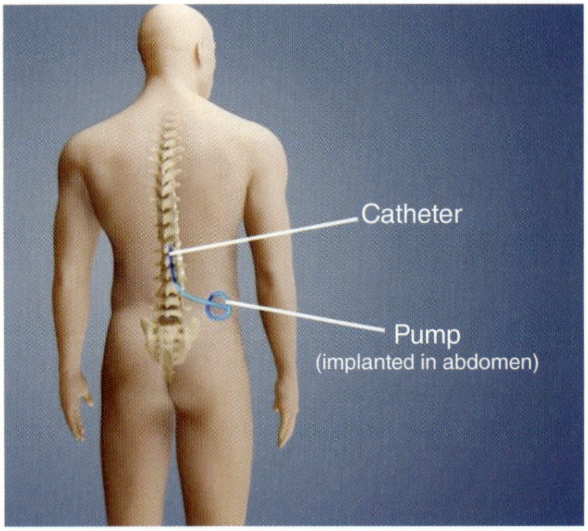

Fig. 21.1 Typical programmable pump intrathecal catheter system with patient controller. (From Medtronic.com. 2021. *Targeted Drug Delivery for Chronic Pain*. September 2020. https://www.medtronic.com/us-en/healthcare-professionals/products/neurological/drug-infusion-systems/synchromed-ii.html)

TABLE 21.1 FDA Approved Medicines for Use in Implanted Pain Pumps

The only approved medicines identified in implanted pump labeling for intrathecal infusion to treat or manage pain	Examples of medicines not identified in the implanted pump labeling for intrathecal infusion to treat or manage pain
Infumorph (morphine sulfate), preservative-free, injectable solution *Prialt (preservative-free ziconotide sterile solution)	Medicines not FDA approved for intrathecal administration or intrathecal implanted pump use (e.g., hydromorphone, bupivacaine, fentanyl, clonidine) Any mixture of two or more different kinds of medicines Any compounded medicine (e.g., to achieve higher concentration or different formulation of an FDA-approved medicine)

***The current labeling (instructions for use) of the implanted pump should be reviewed because not all pumps are currently approved for use with Prialt.**

From U.S. Food and Drug Administration. FDA Safety Communication: Use caution with implanted pumps for intrathecal administration of medicines for pain management. *Safety Communications*, November 2018. https://wayback.archive-it.org/7993/20190207180535/https://www.fda.gov/MedicalDevices/Safety/AlertsandNotices/ucm625789.html

What Does Off-Label Mean?

In the United States, the FDA has the responsibility to regulate foods, medical drugs and medical devices to protect the public. The FDA requires drug manufacturers to perform rigorous scientific studies to prove that a new drug will safely and effectively treat the disease for which it is intended. If scientific studies prove the product to be safe and effective for the disease or condition, then the FDA will issue a label that allows the company to market and sell the product for the labelled indication. The drug label is highly restrictive, however, allowing the company to market the drug to treat only the specific disease or condition for which it was studied. If the company wants to promote the product to treat a different disease or condition, it needs to perform additional scientific studies to prove safety and effectiveness for that specific disease. This system protects patients in the sense that it prevents companies from recklessly promoting drugs or devices for financial benefit to treat conditions for which they have not been proven safe and effective.

Once a drug or device is approved by the FDA for a specific indication and released into the marketplace, doctors begin to use this drug to treat their patients. During medical practice, doctors may learn that the product is effective in treating diseases or conditions for which it has not been thoroughly studied and for which it has not been approved by the FDA. The doctor is then faced with a dilemma: *Should I use the product to treat a condition for which it is not yet approved, or should I wait until the studies are done and the FDA changes the label to approve the product for this new use?*

However, randomized controlled trials are time-consuming and expensive. It may take years before additional studies on any drug or device are completed or studies may never be done, in which case the FDA may or may not change the label. In waiting for FDA approval, the doctor may be depriving the patient of a beneficial treatment. Since doctors are scientists who are trained to think critically and are primarily concerned with helping their patients, they may evaluate the existing scientific evidence regarding an available drug or device and make their own determination of safety and effectiveness to treat their patients. A doctor who decides that it is in a patient's best interest may prescribe a drug or device "off-label" to give the patient immediate benefit, before any formal approval by the FDA. There are many examples in medicine of drugs and devices being prescribed safely and effectively for off-label uses and this is often how new indications for approved drugs are discovered. Off-label prescribing is a time-tested and accepted medical practice; our American medical system considers it to be in the best interest of patients to allow physicians to prescribe medications off-label. The FDA does not regulate doctors or the practice of medicine. The FDA mission is to:

Protect the public health by ensuring the safety, efficacy, and security of human and veterinary drugs, biological products, and medical devices; and by ensuring the safety of our nation's food supply, cosmetics, and products that emit radiation. FDA is responsible for advancing the public health by helping to speed innovations that make medical products more effective, safer, and more affordable and by helping the public get the accurate, science-based information they need to use medical products and foods to maintain and improve their health.[5]

Although the FDA does not regulate doctors or the practice of medicine, it can certainly issue statements and warnings that influence health care payers and impact doctors and the patients they treat. For example, on November 14, 2018, the FDA issued a safety communication titled *Use Caution with Implanted Pumps for Intrathecal Administration of Medicines for Pain Management*[6] that has impacted the ability of pain specialists to effectively manage pump patients. FDA concerns about the use of off-label medications in pain pumps outlined in this communication include dosing errors, mechanical pump failures, and lack of safety and effectiveness data for compounded pump medications. The communication was met with widespread concern among the pain specialist community and resulted in a multispecialty letter signed by 21 specialized physicians representing leadership of the major pain and surgical societies, including the North American Neuromodulation Society (NANS), American Association of Neurological Surgeons (AANS), American Society of Interventional Pain Physicians (ASIPP), American Society of Pain and Neuroscience, American Society of Regional Anesthesia, and the International Neuromodulation Society. The multi-society response letter commented on each FDA concern as follows:

1. **Dosing errors:** Dosage errors occur equally with FDA-approved and non–FDA-approved medications. Errors can occur when there is inadequate vigilance regarding ordering the drug, dosage entry, and the subsequent programming of the IT device. The Polyanalgesia Consensus Conference (PACC) publications address the need for protocols to mitigate such errors.
2. **Mechanical pump failures:** In a registry specific to targeted drug delivery, 60 centers enrolled and included data for 7459 patients, with data collected between August 7, 2003 and July 31, 2016.[7] A total of 2330 programmable rotor pumps were classified as on-label, while a total of 5189 pumps were classified as off-label with exposure to an off-label drug/admixture. Thus, 69% of IT pumps were exposed to and used off-label drugs/admixtures. There was no statistically significant difference in the risk of failure between the on-label and off-label pumps implanted for the treatment of pain ($P = 0.31$). Further, in a valve-gated IT pump post-marketing study, the majority of patients maintained on IT therapy received off-label IT medications.[8] Another valve-gated IT pump post-marketing study showed that patients who received compounded versus commercially prepared IT morphine experienced improved efficacy with no difference in device-related failures, including pump failure and granuloma formation.[9]
3. **Safety and effectiveness of compounded pump medications:** The most recent PACC guidelines applied a validated evidence-ranking system from the US Preventive Services Task Force (USPSTF) to establish the hierarchy of studies, along with degrees of recommendation and level of consensus.[10] The panel's focus on safety, quality, efficacy, and transparency has not changed over the past 2 decades. To that end, it has been unequivocally established that the standard of care for IT therapy is to employ on-label and off-label medications for pain pump management

Regarding pump failure in pumps with off-label medications, more recent data discussed in the 2020 Medtronic PSR publication for targeted drug delivery[11] explained the following:

Design changes to the SynchroMed II pump models were implemented in 2016 to reduce the likelihood of nonrecoverable motor stalls due to component wear or corrosion, a failure in some circumstances associated with off-label drug exposure. Analysis of data from the first 21 months available presented at 2019 North American Neuromodulation Society Meeting (4) indicated a 21-month overall survival from product performance-related events with an underlying reported etiology related to pump function of 99.9%. (See **Table 21.2.***)*

In the United States, compounded morphine, hydromorphone, fentanyl, bupivacaine and clonidine, alone or in combination, are commonly used in pain pumps for targeted IT drug delivery. Each of these off-label spinal medications have a long track record of safety with IT use. In addition, numerous clinical studies have demonstrated the safety and effectiveness of these drugs and drug combinations for long-term IT infusion. The FDA has not yet approved any of these drugs for IT use in pain pumps and there is little hope for approval since these drugs are all generic, thus, not proprietary to any pharmaceutical company. It is unlikely that any company would spend the millions of dollars necessary to fund the scientific research required by the FDA to approve a generic medication for a new use without a financial incentive to do so based on future profits. Without FDA approval, how do doctors determine which pump medications are safe and effective?

The Advent of the Polyanalgesia Consensus Conference: A Living Document to Guide Targeted Drug Delivery Practitioners

After FDA approval of preservative-free morphine for IT use in 1984, physicians began to use IT morphine for the treatment of intractable chronic pain. In subsequent years, multiple untested IT medications were used in pain pumps by some practitioners when IT morphine proved ineffective or caused intolerable side effects. In the 1990s, a variety of drugs intended for other uses were employed for IT injection or infusion, causing unpredictable results and occasional neurotoxicity.

The haphazard use of untested IT medications underscored the need for scientific, evidence-based guidance in the form of an algorithm for safe and effective IT drug delivery. In 2000, neurosurgeon Sam Hassenbush, MD convened an international panel of expert pain pump physicians to discuss best practices for targeted IT drug delivery and to create written evidenced-based guidelines for practitioners. The resulting consensus publications, called the Polyanalgesia Consensus Conference (PACC), summarized available scientific evidence to provide guidelines in the use of off-label TDD medications. The PACC is an international group

TABLE 21.2 Failure Summary Table: All Therapies

Category	Survival at 1 y, Sample Size	Survival at 2 y, Sample Size	Survival at 3 y, Sample Size	Survival at 4 y, Sample Size	Survival at 5 y, Sample Size	Survival at 6 y, Sample Size	At 81 Mo Survival at 81 mo, Sample Size	Survival at 7 y, Sample Size
Overall	99.5% 6174	99.1% 4924	98.3% 3807	96.9% 2831	93.8% 2017	89.1% 1334	79.9% 161	77.7% 25
On-label	99.7% 1929	99.5% 1497	99.0% 1114	98.2% 824	96.9% 586	95.2% 413	86.8% 38	
Off-label	99.5% 4245	98.9% 3427	98.0% 2693	96.4% 2007	92.6% 1431	86.7% 921	77.2% 123	

Data from 2019 Medtronic study shows that out of 6174 patients, more than 65% of patients had off-label drugs in their intrathecal pain pumps. It also compares the survival rates of pumps with on-label versus off-label medications. (https://www.medtronic.com/content/dam/medtronic-com/products/product-performance/ppr-reports/2019-product-performance-report-combined.pdf.)

of pain physician experts who met first in 2000 and then again in 2003, 2007, 2012, and 2017 to review current published data on IT drugs and to update guidelines. The consensus panel focused on current expert practice, with the goal of creating an evolving document that would generate consensus publications, updated over time, to guide clinicians in the selection of appropriate candidates for IT therapy, the choice of appropriate medications with starting doses and concentrations, and the ongoing management of devices used to deliver IT therapy. The most recent PACC guidelines (2017) applied a validated evidence-ranking system from the USPSTF to establish the hierarchy of studies, along with degrees of recommendation and level of consensus. The panel's focus on safety, quality, efficacy, and transparency has been consistent over the past 2 decades. The PACC has established that the standard of care in the United States for IT pain therapy is to employ both on-label and off-label medications.

The Evolution of the Polyanalgesia Consensus Conference Guidelines

PACC 2003 focused on reviewing published scientific literature on IT medications from 1999 to 2003, developing guidelines for optimizing drug dosage and concentration, creating a process for documenting minimum evidence supporting the use of a drug for spinal infusion, and clarifying recommendations for compounding IT medications.[12] The following IT medications were used in the PACC 2003 study[12]:

- Opioids
  - Morphine
  - Hydromorphone
  - Fentanyl
  - Sufentanil
  - Methadone
  - Meperidine
- Local Anesthetics
  - Bupivacaine
  - Ropivacaine
  - Tetracaine
- Adrenergic Agonists
  - Clonidine
  - Tizanidine
- *N*-methyl-D-aspartate (NMDA) Antagonist
  - Ketamine
- Other Agents
  - Adenosine
  - Aspirin
  - Baclofen
  - Droperidol
  - Gabapentin
  - Ketorolac
  - Midazolam
  - Neostigmine
  - Octreotide
  - Ziconotide

Based on a review of literature, PACC 2003 recommended maximum daily dosages and concentrations for the four IT medications they considered to be initial choices[12]:

- 15 mg/day of morphine at 30 mg/mL
- 10 mg/day of hydromorphone at 30 mg/mL
- 30 mg/day of bupivacaine at 38 mg/mL
- 1.0 mg/day of clonidine at 2.0 mg/mL

For future research, the authors summarized a framework for evidence review[12]:

- Preclinical Studies
  - Essential Criteria
    - Solubility
    - pH
    - Stability at room temperature in solution
    - Stability at room temperature in device
    - Stability at body temperature in solution
    - Compatibility with delivery device
    - Animal Studies
  - Essential Criteria
    - Toxicity (side effects and neurotoxicity)
  - Desirable Criteria
    - Mechanism/site of action
    - Pharmacokinetics
    - Efficacy
- Clinical Studies
  - Essential Criteria
    - Side effects
    - Safety
  - Desirable Criteria
    - Pharmacokinetics
    - Existence of FDA labelling
- Efficacy Studies
  - Desirable Criteria
    - Case report
    - Case series

- Historical case control
- Randomized controlled trial
- Database
  - Desirable Criteria
    - Registry of patients
    - Receiving treatment
    - Safety

PACC 2003 came up with an algorithmic recommendation for IT medications that focused on morphine, hydromorphone, bupivacaine, and clonidine, all drugs commonly used today and supported by cumulative data. In 2003, fentanyl, sufentanil, midazolam, and baclofen were considered fourth-line options whereas neostigmine, adenosine, ketorolac, ropivacaine, meperidine, gabapentin, buprenorphine, and octreotide were considered investigational and only for "selected patients"[12]:

Line 1[a]: Morphine or hydromorphone[e]

Line 2[b,c]: Morphine (or hydromorphone) + bupivacaine *or* morphine (or hydromorphone) + clonidine[d]

Line 3: Morphine (or hydromorphone) + bupivacaine + clonidine

Line 4: Fentanyl, sufentanil, midazolam, baclofen Ziconotide[h]

For Selected Patients Only

Line 5[f]: Neostigmine, adenosine, ketorolac

Line 6[g]: Ropivacaine, meperidine, gabapentin, buprenorphine, octreotide, other[i]

[a] If side effects occur, switch to the other opioid.

[b] If maximum dosage is reached without adequate analgesia, add adjuvant medication (Line 2).

[c] If patient has neuropathic pain, consider starting with opioid monotherapy (morphine or hydromorphone) or, in selected patients with pure or predominant neuropathic pain, consider opioid plus adjuvant medication (bupivacaine or clonidine; Line 2).

[d] Some of the panel advocated the use of bupivacaine first because of concern about clonidine-induced hypotension.

[e] If side effects or lack of analgesia on second first-line opioid, may switch to fentanyl (Line 4).

[f] There are limited preclinical data and limited clinical experience; therefore, caution in the use of these agents should be considered.

[g] There are insufficient preclinical data and limited clinical experience; therefore, extreme caution in the use of those agents should be considered.

[h] The specific line to be determined after FDA review

[i] Potential spinal analgesics: Methadone, oxymorphone, NMDA antagonists

Over the next decade, new information and data became available. PACC 2012 authors summarized their mission as follows:

The use of intrathecal (IT) infusion of analgesic medications to treat patients with chronic refractory pain has increased since its inception in the 1980s, and the need for clinical research in IT therapy is ongoing. The Polyanalgesic Consensus Conference (PACC) panel of experts convened in 2000, 2003, and 2007 to make recommendations on the rational use of IT analgesics based on preclinical and clinical literature and clinical experiences.

The PACC panel convened again in 2011 to update the standard of care for IT therapies to reflect current knowledge gleaned from literature and clinical experience. A thorough literature search was performed, and information from this search was provided to panel members. Analysis of published literature was coupled with the clinical experience of panel members to form recommendations regarding the use of IT analgesics to treat chronic pain.

After a review of literature published from 2007 to 2011 and discussions of clinical experience, the panel created updated algorithms for the rational use of IT medications for the treatment of neuropathic pain and nociceptive pain.[13]

PACC 2012 recommendations refined the 2003 recommendations as follows:

1. The authors updated the list of recommended medications with FDA approved (first line) as well as non–FDA approved (second-fifth line) IT pain pump medications.[13]

   Line 1: Morphine *or* hydromorphone *or* ziconotide *or* fentanyl

   Line 2: Morphine + bupivacaine *or* ziconotide + opioid *or* hydromorphone + bupivacaine *or* fentanyl + bupivacaine

   Line 3: Opioid (morphine, hydromorphone, or fentanyl) + clonidine *or* sufentanil

   Line 4: Opioid + clonidine + bupivacaine *or* sufentanil + bupivacaine *or* clonidine

   Line 5: Sufentanil + bupivacaine + clonidine

   Commentary:

   Line 1: Morphine and ziconotide are approved by the FDA for IT therapy and are recommended as first-line therapy for nociceptive pain. Hydromorphone is recommended based on widespread clinical use and apparent safety. Fentanyl has been upgraded to first-line use by the consensus conference. **Line 2:** Bupivacaine in combination with morphine, hydromorphone, or fentanyl is recommended. Alternatively, the combination of ziconotide and an opioid drug can be employed. **Line 3:** Recommendations include clonidine plus an opioid (i.e., morphine, hydromorphone, or fentanyl) or sufentanil monotherapy. **Line 4:** The triple combination of an opioid, clonidine, and bupivacaine is recommended. An alternative recommendation is sufentanil in combination with either bupivacaine or clonidine. **Line 5:** The triple combination of sufentanil, bupivacaine, and clonidine is suggested.

2. They recommended against using certain drugs based on concerns about potential neurotoxicity. The drugs that have demonstrated neurotoxicity and are not recommended for IT use (except for specific cases) included[13]:
   - Opioids
     - Meperidine
     - Methadone
     - Tramadol
   - Local anesthetic
     - Tetracaine
   - Adrenergic agonist
     - Dexmedetomidine
   - *N*-methyl-D-aspartate (NMDA) antagonist
     - All agents in this group
   - Other nonopioids
     - Droperidol
     - Midazolam
     - Methylprednisolone
     - Ondansetron
3. They categorized various drugs as probably safe but without proven efficacy[13]:
   - GABA analogs
     - Gabapentin
     - Baclofen
   - Peptidomimetic
     - Octreotide
   - Local anesthetic
     - Ropivacaine
4. They provided separate recommendations for drugs to be used for neuropathic pain vs. nociceptive pain with ziconotide as a potential first-line drug for either indication. Of note is that the mainstay drugs morphine, hydromorphone, bupivacaine, and clonidine from PACC 2003 continue to be primary choices in PACC 2012. In addition, fentanyl and sufentanil moved up in the algorithmic hierarchy.[13]

Recommendations for IT medications for neuropathy include:

Line 1: Morphine *or* ziconotide *or* morphine + bupivacaine

Line 2: Hydromorphone *or* hydromorphone + bupivacaine or hydromorphone + clonidine *or* morphine + clonidine

Line 3: Clonidine *or* ziconotide + opioid *or* fentanyl *or* fentanyl + bupivacaine *or* fentanyl + clonidine

Line 4: Opioid + clonidine + bupivacaine *or* bupivacaine + clonidine

Line 5: Baclofen

Commentary:

Line 1: Morphine and ziconotide are approved by the FDA for IT therapy and are recommended as first-line therapy for neuropathic pain. The combination of morphine and bupivacaine is recommended for neuropathic pain because of clinical use and apparent safety. **Line 2:** Hydromorphone, alone or in combination with bupivacaine or clonidine, is recommended. Alternatively, the combination of morphine and clonidine may be used. **Line 3:** Third-line recommendations for neuropathic pain include clonidine, ziconotide plus an opioid, and fentanyl alone or in combination with bupivacaine or clonidine. **Line 4:** The combination of bupivacaine and clonidine (with or without an opioid drug) is recommended. **Line 5:** Baclofen is recommended based on safety, although reports of efficacy are limited.

The following is an updated list of recommended medications for IT pain pumps:

Line 1: Morphine *or* hydromorphone *or* ziconotide *or* fentanyl

Line 2: Morphine + bupivacaine *or* ziconotide + opioid *or* hydromorphone + bupivacaine *or* fentanyl + bupivacaine
Line 3: Opioid (morphine, hydromorphone, or fentanyl) + clonidine *or* sufentanil
Line 4: Opioid + clonidine + bupivacaine *or* sufentanil + bupivacaine or clonidine
Line 5: Sufentanil + bupivacaine + clonidine
Commentary:
Line 1: Morphine and ziconotide are approved by the FDA for IT therapy and are recommended as first-line therapy for nociceptive pain. Hydromorphone is recommended based on widespread clinical use and apparent safety. Fentanyl has been upgraded to first-line use by the consensus conference. **Line 2:** Bupivacaine in combination with morphine, hydromorphone, or fentanyl is recommended. Alternatively, the combination of ziconotide and an opioid drug can be employed. **Line 3:** Recommendations include clonidine plus an opioid (i.e., morphine, hydromorphone, or fentanyl) or sufentanil monotherapy **Line 4:** The triple combination of an opioid, clonidine, and bupivacaine is recommended. An alternative recommendation is sufentanil in combination with either bupivacaine or clonidine. **Line 5:** The triple combination of sufentanil, bupivacaine, and clonidine is suggested.

In addition, PACC 2012 recommended starting dosages and dose ranges for both trialing and continuous infusion after implantation for the commonly used IT drugs.[13]

The recommended starting dosage ranges of IT medications included:

- Morphine: 0.1–0.5 mg/day
- Hydromorphone: 0.02–0.5 mg/day
- Ziconotide: 0.5–2.4 μg/day
- Fentanyl: 25–75 μg/day
- Bupivacaine: 1–4 mg/day
- Clonidine: 40–100 μg/day
- Sufentanil: 10–20 μg/day

The recommended doses for IT bolus trialing included:

- Morphine: 0.2–1.0 mg
- Hydromorphone: 0.04–0.2 mg
- Ziconotide: 1–5 μg
- Fentanyl: 25–75 μg
- Bupivacaine: 0.5–2.5 mg
- Clonidine: 5–20 μg
- Sufentanil: 5–20 μg

Finally, PACC 2012 recommended maximum concentrations and maximum doses of the commonly used IT drugs to reduce the incidence of precipitation and catheter tip granuloma.[13]

- Morphine
  - Maximum concentration: 20 mg/mL
  - Maximum dose per day: 15 mg
- Hydromorphone
  - Maximum concentration: 15 mg/mL
  - Maximum dose per day: 10 mg
- Fentanyl
  - Maximum concentration: 10 mg/mL
  - Maximum dose per day: No known upper limit
- Sufentanil
  - Maximum concentration: 5 mg/mL
  - Maximum dose per day: No known upper limit
- Bupivacaine
  - Maximum concentration: 30 mg/mL
  - Maximum dose per day: 10 mg
- Clonidine
  - Maximum concentration: 1000 μg/mL
  - Maximum dose per day: 40–600 μg
- Ziconotide
  - Maximum concentration: 100 μg/mL
  - Maximum dose per day: 19.2 mg

In the most recent conference, PACC 2017, the focus was expanded to address three separate aspects of TDD with three separate publications: IT Infusion Best Practices, IT Trialing Best Practices, and IT Infusion Risk Mitigation.

PACC 2017 authors explained their approach as follows:

Pain treatment is best performed when a patient-centric, safety-based philosophy is used to determine an algorithmic process to guide care. Since 2007, the International Neuromodulation Society has organized a group of experts to evaluate evidence and create a Polyanalgesic Consensus Conference (PACC) to guide practice.

The current PACC update is designed to address the deficiencies and innovations emerging since the previous PACC publication of 2012. An extensive literature search identified publications between January 15, 2007 and November 22, 2015 and authors contributed additional relevant sources. After reviewing the literature, the panel convened to determine evidence levels and degrees of recommendations for intrathecal therapy. This meeting served as the basis for consensus development, which was ranked as strong, moderate or weak. Algorithms were developed for intrathecal medication choices to treat nociceptive and neuropathic pain for patients with cancer, terminal illness, and noncancer pain, with either localized or diffuse pain.

The PACC has developed an algorithmic process for several aspects of intrathecal drug delivery to promote safe and efficacious evidence-based care. Consensus opinion, based on expertise, was used to fill gaps in evidence. Thirty-one consensus points emerged from the panel considerations.[14]

PACC 2017 made recommendations as to disease indications in patient selection for TDD[14]:

- Axial neck or back pain; not a surgical candidate
  - Multiple compression fractures
  - Discogenic pain
  - Spinal stenosis
  - Diffuse multiple-level spondylosis
- Failed back surgery syndrome
- Abdominal/pelvic pain
  - Visceral
  - Somatic
- Extremity pain
  - Radicular pain
  - Joint pain
- Complex regional pain syndrome (CRPS)
- Trunk pain
  - Postherpetic neuralgia
  - Post-thoracotomy syndrome
- Cancer pain, direct invasion and chemotherapy related
- Analgesic efficacy with systemic opioid delivery complicated by intolerable side effects

With regard to medication recommendations and an updated treatment algorithm, PACC 2017 continued to recommend morphine, ziconotide, hydromorphone, bupivacaine, clonidine, and fentanyl as reasonable choices with slight differences in the algorithmic hierarchy for localized versus diffuse cancer pain and localized versus diffuse noncancer pain. Recommendations did not differ based on whether pain was nociceptive or neuropathic.[14]

IT medication recommendations for cancer or other terminal condition-related pain with localized nociceptive or neuropathic pain include:

<u>Line 1A:</u> Ziconotide *or* morphine
<u>Line 1B:</u> Fentanyl *or* morphine or fentanyl + bupivacaine
<u>Line 2:</u> Hydromorphone *or* hydromorphone + bupivacaine *or* hydromorphone or fentanyl or morphine + clonidine *or* morphine or hydromorphone or fentanyl + bupivacaine + ziconotide
<u>Line 3:</u> Hydromorphone or morphine or fentanyl + bupivacaine + clonidine *or* ziconotide + bupivacaine *or* ziconotide + clonidine *or* Hydromorphone or morphine or fentanyl + bupivacaine + ziconotide *or* sufentanil
<u>Line 4:</u> Sufentanil + ziconotide *or* sufentanil + bupivacaine *or* baclofen *or* sufentanil + clonidine *or* bupivacaine + clonidine + ziconotide *or* Bupivacaine + clonidine
<u>Line 5:</u> Sufentanil + bupivacaine + clonidine
<u>Line 6:</u> Opioid* + bupivacaine + clonidine + adjuvants**

IT medication recommendations for cancer or other terminal condition–related pain with diffuse nociceptive or neuropathic pain include:

<u>Line 1A:</u> Ziconotide *or* morphine
<u>Line 1B:</u> Hydromorphone *or* morphine or hydromorphone + bupivacaine
<u>Line 2:</u> Hydromorphone or morphine + clonidine *or* morphine or hydromorphone + ziconotide
<u>Line 3:</u> Hydromorphone or morphine or fentanyl + bupivacaine + clonidine *or* ziconotide + bupivacaine *or* ziconotide + clonidine *or* hydromorphone or morphine or fentanyl + bupivacaine + ziconotide *or* sufentanil
<u>Line 4:</u> Sufentanil + ziconotide *or* baclofen *or* sufentanil + bupivacaine *or* sufentanil + clonidine *or* bupivacaine + clonidine + ziconotide *or* bupivacaine + clonidine

*All known IT opioids
**Adjuvants include midazolam, ketamine, and octreotide

Line 5: Sufentanil + bupivacaine + clonidine *or* sufentanil + bupivacaine + ziconotide

Line 6: Opioid* + bupivacaine + clonidine + adjuvants**

IT medication recommendations for noncancer-related pain with localized nociceptive or neuropathic pain include:

Line 1A: Ziconotide *or* morphine

Line 1B: Fentanyl *or* fentanyl + bupivacaine

Line 2: Fentanyl + clonidine *or* hydromorphone or morphine + bupivacaine *or* fentanyl + bupivacaine + clonidine *or* bupivacaine

Line 3: Fentanyl + ziconotide + bupivacaine **or** Morphine or hydromorphone + clonidine **or** Ziconotide + clonidine or bupivacaine or both **or** Bupivacaine + clonidine

Line 4: Sufentanil + bupivacaine + clonidine *or* baclofen *or* bupivacaine + clonidine + ziconotide

Line 5: Sufentanil + bupivacaine + clonidine *or* sufentanil + ziconotide

IT medication recommendations for noncancer-related pain with diffuse nociceptive or neuropathic pain include:

Line 1A: Morphine *or* ziconotide*

Line 1B: Hydromorphone *or* morphine or hydromorphone + bupivacaine

Line 3: Hydromorphone or morphine + clonidine *or* fentanyl + bupivacaine *or* ziconotide + morphine or hydromorphone

Line 4: Hydromorphone or morphine + bupivacaine + clonidine *or* fentanyl + ziconotide *or* sufentanil + bupivacaine or clonidine *or* ziconotide + clonidine or bupivacaine or both

Line 5: Fentanyl or sufentanil + bupivacaine + clonidine *or* sufentanil + ziconotide *or* baclofen

Line 6: Opioid + ziconotide + bupivacaine or clonidine

*All known IT opioids

**Adjuvants include midazolam, ketamine, and octreotide

*Ziconotide should be first choice in patients with >120 morphine equivalents or fast systemic dose escalation, in the history of psychosis.

PACC 2017 also updated recommendations as to starting doses and concentrations, trial bolus doses, and maximum continuous infusion doses and concentrations as follows.[14]*

The recommended starting dosage ranges of IT medications for long-term therapy delivery include:

- Morphine: 0.1–0.5 mg/day
- Hydromorphone: 0.001–0.15 mg/day
- Ziconotide: 0.5–1.2 μg/day (to 2.4 μg/day per product labeling)
- Fentanyl: 25–75 μg/day
- Bupivacaine: 0.01–4 mg/day
- Clonidine: 20–100 μg/day
- Sufentanil: 10–20 mg/day

The recommended doses for IT bolus trialing include the following.

- Morphine: 0.1–0.5 mg/day
- Hydromorphone: 0.025–0.1 mg/day
- Ziconotide: 1–5 μg/day
- Fentanyl: 15–75 μg/day
- Bupivacaine: 0.5–2.5 mg/day
- Clonidine: 5–20 μg/day
- Sufentanil: 5–20 mg/day

Maximum concentrations and daily doses of IT agents as recommended by PACC 2012[8] and 2016 include:*

- Morphine
  - Maximum concentration: 20 mg/mL
  - Maximum dose per day: 15 mg
- Hydromorphone
  - Maximum concentration: 15 mg/mL
  - Maximum dose per day: 10 mg
- Fentanyl
  - Maximum concentration: 10 mg/mL
  - Maximum dose per day: 1000 μg
- Sufentanil
  - Maximum concentration: 5 mg/mL
  - Maximum dose per day: 500 μg
- Bupivacaine

*Starting doses of continuous IT delivery should be half of the trial dose for opioid-based medications.

*Starting doses of medication in the opioid-naïve patient for outpatient bolus delivery do not exceed 0.15 mg morphine, 0.04 mg hydromorphone, or 25 μg fentanyl.

- Maximum concentration: 30 mg/mL
- Maximum dose per day: 15–20 mg*

- Clonidine
  - Maximum concentration: 1000 μg/mL
  - Maximum dose per day: 600 μg
- Ziconotide
  - Maximum concentration: 100 μg/mL
  - Maximum dose per day: 19.2 mg

Pharmacy and Compounding Information

At present, IT pump drugs that are commonly used and widely accepted include morphine, ziconotide, hydromorphone, fentanyl, baclofen, bupivacaine, and clonidine. All of these medications must be compounded except for morphine and ziconotide, which are available as on-label commercial preparations. The FDA-approved, commercially prepared morphine and ziconotide are available in limited concentrations and, therefore, restrict the ability of physicians to customize dosages for their patients while maintaining on-label use.

Lioresal and Gablofen (commercial preparations of baclofen) are FDA approved for spasticity but not for pain. Baclofen is sometimes used as an adjunct medication in pump admixtures, particularly if the patient has pain associated with spasticity or muscle spasm. It is off-label when used for pain or when combined with any other medication. Ketamine is also compounded for use in pain pumps but is typically reserved for terminal cancer patients with short life expectancy since ketamine may be neurotoxic with prolonged use.

FDA-approved drugs must go through rigorous phase 1, phase 2, and phase 3 clinical trials to prove safety and efficacy for the condition they are intended to treat. Once approved, the manufacturing process for these drugs is governed by federal regulations and drug manufacturing must occur in 503B-compliant facilities that are subject to rigorous monitoring and inspection by the FDA. 503B pharmacies are typically large, commercial operations that cost millions of dollars to build and are subject to FDA regulations and inspections. 503B facilities are allowed to compound large quantities of medication for sale with or without patient-specific prescriptions. Regardless of facility, United States Pharmacopeia (USP) 797 requires every compounded product to have a Beyond Use Date (BUD) assigned to it. The BUD takes into consideration how the product should be stored, whether the products used to compound were sterile or nonsterile, and how the final product was eventually sterilized if nonsterile products were used to compound.

Compounding pharmacies, on the other hand, are under less rigorous control and are monitored and overseen by state boards of pharmacy. Rules for compounding pharmacies are less stringent than rules for manufacturing pharmacies and concerns about safety with sterile-compounded IT medications are well founded, especially after the New England Compounding Pharmacy contamination disaster of 2012. PACC 2012 addresses these compounding safety concerns as follows.

1. ***Training of personnel:*** *Compounding personnel should be adequately trained in aseptic technique and manipulation of compounded sterile preparations. Personnel should undergo scheduled and periodic evaluations, appropriately use gowns and gloves, have a thorough understanding of compounded pharmaceuticals, and perform aseptic media fill unit testing. Training and evaluations should be documented.*
2. ***Segregated sterile compounding area:*** *The compounding environment must be a dedicated, enclosed area segregated from surrounding spaces to reduce the risk of contamination. Proper temperature, humidity, and air filtration controls must be used for activities and work within the sterile compounding area should be conducted only by those individuals who are directly involved with sterile compounding. The sterile compounding area should be physically designed and environmentally controlled to reduce the risk of airborne contamination.*
3. ***Air quality of the compounding area:*** *The sterile compounding area should be certified every six months. Primary engineering controls (i.e., IV hoods) and devices should be placed in the sterile compounding area, and the air quality should be no less than International Standards for Organization (ISO) 7 standards. Equipment must be procured and maintained as necessary to safely compound and monitor*

*May be exceeded in end-of-life care and complicated cases as determined by medical necessity

the environment. Primary laminar airflow workbenches should provide an environment of ISO 5 or better; ISO 5 represents an air quality not exceeding 3520 particles of 0.5 microns per cubic meter. Air changes per hour must be maintained per USP standards; air pressure differential should be monitored. Environmental monitoring should be implemented to demonstrate that primary engineering controls will maintain air quality. Such monitoring consists of assessment of viable (bacteria) and nonviable (particulates) levels. Environmental air sampling should occur as an integral component of a comprehensive quality assurance program. Active air sampling should occur at least every six months to properly assess the air quality and cleaning program. An appropriate sampling plan should be developed based on the size and design of the compounding area. Action levels and alerts should be established.

4. **Equipment should be certified and calibrated** *annually, and staff must be trained and knowledgeable in its operation.*
5. **A cleaning and disinfection program** *must be implemented with attention to the agents used in the compounding area.*
6. ***Quality assurance program:*** *A comprehensive quality assurance program should be in writing and implemented to include monitoring and evaluation of the compounding staff and the compounding environment. All factors associated with preparations and dispensing of products should be considered. Policies should describe specific monitoring and evaluation. A robust random sampling program to assess final product accuracy is imperative. The quality assurance program must be continuous in activity to ensure optimal outcomes. Generally, the identification of indicators and the effectiveness of the quality assurance program should be reassessed yearly. The long-term goal is to have this be the benchmark for quality in all countries where IT therapy is utilized.*

One advantage to compounded pump medications is that they can be tailored to the patient's specific needs based on the managing physician's order. With compounded pump medications, the pharmacist makes a customized syringe by calculating the amount of USP powder to achieve the physician-specified concentrations and dosages.

As to regulation of compounding pump medications, most compounding pharmacies are 503A facilities, which are regulated by the state and not subject to routine FDA inspections. For compounded IT pump medications, one of the issues is the BUD. Unlike manufactured drugs which have a prolonged shelf life, sterilely compounded medications have a relatively short shelf life measured in hours or days. The BUD can sometimes be extended if sterility testing is performed and passed (Fig. 21.2).

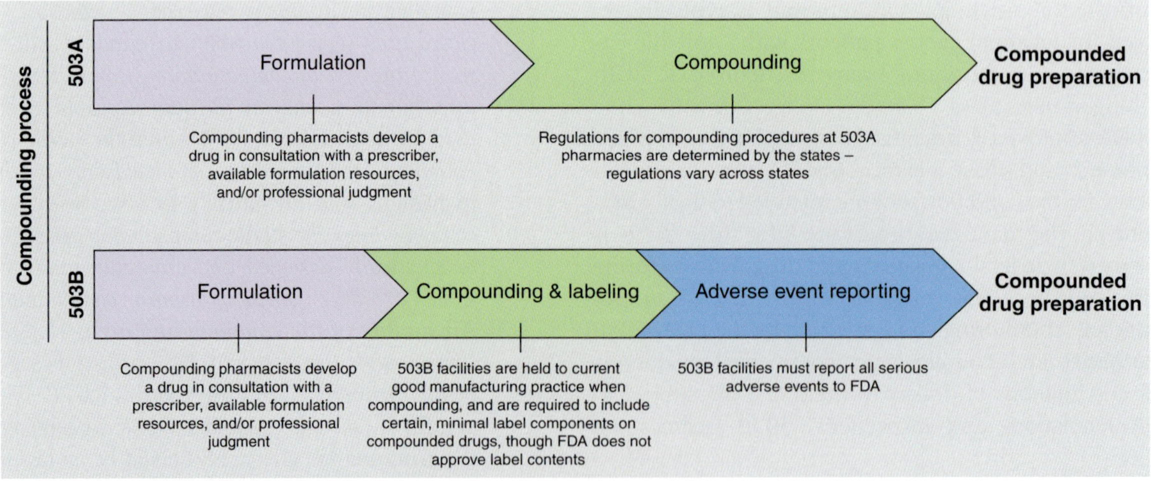

Fig. 21.2 Compounding processes for 503A and 503B facilities. (National Academies of Sciences, Engineering, and Medicine. 2020. Compounded Topical Pain Creams: Review of Select Ingredients for Safety, Effectiveness, and Use. https://doi.org/10.17226/25689. Adapted and reproduced with permission from the National Academy of Sciences, Courtesy of the National Academies Press, Washington, D.C.)

With regard to compounded IT pump medications, a typical physician's order might be:

- Fentanyl 100 μg/day
- Bupivacaine 1 mg/day
- Clonidine 50 μg/day

Continuous IT infusion to run at 100 μg fentanyl per day with 4 patient-administered bolus doses of 25 μg fentanyl each, with a 2-hour lockout period. Total volume = 41 mL.

The compounding pharmacist must know the patient's history to ensure that the patient is not allergic to any of the ordered medications and the physician's order must be scrutinized to ensure that there are no drug interactions. The pharmacy prescription system (typically, electronic and software driven) processes the order, and the pharmacist decides which medication concentrations to compound. Multiple factors go into concentration selection, including how long the patient has been on pump therapy, the institution's maximum concentration guidelines, and the flow rate of the pump. With the example order, if all programmed boluses are used, the patient's total possible daily dose is 200 μg fentanyl/day. The pharmacist may decide to concentrate the fentanyl to 1000 μg/mL. This makes the bupivacaine 10 mg/mL and clonidine 500 μg/mL. The pharmacist then calculates how much active pharmaceutical ingredient medication powder is needed to make the 41-mL syringe for the pump fill. This calculates to fentanyl 41 mg, bupivacaine 410 mg, and clonidine 20.5 mg. During this process, a pump syringe label and compounding worksheet are completed. A second pharmacist then double checks the order entry and calculations. The compounded medications are weighed once the order is approved by both pharmacists. The weighed powders are then compounded in a clean room and sterilized with filter sterilization. To ensure filter integrity, the filter is tested, and a limulus amebocyte lysate (LAL) test is performed for bacterial endotoxin. A third pharmacist does a visual check and triple checks the order entry and calculations. The syringe is then labeled, and the pharmacist assigns the appropriate BUD to the product based on USP 797 regulations and how the product will be stored. The product in our example is given a 3-day BUD since it will be stored in the refrigerator (Figs. 21.3–21.5).

The main risks of compounding include order entry error, compounding errors, and contamination of the clean room. Most compounding pharmacies use a total of five checks done on each compounded syringe and assess pharmacy staff compounding competency twice per year. The pharmacy clean room should be tested and certified every 6 months by a third party. These measures are taken to prevent error and ensure patient safety. Failure to ensure staff competency can lead to disasters such as the 2012 New England

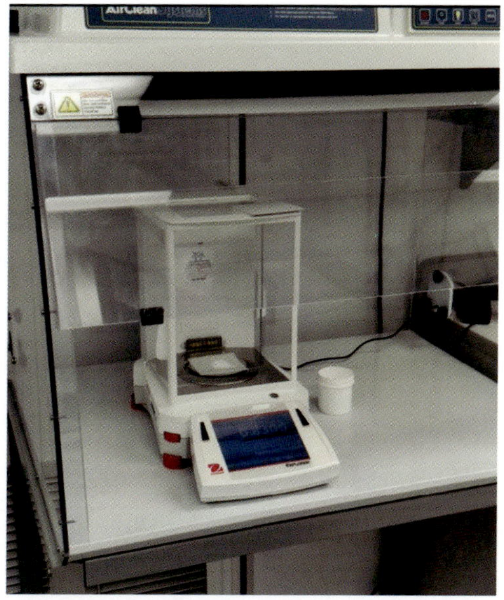

Fig. 21.3 Compounded medication being made and weighed at Nura Pain Clinic Pharmacy. (Courtesy Nura Pain Clinics, Minneapolis, MN)

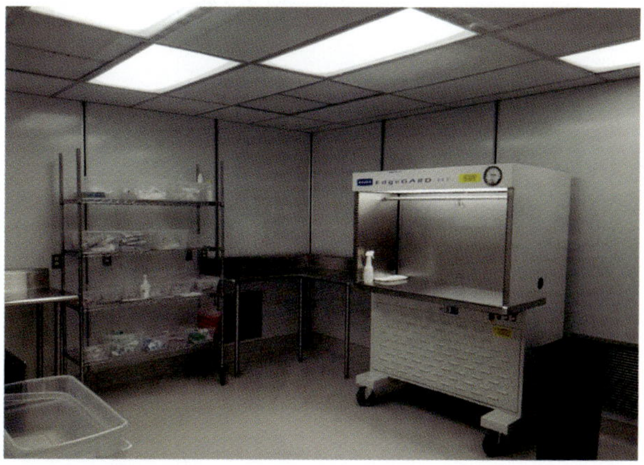

Fig. 21.4 Clean room in a pharmacy. (Courtesy Nura Pain Clinics, Minneapolis, MN)

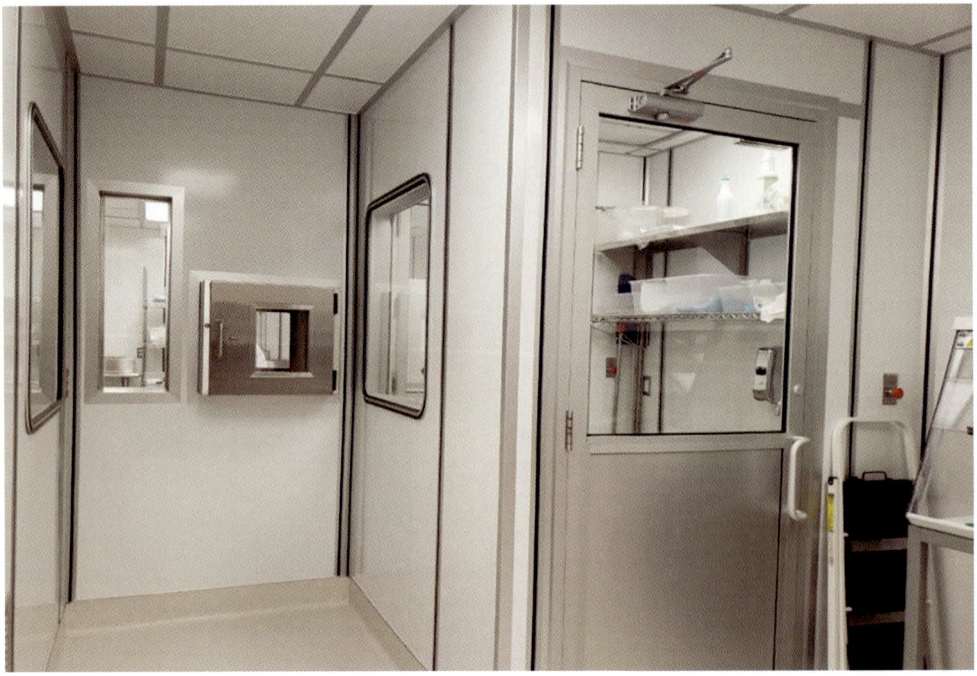

Fig. 21.5 Interior of a sterile compounding pharmacy. (Courtesy Nura Pain Clinics, Minneapolis, MN)

Compounding Center (NECC) meningitis outbreak. In this debacle, lack of compounding competency and standard safety measures led to the death of 64 patients. The federal investigation revealed that the NECC was acting as a drug manufacturer and bulk compounding without patient-specific prescriptions. An FDA inspection found many unsanitary practices, including shutting off the clean room air conditioning system at night and lack of proper cleaning using ISO class environments.[15] This disaster caused Congress to pass the Drug Quality and Security Act (DQSA). The DQSA requires large-scale compounders producing in bulk and shipping across state lines without patient-specific prescriptions to register with the FDA as an outsourcing facility.

Questions the implanter should ask before ordering compounded pump medications from a compounding pharmacy include:

1. Is the pharmacy accredited?
2. Does the pharmacy perform sterility testing on the final product?
3. How does the pharmacy sterilize the final product?
4. Does the pharmacy have a license in its home state and in the state where the managing pain clinic is located?

If an implanter decided to build a private compounding pharmacy to personally control quality and price, the doctor would need to hire a full-time pharmacist and work with the pharmacist's state board of pharmacy to determine regulatory requirements. A clinic with 500 pump patients could reasonably assume that a 2000-square-foot pharmacy would be necessary to supply the medications for this number of pump patients. A pharmacy of this size might typically cost $600,000 to $1,000,000 to build and equip with hoods, scales, and testing equipment. There would be additional annual costs to hire and manage an experienced compounding pharmacist, pharmacy technicians, support personal and for insurance, utilities and ongoing maintenance.

REFERENCES

1. Wang JK, Nauss LA, Thomas JE. Pain relief by intrathecally applied morphine in man. *Anesthesiology*. 1979;50(2):149-151.
2. West-Ward Pharmaceuticals Corp. Infumorph (Morphine Sulfate), preservative-free, injectable solution, for intrathecal or

epidural infusion, using a continuous micro infusion device, CII Initial U.S. Approval: 1941. https://dailymed.nlm.nih.gov/dailymed/fda/fdaDrugXsl.cfm?setid=db9ac9e3-d761-4a99-9f34-4946ebe8f255&type=display.
3. Elan Pharmaceuticals. *Prialt (Ziconotide Intrathecal Infusion)*. U.S. Food and Drug Administration Website. Dec. 2004. May 2021. https://www.accessdata.fda.gov/drugsatfda_docs/nda/2004/21-060_Prialt.cfm.
4. Medtronic. *PRODUCT PERFORMANCE REPORT SUMMARY of DATA from the MEDTRONIC POST-MARKET REGISTRY*. https://www.medtronic.com/content/dam/medtronic-com/products/product-performance/ppr-reports/2019-product-performance-report-combined.pdf.
5. U.S. Food and Drug Administration. *What We Do*. Spring, MD: Silver; 2018. https://www.fda.gov/about-fda/what-we-do.
6. U.S. Food and Drug Administration. *Use Caution with Implanted Pumps for Intrathecal Administration of Medicines for Pain Management*. FDA Safety Communication; November 14, 2018. https://wayback.archive-it.org/7993/20190207180535/https://www.fda.gov/MedicalDevices/Safety/AlertsandNotices/ucm625789.htm.
7. Konrad PE, Huffman JM, Stearns LM, et al. Intrathecal drug delivery systems (IDDS): The Implantable Systems Performance Registry (ISPR). *Neuromodulation*. 2016;19(8):848-856. doi:10.1111/ner.12524.
8. Pope J, Rosen S, Vinayakan A, et al. *Updated Results of a Long-Term, Open Label, Multi-Center Prospective Safety Study for a Novel Valve-Gated Implantable Infusion Pump*. Santa Barbara, California: California Society of Interventional Pain Physicians Annual Meeting November 2–4, 2018; 2018.
9. Rosen SM, Bromberg TA, Padda G, et al. Intrathecal administration of Infumorph® vs compounded morphine for treatment of intractable pain using the Prometra® programmable pump. *Pain Med*. 2013;14(6):865-873. doi:10.1111/pme.12077.
10. Deer TR, Pope JE, Hayek SM, et al. The Polyanalgesic Consensus Conference (PACC): recommendations on intrathecal drug infusion systems best practices and guidelines. *Neuromodulation*. 2017;20(2):96-132. doi:10.1111/ner.12538.
11. Schultz DM, Abd-Elsayed A, Calodney A, et al. Targeted drug delivery for chronic nonmalignant pain: longitudinal data from the Product Surveillance Registry. *Neuromodulation*. 2021;24(7):1167-1175. doi:10.1111/ner.13353.
12. Hassenbusch SJ, Portenoy RK, Cousins M, et al. Polyanalgesic Consensus Conference 2003: an update on the management of pain by intraspinal drug delivery—report of an expert panel. *J Pain Symptom Manage*. 2004;27(6):540-563.
13. Deer TR, Prager J, Levy R, et al. Polyanalgesic Consensus Conference 2012: recommendations for the management of pain by intrathecal (intraspinal) drug delivery: report of an interdisciplinary expert panel. *Neuromodulation*. 2012;15(5):436-464; discussion 464-466.
14. Deer TR, Pope JE, Hayek SM, et al. The Polyanalgesic Consensus Conference (PACC): recommendations on intrathecal drug infusion systems best practices and guidelines. *Neuromodulation*. 2017;20(2):96-132.
15. Office of Regulatory Affairs. *Owner and Four Former Employees of New England Compounding Center Convicted Following Trial. FDA*. U.S. Food and Drug Administration; February 27, 2019. https://www.fda.gov/inspections-compliance-enforcement-and-criminal-investigations/press-releases/december-13-2018-owner-and-four-former-employees-new-england-compounding-center-convicted-following. [Accessed 27 May 2021].

Chapter 22

Intrathecal Pump Trial

Shashank Vodapally, Neal Rakesh, and Amitabh Gulati

Chapter Outline

Introduction

After patients have failed conservative treatment options for intractable chronic pain, cancer-related pain, spasticity, pain stemming from failed back surgery syndrome/persistent spinal pain syndrome, and complex regional pain syndrome (CRPS), clinicians may turn to implantable intrathecal drug delivery systems (IDDSs). Only three neuraxial medications, which include morphine and ziconotide for pain and baclofen for spasticity, have been approved by the US Food and Drug Administration (FDA). There are also several others—such as hydromorphone, fentanyl, clonidine, and bupivacaine—that are commonly used in practice.[1]

Prior to initiating any of these therapies with a permanently implanted device, an intrathecal trial is recommended to provide clinicians a snapshot of how these medications may impact their patients. There is some controversy over the use of intrathecal trials. In 2016, however, the Polyanalgesic Consensus Conference (PACC) created a set of guidelines to help clinicians decide when it should be performed[2]:

- When should a patient be trialed?
  - If considering ziconotide as a first-line chronic infusion to monitor for positive response and side effects.
  - If considering the use of baclofen to monitor for improvement in spasticity and side effects from medication.
  - If utilizing a combination of medication, such as an opioid and local anesthetic.
  - If a patient may have increased risk of respiratory depression as a result of underlying pulmonary pathology, obesity, history of smoking and if being considered for intrathecal opioid medication.
  - If assessing for functional improvement or behavioral changes over a period of time.

General Considerations

When planning to perform an intrathecal trial, either an intrathecal or epidural trialing method can be considered. The predetermined medication can be administered as a single bolus, intermittent boluses, or continuous infusion. In a prospective study performed by Deer et al.[3] looking at the long-term outcomes of chronic low back pain patients treated with IDDSs, the group found significant functional improvement and improved quality of life regardless of whether continuous epidural infusion, continuous intrathecal infusion, single intrathecal bolus injection, or multiple intrathecal bolus injections were used during the trialing period.

Hamza et al.[4] later performed a prospective study to compare intermittent intrathecal bolusing with continuous intrathecal infusions when trialing patients and found that there was no difference in long-term outcomes. In addition, neither of the two techniques was found to be better at predicting trial success or long-term outcomes once a permanent IDDS was implanted. The 2016 PACC guidelines also concluded there is no evidence showing that the continuous trial method is superior to other trialing methods. Deciding which trial method to use should be based on the acuity of the patient, the diagnosis, the preference of the physician, and which medication is being administered. To provide some guidance on dose ranges for analgesic medications, the PACC also provided dosing parameters for both infusion and bolus trials based on which medications are being used. Boster et al.[5] provided other guidelines reviewing best practice recommendations when trialing with intrathecal baclofen for spasticity. Both groups of guidelines are summarized in Table 22.1.

If considering an epidural trial prior to permanent implantation of an IDDS, it is important to note that epidural trials may overestimate the intrathecal dosage needed once the permanent implant is in place.[6] When comparing epidural infusion to intrathecal bolus trials, however, Anderson et al. found an increased risk of opioid-induced adverse events—such as nausea, vomiting, and urinary retention—in the intrathecal group.[7] It is also important to note that no patients in either group of this study experienced respiratory depression, one of the most concerning side effects that is monitored when performing an intrathecal trial with opioids.

TABLE 22.1 Best Practice for Trialing

Drug	Intrathecal Bolus Trialing Starting Dose Ranges[a]	Intrathecal Infusion Trialing Starting Dose Ranges[b]
Bupivacaine	0.5–2.5 mg	0.01–4 mg/day
Clonidine	5–20 μg	20–100 μg/day
Fentanyl	15–75 μg	25–75 μg/day
Hydromorphone	0.025–0.1 mg	0.01–0.15 mg/day
Morphine	0.1–0.5 mg	0.1–0.5 mg/day
Sufentanil	5–20 μg	10–20 μg/day
Ziconotide	1–5 μg	0.5–2.4 μg/day
Baclofen[c]	50 μg, 75 μg, 100 μg	

[a]For opioid-naïve patients receiving outpatient bolus trials, it is important not to exceed 0.15 mg morphine, 0.04 mg hydromorphone, or 25 μg fentanyl.

[b]For opioid medications, the initial dosing of continuous intrathecal therapy should be half of the dose used during the trial.

[c]Standard starting dose is 50 μg intrathecal bolus. However, if predetermined goals are not achieved and spasticity does not improve, another bolus of 75 μg and 100 μg may be required to see full effect (must wait minimum 24 hours between boluses)[5]

Clinicians may also combine various classes of analgesic medications while trialing and after permanently implanting the IDDS with the goal of achieving long-term outcomes. One of the most common medications used as an adjunct is bupivacaine. A retrospective study performed by Galica et al.[8] looked at patients with intractable pain following laminectomy who subsequently underwent an intrathecal trial with hydromorphone and bupivacaine and eventually had an IDDS implanted with the same medications. His team concluded that trialing with these medications significantly decreased patients' pain Numeric Rating Scale scores and appeared to be predictive of patients' response following permanent implantation of an intrathecal device. The benefit of combination therapy with bupivacaine can be seen in a study by Veizi et al.,[9] who found that concurrent administration of bupivacaine and opioids required a lower rate of opioid escalation during the first year following IDDS implantation. In another study looking at satisfaction in patients with an IDDS, a majority of whom were being treated with intrathecal fentanyl and bupivacaine, 357 of 413 patients reported improved quality of life compared with pre-IDDS implantation. In addition, 88.4% of these patients were taking less oral opioids and 38.9% of patients completely stopped all oral opioids after the IDDS was implanted.[10]

The lipophilicity of the medications has an impact on deciding whether to perform the trial using an epidural or intrathecal method. Fentanyl, a more lipophilic opioid, is known to clear from the intrathecal space faster than hydrophilic opioids, such as morphine.[11] Ummenhofer et al.[12] compared the distribution and clearance of opioid medications, such as morphine and fentanyl, after injecting 100 μL over

2 minutes into the intrathecal space at the L4 to L5 level in bovine specimens. His team found varying pharmacokinetic behaviors between the drugs. The intrathecal concentrations of these medications were checked at varying spinal levels; they consistently found morphine to have the highest concentration intrathecally. They also found that intrathecal fentanyl concentrations were statistically significantly lower at higher spinal levels than intrathecal morphine concentrations. Not only was there decreased cephalad spread of fentanyl compared to morphine when checked at the L2 to L3, T11, and T7 spinal levels, but they also found that fentanyl had distributed into the largest volume of epidural fat compared to any of the other opioids tested, including morphine. These findings demonstrated that fentanyl was cleared from the cerebrospinal fluid (CSF) faster than morphine, likely due to its highly lipophilic nature. These characteristics of fentanyl can be used to the clinician's advantage if choosing to perform the intrathecal trial with fentanyl prior to permanently implanting the intrathecal pump with morphine. As discussed in the PACC 2016 guidelines, the risk for delayed respiratory depression using fentanyl, one of the known fatal side effects for opioids during intrathecal trial, is decreased while still maintaining the ability to evaluate a patient's response to intrathecal opioids.[2]

Ziconotide, which is a nonopioid medication, has been FDA approved to be administered intrathecally for managing moderate to severe pain. Although it is known to have a narrow therapeutic window, requires slow titration to avoid neuropsychiatric adverse events, can cause elevation in creatinine kinase, and is contraindicated in patients with a history of psychosis, it has been shown to have several advantages over morphine for managing pain. It has no cardiopulmonary side effects if delivered intrathecally, no risk of tolerance, and may be discontinued abruptly without concern for withdrawal.[13] Although Deer et al.[14] found both morphine and ziconotide to be first-line monotherapy treatments for treating cancer and non–cancer-related pain in patients, the advantages of ziconotide must be weighed in opioid-experienced patients as they may become tolerant of morphine and risk respiratory depression at the higher doses needed for therapeutic effect. If considering ziconotide, there was a strong level of consensus in the 2016 PACC guidelines for trialing the medication with an intrathecal bolus method prior to permanently implanting an intrathecal device. Ziconotide is one medication that must be trialed intrathecally due to its large molecular structure, which limits its ability to enter the CSF if injected into the epidural space.[15] Regardless of which trialing method and medication is used by the clinician, a similar stepwise approach is needed, which we will further discuss in this chapter.

Step-by-Step Description of the Procedure

Prior to initiating the procedure, the patient is asked to lie prone, appropriately draped to expose the lumbar region and then prepped using sterile technique. Subsequently, an anteroposterior (AP) image of the lumbosacral region is taken using fluoroscopy. Typically, a cephalocaudal tilt must be introduced to form an image where the inferior endplate of the superior vertebrae, forming the target interlaminar space, is parallel with the axis formed between the image intensifier and X-ray generator of the C-arm. This will prevent the anterior and posterior regions of the endplate from overlapping on the fluoroscopic image.[16]

Most individuals have termination of the conus medullaris at the level of the L1/L2 intervertebral disk.[17-19] Thus, typically, the interlaminar target level is at the L2 to L3 or L3 to L4 level. It is important to note that this targeted area will be the point of entry into the epidural/intrathecal space for the needle tip when performing needle placement with the paramedian technique. However, initial entry of the needle through the skin is performed about 2 vertebral body segments caudal to this targeted entry site. The clinician should also attempt to position the spinous process of that vertebrae midline. Ideally, this should create a "boxed" appearance of the vertebral body with the spinous process lying in the middle. If visualization of the interlaminar space is difficult, then decreasing lordosis of the lumbar spine with the use of pillows under the patient's abdomen/pelvis may be helpful.[15,16]

The paramedian technique is used for needle placement in both bolus and catheter intrathecal trials. The trajectory of the needle should be caudad to cephalad, dorsal to ventral, and lateral to medial, with a needle trajectory that is about 30 degrees above the coronal plane (Fig. 22.1). Once the target interlaminar space

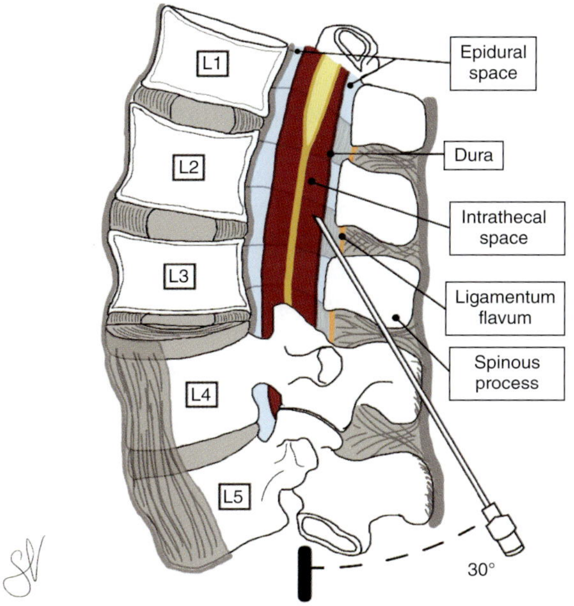

Fig. 22.1 Sagittal view illustration showing intrathecal injection. The spinal needle can be seen entering the target L2 to L3 intrathecal space after passing through the ligamentum flavum (*orange*) and dura (*red*). If an epidural trial is considered, the spinal needle is advanced through the ligamentum flavum only and trial injectate is administered into the epidural space (*light blue*).

is identified under fluoroscopy using the previously described technique, the needle entry site through the skin can be identified and marked about 2 vertebral levels caudal to the interlaminar site, just medial to the pedicle. After appropriately identifying these two locations, 5 to 10 cc of 1% lidocaine can be injected in the local subcutaneous tissue underlying the needle entry site. Either a No. 11 or No. 15 blade scalpel can then be used to create a small stab incision at the site of needle insertion. A 17-gauge spinal needle or Tuohy needle is then advanced under fluoroscopy through the locally anesthetized area in the previously described trajectory until the needle tip contacts the ipsilateral laminae at the inferior border of the target interlaminar space (lamina approach). The needle tip can also be directed toward the target interlaminar space just inferior to the spinous process below the spino-laminar junction. Lateral fluoroscopic images can then be taken to help confirm placement.[15,16]

The epidural space is then entered by advancing the needle through the ligamentum flavum (Fig. 22.2) while using the loss-of-resistance technique. If the lamina approach is used, the needle must first be walked off superiorly into the interlaminar space. If

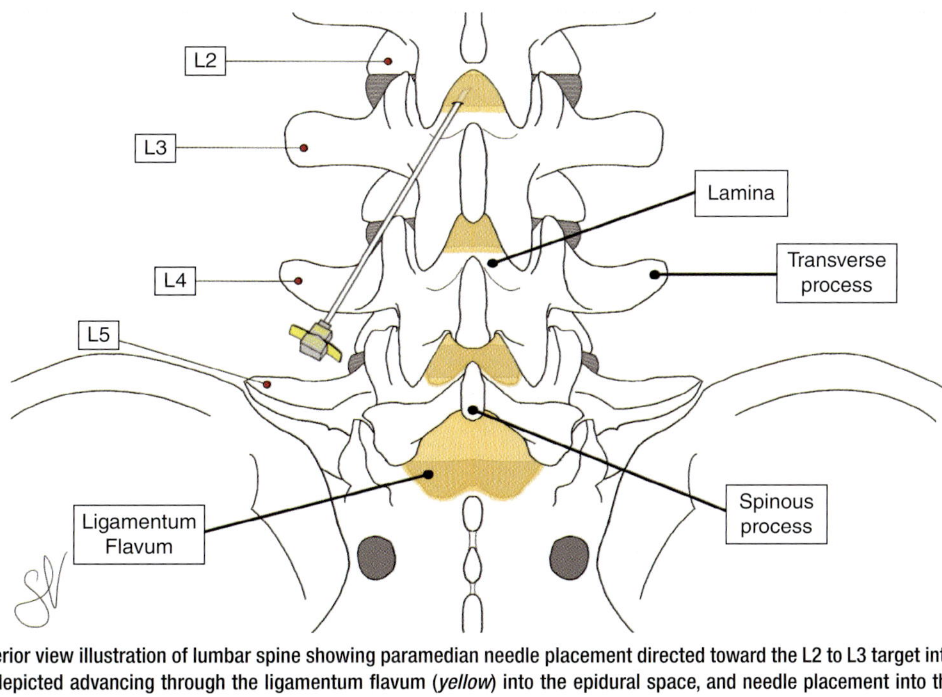

Fig. 22.2 Posterior view illustration of lumbar spine showing paramedian needle placement directed toward the L2 to L3 target interlaminar region. The needle is depicted advancing through the ligamentum flavum (*yellow*) into the epidural space, and needle placement into the epidural space is confirmed using loss-of-resistance technique.

the clinician plans to perform an epidural trial, this is the final needle placement. Either the bolus injection may be administered or the epidural trial catheter can be advanced to the desired level through the needle. The catheter should travel in the cephalad direction in the dorsal epidural space, which can be confirmed with lateral fluoroscopic images. Contrast medium can be injected at this time to confirm location and patency of the catheter tip.[15]

If an intrathecal trial is planned, the needle must be further advanced through the dura until CSF return is observed spontaneously. When performing a continuous infusion intrathecal trial, the needle tip is further advanced through the dura mater, as described previously. Then, an intrathecal catheter is passed through under fluoroscopic guidance until the catheter tip is in the appropriate desired position in the spinal canal on both AP and lateral images.[15]

To evaluate whether performing an intrathecal trial for pain control has been effective, it is important for the clinician to have a baseline pain score for the patient prior to the procedure. An improvement of 50% from the baseline pain score equates with a successful trial.[20] When considering the trial for spasticity, having a pretrial Modified Ashworth Score as well as baseline assessment from physical and occupational therapy is helpful. A reduction by 2 points in a patient's Modified Ashworth Score may indicate a successful trial. However, assessing the patient's functional improvement with intermittent therapy evaluations on the screening day may offer further insight into the trial's success.[5,15]

Intraoperative Complications and How to Handle Them

In 2016, the PACC released guidelines to help improve safety surrounding intrathecal drug therapy.[13] Some of their recommendations with the strongest level of evidence and consensus support are the following:

- Closely monitoring for respiratory depression when administering intrathecal opioid medication and making sure to carefully dose the medication based on whether intrathecal or epidural trial is being performed.
- Avoiding concurrent sedative medications when trialing with opioids.
- Not trialing intrathecal ziconotide in patients who have a history of psychosis.
- Monitoring for any endocrine-related side effects that present following intrathecal opioid administration.
- Monitoring for cardiac side effects when administering intrathecal clonidine.
- At higher doses of intrathecal bupivacaine, patients may experience urinary incontinence, numbness, and weakness.

In addition to these guidelines, it is also important to monitor for allergic reactions to medications, contrast medium, or any instrumentation used during the trial.

REFERENCES

1. Choi KS, Hayek SM. Intrathecal Drug Delivery: Pharmacokinetics and Dynamics. In: Diwan S, Deer TR, eds. *Advanced Procedures for Pain Management*. Springer International Publishing; 2018:347-358. doi:10.1007/978-3-319-68841-1.
2. Deer TR, Hayek SM, Pope JE, et al. The Polyanalgesic Consensus Conference (PACC): recommendations for trialing of intrathecal drug delivery infusion therapy. *Neuromodulation*. 2017;20(2):133-154. doi:10.1111/ner.12543.
3. Deer T, Chapple I, Classen A, et al. Intrathecal drug delivery for treatment of chronic low back pain: report from the National Outcomes Registry for Low Back Pain. *Pain Med*. 2004;5(1): 6-13. doi:10.1111/j.1526-4637.2004.04011.x.
4. Hamza M, Doleys DM, Saleh IA, Medvedovsky A, Verdolin MH, Hamza M. A prospective, randomized, single-blinded, head-to-head long-term outcome study, comparing intrathecal (it) boluses with continuous infusion trialing techniques prior to implantation of drug delivery systems (DDS) for the treatment of severe intractable chronic nonmalignant pain. *Neuromodulation*. 2015;18(7):636-648; discussion 649. doi:10.1111/ner.12342.
5. Boster AL, Bennett SE, Bilsky GS, et al. Best practices for intrathecal baclofen therapy: screening test. *Neuromodulation*. 2016;19(6):616-622. doi:10.1111/ner.12437.
6. Maniker AH, Krieger AJ, Adler RJ, Hupert C. Epidural trial in implantation of intrathecal morphine infusion pumps. *N J Med*. 1991;88(11):797-801.
7. Anderson VC, Burchiel KJ, Cooke B. A prospective, randomized trial of intrathecal injection vs. epidural infusion in the selection of patients for continuous intrathecal opioid therapy. *Neuromodulation*. 2003;6(3):142-152. doi:10.1046/j.1525-1403.2003.03023.x.
8. Galica RJ, Hayek SM, Veizi E, et al. Intrathecal trialing of continuous infusion combination therapy with hydromorphone and bupivacaine in failed back surgery patients. *Neuromodulation*. 2018;21(7):648-654. doi:10.1111/ner.12737.
9. Veizi IE, Hayek SM, Narouze S, Pope JE, Mekhail N. Combination of intrathecal opioids with bupivacaine attenuates opioid dose escalation in chronic noncancer pain patients. *Pain Med*. 2011; 12(10):1481-1489. doi:10.1111/j.1526-4637.2011.01232.x.
10. Schultz DM, Orhurhu V, Khan F, Hagedorn JM, Abd-Elsayed A. Patient satisfaction following intrathecal targeted drug delivery for benign chronic pain: results of a single-center survey study. *Neuromodulation*. 2020;23(7):1009-1017. doi:10.1111/ner.13167.

11. Bernards CM. Understanding the physiology and pharmacology of epidural and intrathecal opioids. *Best Pract Res Clin Anaesthesiol*. 2002;16(4):489-505. doi:10.1053/bean.2002.0255.
12. Ummenhofer WC, Arends RH, Shen DD, Bernards CM. Comparative spinal distribution and clearance kinetics of intrathecally administered morphine, fentanyl, alfentanil, and sufentanil. *Anesthesiology*. 2000;92(3):739-753. doi:10.1097/00000542-200003000-00018.
13. Deer TR, Pope JE, Hayek S, et al. The Polyanalgesic Consensus Conference (PACC): Recommendations for intrathecal drug delivery: guidance for improving safety and mitigating risks. *Neuromodulation*. 2017;20:155–176.
14. Deer TR, Pope JE, Hanes MC, McDowell GC. Intrathecal therapy for chronic pain: a review of morphine and ziconotide as firstline options. *Pain Med*. 2019;20(4):784-798. doi:10.1093/pm/pny132.
15. Diwan S, Staats P. *Atlas of Pain Medicine Procedures*. 1st ed. New York: McGraw-Hill Education/Medical; 2015.
16. Cianfoni A, Boulter D, Rumboldt Z, Zapton T, Bonaldi G. Guidelines to imaging landmarks for interventional spine procedures: fluoroscopy and CT anatomy. *Neurographics*. 2011;1(1): 39-48.
17. Liu A, Yang K, Wang D, et al. Level of conus medullaris termination in adult population analyzed by kinetic magnetic resonance imaging. *Surg Radiol Anat*. 2017;39(7):759-765. doi:10.1007/s00276-017-1813-3.
18. Soleiman J, Demaerel P, Rocher S, Maes F, Marchal G. Magnetic resonance imaging study of the level of termination of the conus medullaris and the thecal sac: influence of age and gender. *Spine (Phila Pa 1976)*. 2005;30(16):1875-1880. doi:10.1097/01.brs.0000174116.74775.2e.
19. Wilson DA, Prince JR. John Caffey award. MR imaging determination of the location of the normal conus medullaris throughout childhood. *AJR Am J Roentgenol*. 1989;152(5):1029-1032. doi:10.2214/ajr.152.5.1029.
20. Deer TR, Prager J, Levy R, et al. Polyanalgesic Consensus Conference 2012: recommendation on trialing for intrathecal (intraspinal) drug delivery: report of an interdisciplinary expert panel. *Neuromodulation*. 2012;15:420-435.

Chapter 23

Intrathecal Pump Implant

Alaa Abd-Elsayed, David Abejón González, and Cristina Abad Salom

Chapter Outline

Introduction

The use of epidural and intrathecal analgesia should not be considered a therapeutic novelty considering that, in 1901, the French researchers Sicard and Cathelin[1,2] described, for the first time, the administration of epidural injections of local anesthetics through the sacral hiatus. In 1921, the Spaniard Fidel Pagés[3] described and published for the first time the practical application of the lumbar epidural injection.

One of the most exciting advances in medicine has been the discovery of opioid receptors and their pharmacological targetability. The identification of these opioid receptors in the brain and substantia gelatinosa of the spinal cord led to experiments demonstrating the association between intrathecal administration of morphine and the appearance of a potent and prolonged antinociception effect that is dose dependent and reversible with naloxone. As a result of these findings, the administration of opioids using both spinal routes (epidural and intrathecal) began, with the goal of modulating pain in humans. At first, this modality of opioid administration was used in the treatment of postoperative pain. Later, it was used to treat chronic pain of oncological origin resistant to other treatments. Toward the end of the 1980s, its use was extended to patients with chronic nononcological pain in which other treatment options had failed.

The first patients treated with intrathecal opioids were cancer patients in the late 1970s.[4] The first fully implanted morphine infusion system was used in 1981 in a patient with chronic oncological pain who did not respond to treatment with oral opioids at high doses. He was implanted with a continuous-flow system called Infusaid.[5]

There are different ways to administer drugs intrathecally to treat chronic pain. We classify them in the following very general categories:

1. External systems of simple catheters: Implanted percutaneously in the intrathecal space with subcutaneous tunneling.
2. Partially external systems: The spinal catheter is connected to a reservoir placed subcutaneously.
3. Fully implantable systems (or implantable pumps for intrathecal drug infusion): Both the catheter and the infusion system are completely implanted.

To obtain the desired results in the treatment of pain with this type of implant, as in other neuromodulation techniques, a series of basic principles must be met. First, patient selection must be careful and organized. Second, the surgical technique must be polished and correct. Third, drug choice must be scrupulous and maintenance and filling of the implanted pump must be expertly performed. Each of these principles will be explored in depth throughout the chapter.

Patient Selection (Fig. 23.1)

As in any other surgery, patient selection requires a complete medical history. Lack of comorbidities or physical problems that prevent either the surgery or the implant of the pump, or its subsequent maintenance or filling, are verified. The implantation of an intrathecal pump requires psychosocial evaluation as the patient's psychosocial state must not interfere with the proper functioning or handling of the implanted device. Thus, it is mandatory that there are no psychological or sociological contraindications and that the patient has a stable social situation and a favorable home environment.

For proper patient selection, the type and location of the pain must also be considered, as well as the different modalities used to treat it. The pain must have a clear organic origin and be of a moderate-severe constant or almost constant intensity requiring opioid

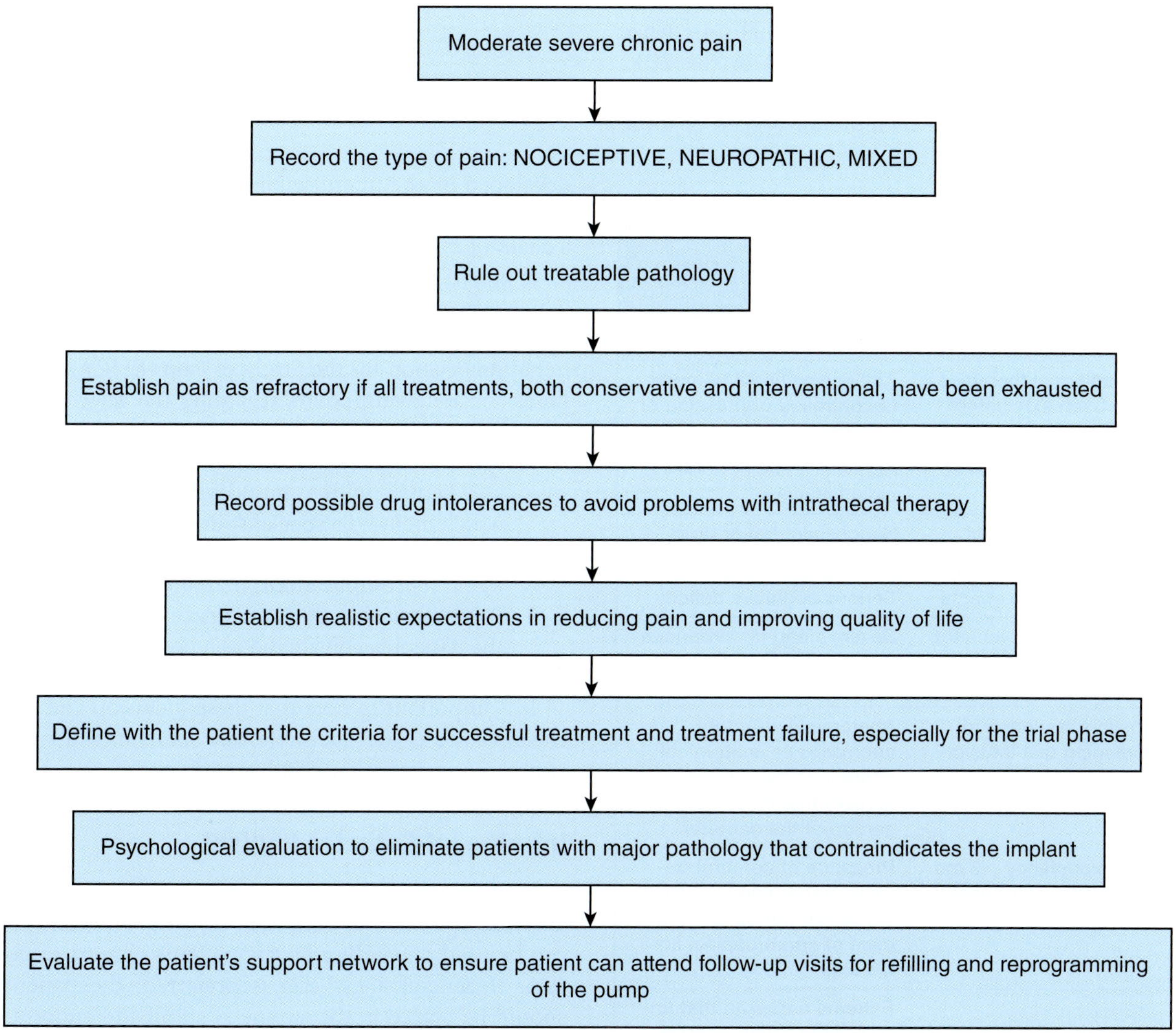

Fig. 23.1 Patient selection algorithm for intrathecal pump implant.

therapy for its control, and the patient should have had a good response previously to opioid treatment, both orally and intravenously, but without achieving the desired results or experiencing side effects that are difficult to control. Finally, oncological patients must have a life expectancy greater than 3 months. It is also advisable to carry out a trial phase (Table 23.1). The main indications for this therapy are chronic pain, of oncological or nononcological origin, and spasticity[6,7] (Table 23.2). Of note, the British Pain Society and the Polyanalgesic Consensus Conference (PACC) have designated special importance to the psychological evaluation of preselected patients to become candidates for the implantation of an internal intrathecal drug infusion pump. This is reflected in the 2012 Recommendations for the Treatment of Pain by Intrathecal Administration, which are an update of those developed by the interdisciplinary panel of experts in 2007. An algorithm has been developed in the form of a chain of evaluations from the selection of the patient as a possible candidate up to the final decision of which system to implant.

TABLE 23.2 Main Intrathecal Pump Treatment Indications

Oncological Pain	Nononcological Pain	Spasticity
Primary tumors Metastatic lesions Neuropathy from chemotherapy treatments Nerve irritation or injury from radiation	Failed back surgery syndrome Spinal canal stenosis Compression fracture Nonsurgical spondylolisthesis Peripheral neuropathy Truncal pain Complex regional pain syndrome Severe osteoarthritis Rheumatoid arthritis Connective tissue disorders	

TABLE 23.1 Inclusion and Exclusion Criteria for an Intrathecal Pump Implant

Inclusion Criteria	Exclusion Criteria
All traditional therapies have been exhausted	Active psychosis or major uncontrolled depression or anxiety
Failure of less-invasive therapies	Active suicidal or homicidal behavior
Inadequate effect of oral opioids	Serious alcohol or drug addiction problems
Intolerable side effects	Serious cognitive deficits
Exclusion of psychiatric disorder or drug-seeking behavior	Severe sleep disturbances
Positive response to screening test infusion	Anatomical structure anomalies or anatomical alterations by a previous surgery that hinder the insertion of the catheter
Life expectancy >3 mo in oncological patients	Presence of cerebral pathology that can lead to cerebellar herniation in the case of cerebrospinal liquid loss
	Extreme cachexia that impedes the pump implant

The European Federation of Chapters of the International Association for the Study of Pain (EFIC) (1998) raises the following points regarding the selection of appropriate patients for a spinal infusion system:

1. The procedure must be carried out in specialized centers with a multidisciplinary approach, which includes a specialist in health psychology.
2. The patient must be informed about the treatment, its complications, and aftercare.
3. Psychological evaluation is necessary as soon as the patient is considered as a possible candidate for the therapy.

It is important to note that these inclusion and exclusion criteria are advisable but sometimes do not apply to certain patients and situations.

Intrathecal Catheter Implant

To perform the intrathecal pump implantation, local anesthesia, conscious sedation, or general anesthesia can be used depending on the patient's clinical situation. If general anesthesia is preferred, the patient should be placed in the supine position and endotracheal intubation should be performed. After anesthetic induction and endotracheal intubation, and before placing the patient in lateral decubitus, the area where the pump will be implanted is marked. The implantation is usually done in the left flank (several other sites have been described as well). Thus, the patient should be placed in right lateral decubitus, keeping the left side up, with slight hip and neck flexion. Placing the patient correctly is important to avoid complications during the procedure, to allow the use of fluoroscopy, and to obtain a quality spine image with X-ray. Before beginning the procedure, a fluoroscopic view should be taken in which the spinous processes are placed in the midline, leaving the pedicles in an equidistant line on both sides of the spinous processes (Fig. 23.2). The most common entrance point to the intradural space is L1 to L2 or L2 to L3. Thus, the incision must be performed in the paravertebral area, in the pedicle line, at the L3 or L4 level. After drawing all incision markings and preparing the surgical field, the skin is infiltrated with local anesthetic. The surgery is performed either under general anesthesia or sedation to avoid postoperative pain. In this case, a mixture of lidocaine 1% with bupivacaine 0.25% with epinephrine, 1:1, is used on the skin for fast onset and long duration. The intrathecal puncture can be performed either before or after the skin incision and preparation of the surgical field up to the fascia. We recommend performing the incision and preparation of the surgical field, with meticulous hemostasis, before the intrathecal puncture so that there is no risk of damaging the catheter. With fluoroscopic guidance, the Tuohy needle is directed to the midline from the paravertebral line, from the ipsilateral pedicle. The desired level to reach is at least one level above where it enters the skin (Figs. 23.3 and 23.4).

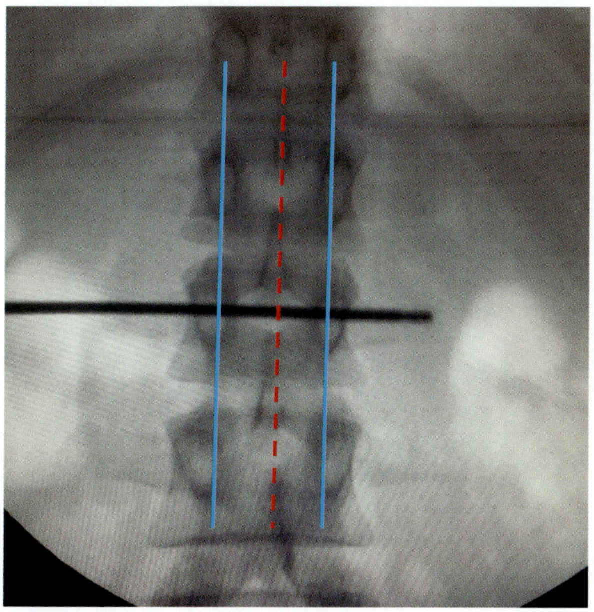

Fig. 23.2 **Marking for catheter implantation. The C-arm should be placed so that the spinous processes can be seen (*broken line in red*) with the equidistant pedicle line (*blue line*).**

The angle at which the needle enters the skin is important in order to avoid complications such as torsion and kinking or stress of the catheter. To avoid repeated dural punctures, an alternative technique can be used on occasion. This technique consists of performing an epidural instead of directly accessing the intradural space so that the entry into the space can be more carefully executed. Some authors suggest using contrast in this step to ensure proper placement in the epidural space,[8] although it may not be necessary. When the epidural space is reached using the loss-of-resistance technique (with air, saline, or pending drop), a 5-cc syringe with 1 cc saline is connected to the needle. Aspiration is performed until the exit of cerebrospinal fluid (CSF) is noted. This technique allows the necessary pressure to obtain the exit of CSF while ensuring that no structures collapse, which might cause confusion. This is completed even though, in most cases, the puncture of the dura obtains a clear view of the CSF.

When the intrathecal space is reached and CSF is observed, the stylet is withdrawn from the needle and the catheter is advanced into the epidural space (Fig. 23.5).

Once the catheter is in the final position, the stylet should be withdrawn and CSF leakage should be clearly observed from the catheter end. Providers must be careful during needle placement in the dural space to minimize the amount of CSF leakage through the needle. This is important because a significant CSF loss during needle placement can reduce the CSF flow through the small-gauge catheter which, in turn, may generate great uncertainty about the correct positioning of the catheter in the

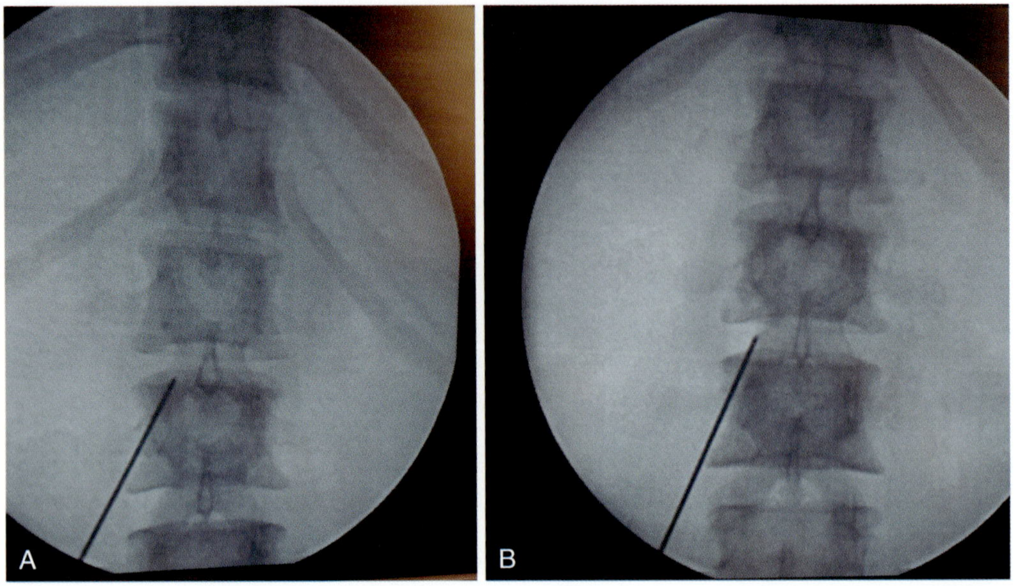

Fig. 23.3 Before performing the dural puncture, we make the incision and prepare the surgical field. The incision is made in the pedicle line (A) ipsilateral to the implant so that we do not cross the midline. We prefer to make the incision before the puncture to have meticulous hemostasis without the risk of breaking the catheter. This also reduces the risk of introducing pathogens in the intradural space. (B) Marking the pedicle line.

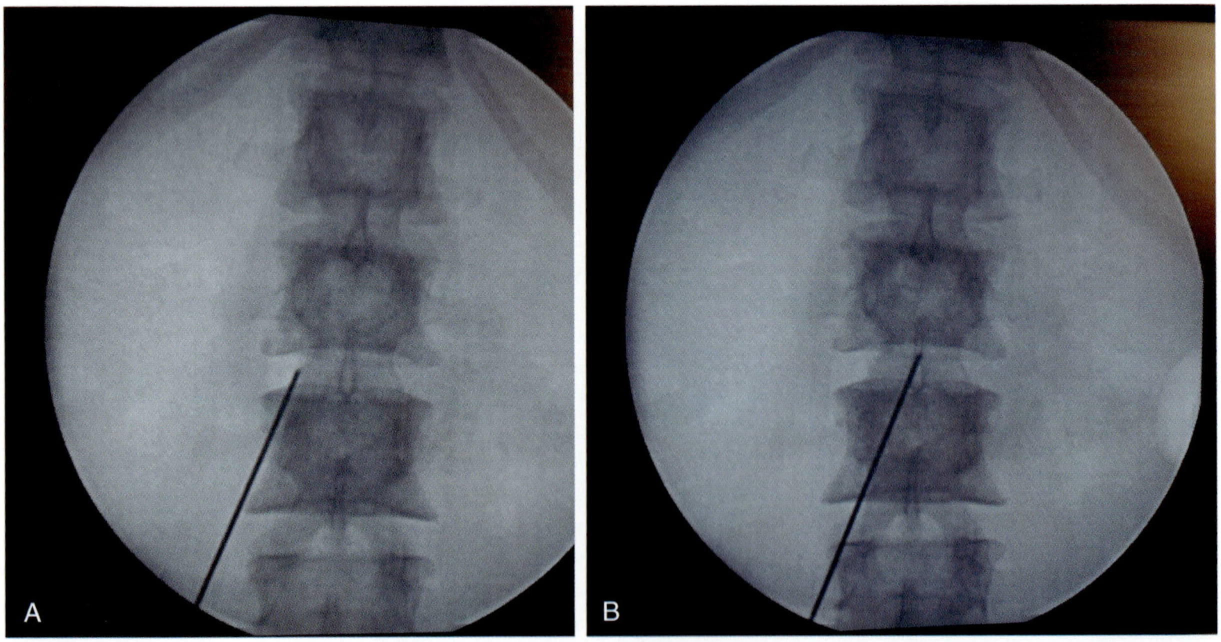

Fig. 23.4 The needle enters the skin one level below the entry to the intrathecal space. It is placed in the pedicle line (A) on the same side in which the pump will be placed to avoid the catheter crossing the midline (B).

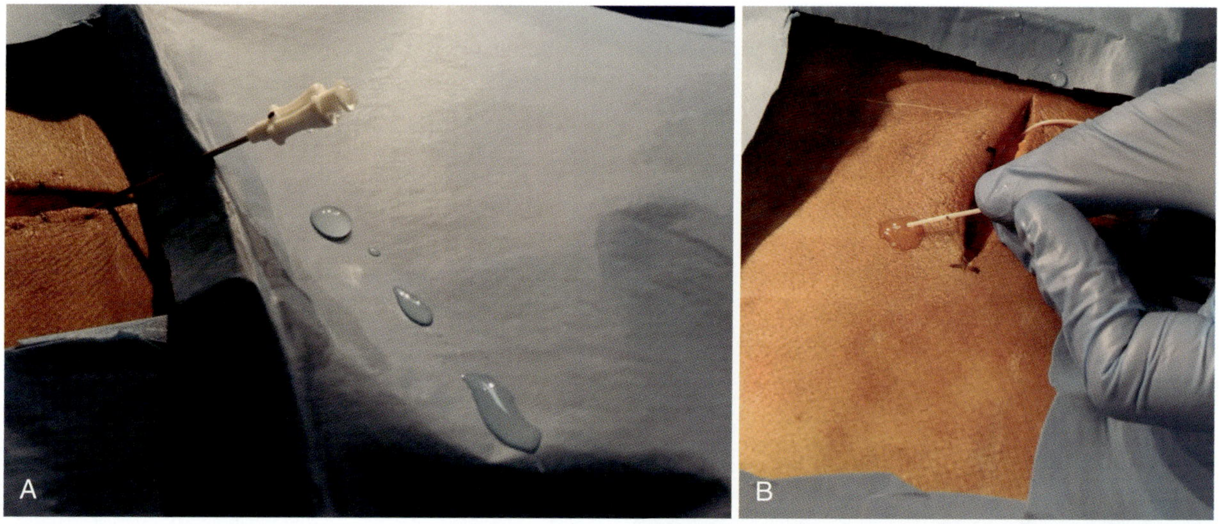

Fig. 23.5 Once the intrathecal space is reached and the leakage of cerebrospinal fluid (CSF) is observed (A), the stylet is withdrawn and the catheter is advanced to the intrathecal space. CSF leakage must be observed through the catheter as well before proceeding to anchor the catheter (B).

dural space and can cause immediate postoperative headache.

Finally, it must be verified that the catheter is in the intrathecal space. The location of the catheter is chosen depending on the drug being used and the location of the pain (Figs. 23.6–23.8).

Catheter Anchoring

Proper and meticulous anchoring is one of the most important steps in this technique. Cranial or rostral migration in this procedure is a very serious concern. Cranial migration can result in loss of effectiveness depending on the drug used. Rostral migration can be even more serious, as it can cause the catheter to leave the intrathecal space, with dire consequences. However, the new anchors that providers currently have at their disposal have drastically reduced this complication and have significantly simplified the procedure.

With the new Medtronic anchor (Injex; Medtronic, Minneapolis, MN), anchoring techniques are safer and easier for the professional to perform. These newer anchors are bi-wing and come preloaded in a syringe-shaped deployment device. The catheter passes through the distal end, where the anchor is loaded, through a metal structure, and exits the handle at the proximal end. This system provides entry to the fascia and, thus, enables clinicians to deposit the anchor deep into the incision site. Once in place, the plunger is pressed. In order to execute this movement

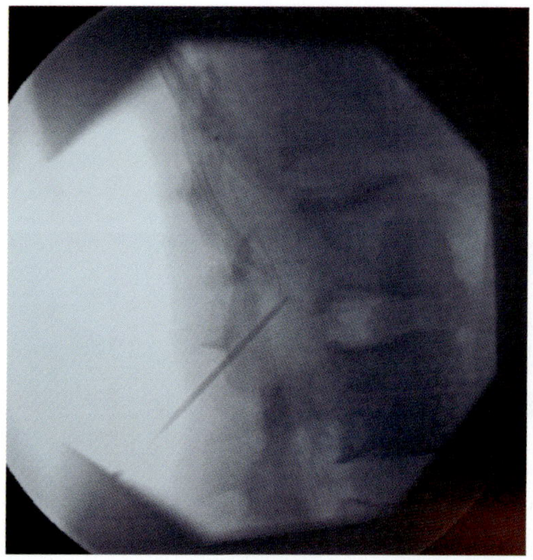

Fig. 23.6 The catheter is advanced into the intrathecal space after verifying a clear and continuous leakage of cerebrospinal fluid.

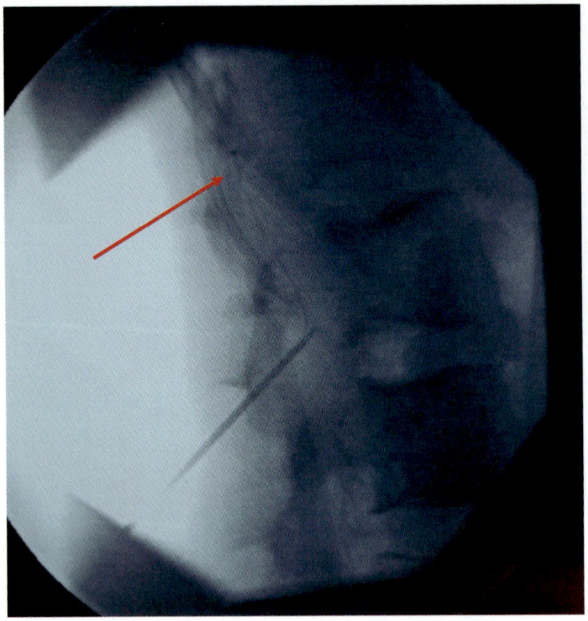

Fig. 23.7 The catheter can be seen in the intrathecal space.

correctly, the opposite movement of pressing the embolus must be performed. This is done by the thumb being left in the distal part and the embolus being retracted with the index and middle fingers until the anchor slides through the device. A layer of Teflon that covers the device helps the process (Figs. 23.9–23.11).

It is important to note that polypropylene sutures, or anything not contained in the anchor kit, such as silicone or glue, should never be used for anchorage. This is important because of the possibility of damaging the catheter or anchorage. Likewise, the suture should not strangle the anchor or the catheter. Thus, suture placement should be done carefully and without squeezing the components of the anchorage. The type of suture that should be used for anchoring the catheter must be nonresorbable; silk is commonly used. Sometimes, however, silk can degrade with time and can break, causing catheter migration or CSF leakage (Table 23.3).

Anchoring the intrathecal catheter properly is very important. A critical step is to place the anchor as close as possible to where the catheter enters the fascia so that injuries and possible migration are avoided. Placing the anchor into the fascia before

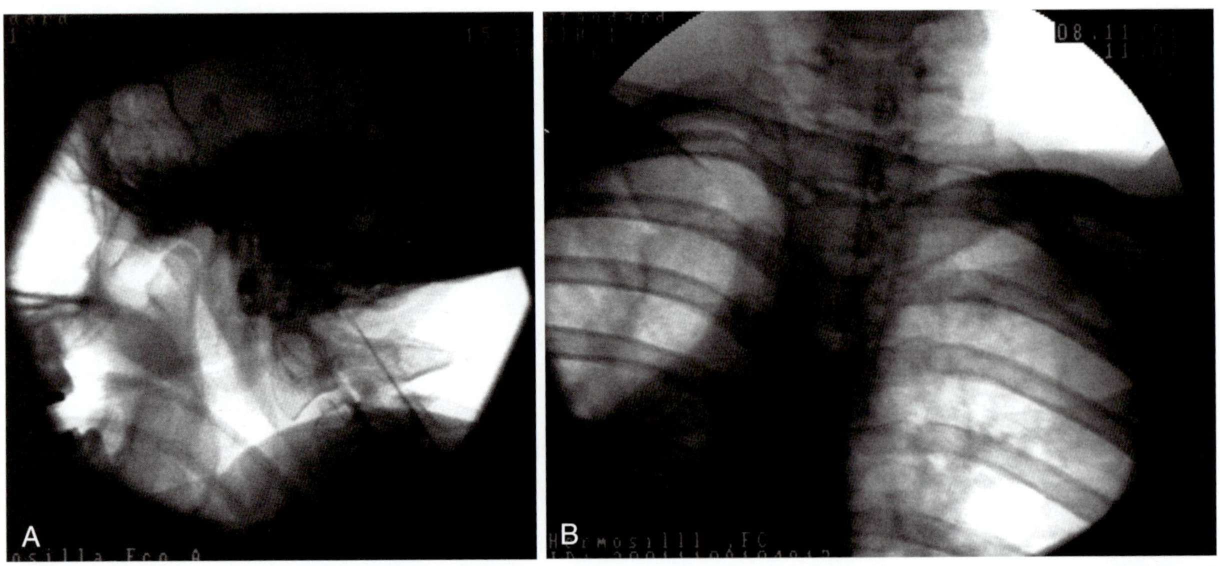

Fig. 23.8 Catheter in the cervical area in posteroanterior (B) and lateral (A) views in a patient with an intrathecal infusion pump to treat face and neck pain produced by an oncological pathology.

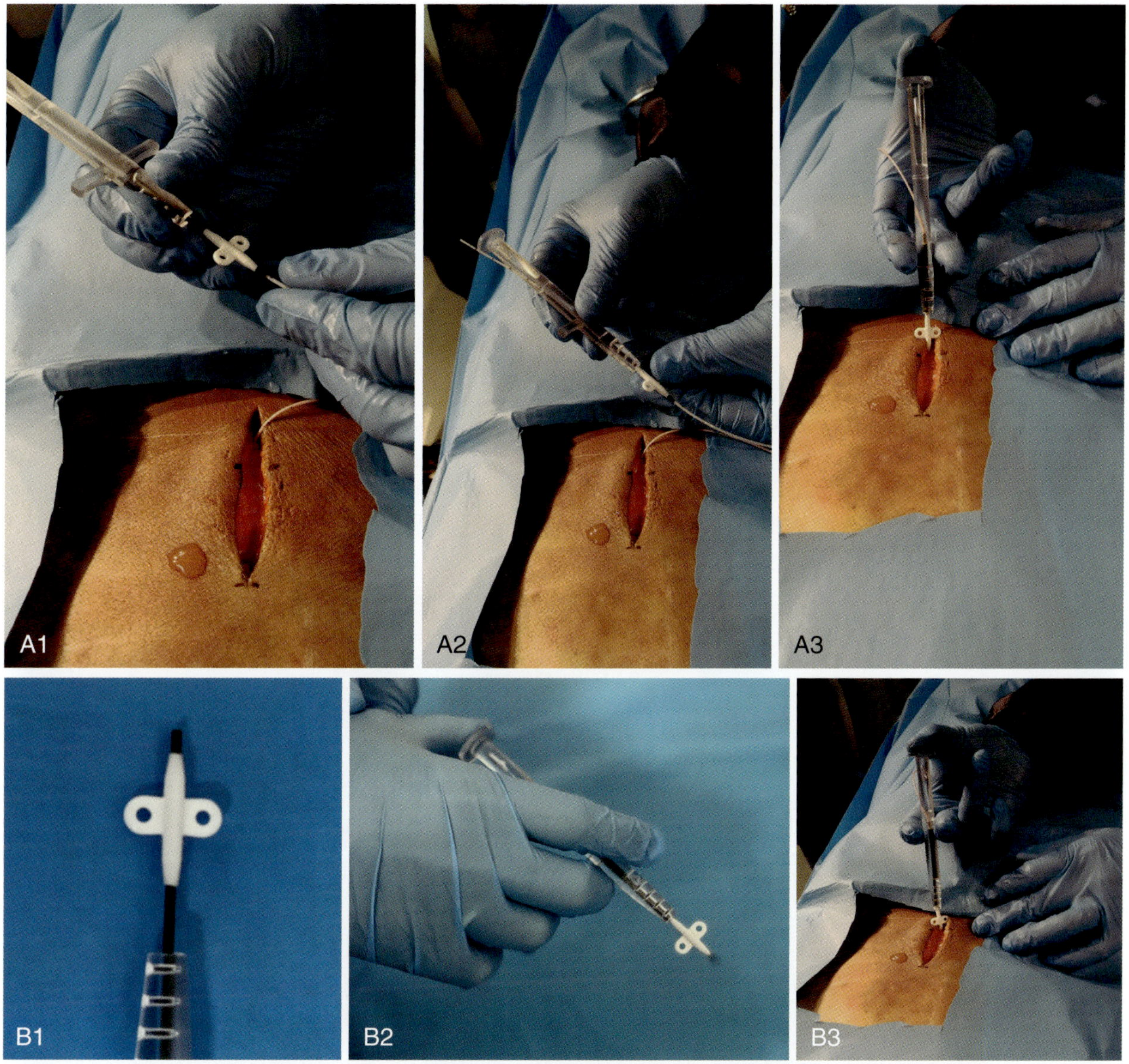

Fig. 23.9 Device that allows the anchor to slide Injex (Medtronic; Minneapolis, MN). The device in the shape of a syringe has a Teflon layer that allows the anchor to slide through it. Note how the catheter is inserted in the proximal part and comes out from the distal part (A1, A2, A3). The anchor injection maneuver is contrary to the one used in a normal syringe—the thumb is kept fixed and the fingers pull toward the thumb (Sequence B1, B2, B3).

anchoring will also avoid distal migrations. It is also preferable to perform the skin opening and establish hemostasis before the dural puncture in order to prevent bleeding or hematoma, which may compress the anchorage.[9,10]

Tunneling and Pocket

Once the catheter has been correctly anchored to the fascia, it should be tunneled from the lumbar area to the pocket in the abdominal area where the pump will

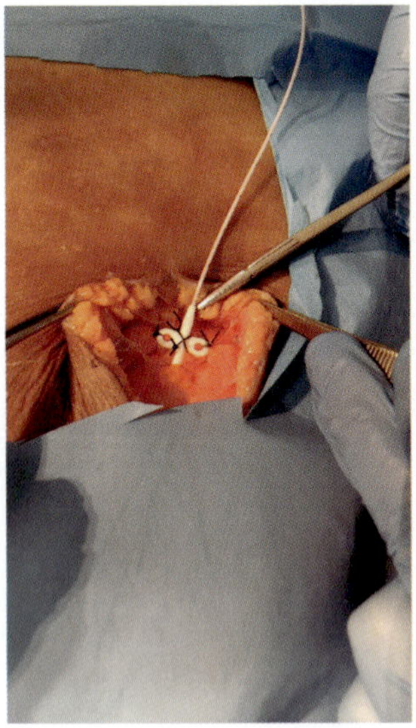

Fig. 23.10 Final appearance of a silicone anchor attached to the fascia with silk.

be implanted. The most frequently used location for the implantation of an intrathecal pump is the left flank. For this, the patient must be placed in the lateral decubitus position with the left side up. Occasionally, other implant sites are chosen, such as the gluteal area/posterior iliac fossa or the lateral thoracic wall under the axilla, with a subpectoral placement. Although tunneling complications might decrease by using these locations, other complications caused by the pump's size and location might increase.

Providers must pay attention to the plane on which they are executing the tunneling. On one hand, too superficial a plane can lead to erosion or decubitus over time. On the other hand, going too deep can cause injuries to internal organs. In the case of an intrathecal pump, with the patient in lateral decubitus, the intestines or lung can be injured. Tunneling the catheter from the lumbar incision can be done in a

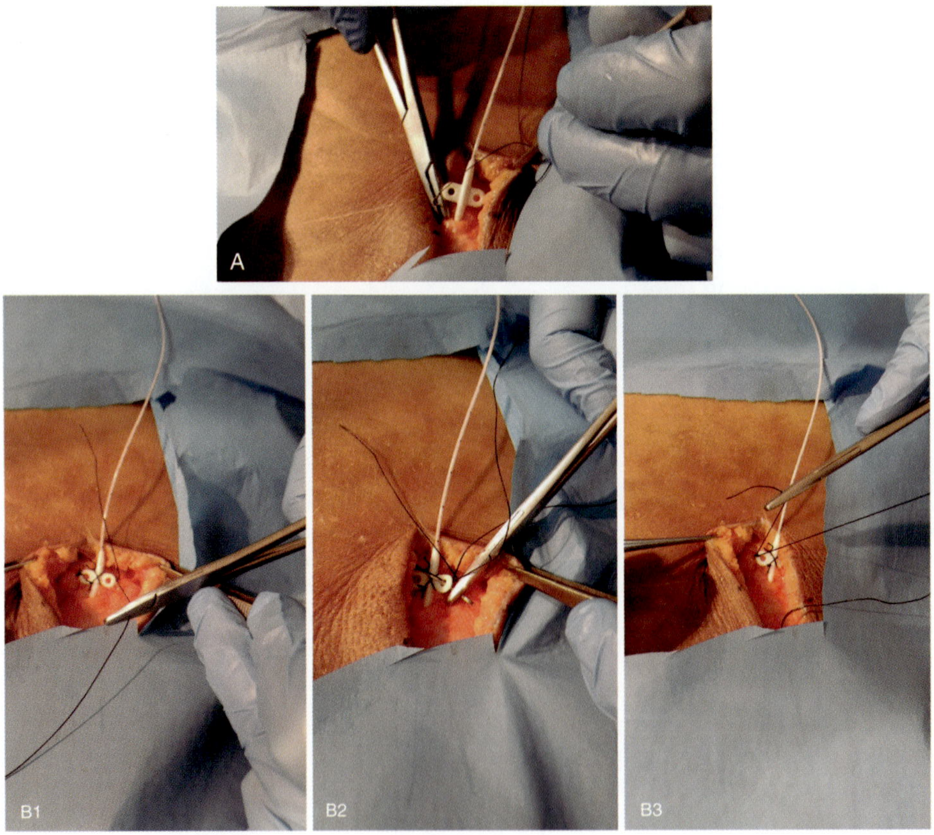

Fig. 23.11 (A) Anchor of an intrathecal catheter. (B) Anchor of an intrathecal catheter (Sequence B1, B2, B3).

TABLE 23.3 Types of Nonabsorbable Sutures

	Silk	Polyester	Polyamide (Nylon)	Polypropylene	Stainless Steel
Composition and structure	Natural multifilament	Synthetic multi/ monofilament	Synthetic multi/ monofilament	Synthetic monofilament	Synthetic monofilament
Size (USP)	11/0 to 7	6/0 to 5	11/0 to 2	10/0 to 1	11/0 to 7
Capillarity	High	Medium	Medium/minimal	Minimal	Minimal
Tissue reaction	High	Moderate	Low	Low	Low
Tensile strength	Good	Very good	Very good	Good	Very good
Thread memory	Low	Medium	High	High	Low
Uses	Skin anastomosis Vascular ligature Ophthalmology Digestive tract General surgery	Plastic surgery Vascular surgery Skin Orthopedic surgery Vascular prosthesis General surgery	Plastic surgery Nerve damage vascular surgery Microsurgery Orthopedic surgery General surgery	Dermatological and plastic surgery Fascia Nerves General surgery Abdominal wall Orthopedic surgery	Abdominal wall Orthopedic surgery Neurosurgery Sternum closure

single step. However, to decrease the rate of potential complications, it is better to do it with two intermediate steps. This way, the depth of the tunnel is easier to control. Tunneling in only one step is used mainly when a high risk of infection exists. In this case, not having intermediate steps decreases the risk of infection (Fig. 23.12).

As with other medical implants, the size of the pocket for the implant depends on the size of the device. It is recommended that the size of the pocket should exceed the size of the pump by 10% to 20% (Figs. 23.13 and 23.14). When implanting an intrathecal pump, the pocket should have a depth of 1 to 3 cm to allow for correct refilling and connection to the programmer. The implant must not be too deep or it will not allow adequate refilling, but it should also not be too superficial, as that would cause decubitus or erosions.

Once the pocket has been correctly constructed, the pump has been tested and properly adjusted, and the catheter has been tunneled into the pocket, the pump can be connected to the catheter (Fig. 23.15). Once everything is connected, the pump can be inserted into the pocket, paying attention to the location of the side port and the pump catheter connector. When everything has been checked, closing can begin. Closing must be done by planes, closing the inner planes with resorbable suture. It is recommended to use nonabsorbable sutures for the skin (Figs. 23.16–23.19).

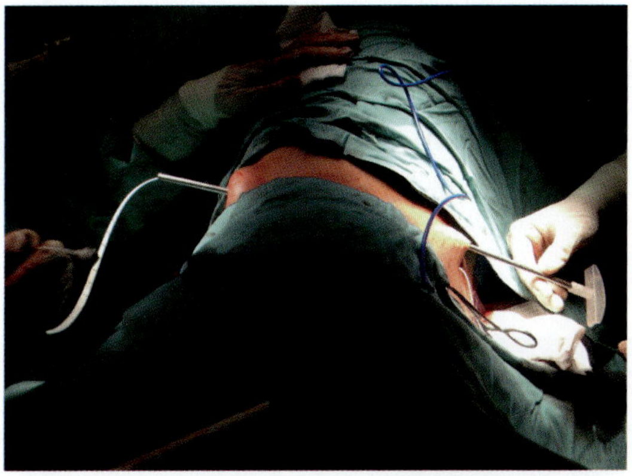

Fig. 23.12 One step intrathecal catheter tunneling from the lumbar incision to the pump placed in the abdominal area. Tunneling in two steps can be performed, passing from the lumbar area to the flank and from there to the abdominal area where the pump is located. To decrease the risk of infection, however, it should be done in one step. (Courtesy Dra. Canos, Department of Anesthesiology, Hospital Universitario y Politécnico La Fe, Valencia, Spain.)

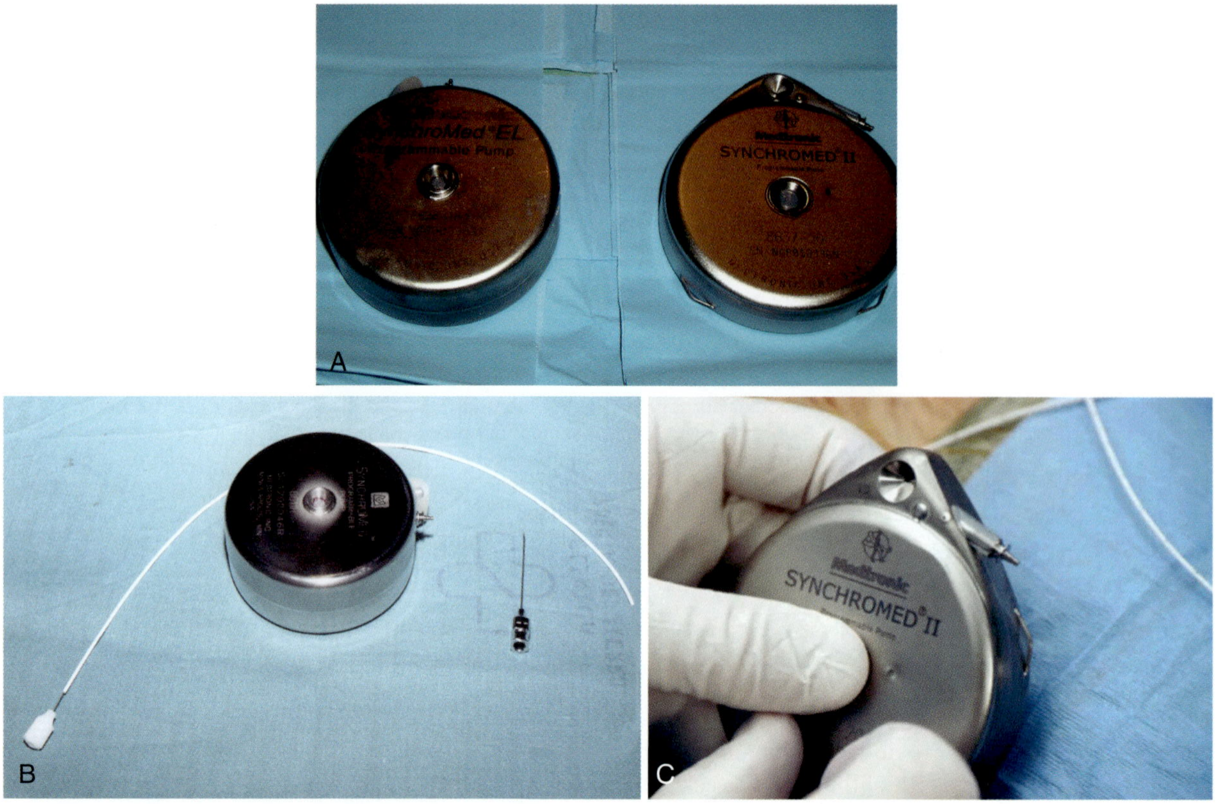

Fig. 23.13 (A) Intrathecal pump. Note the difference in size between the two pumps. (B, C) Intrathecal pump. Note the size of the implant.

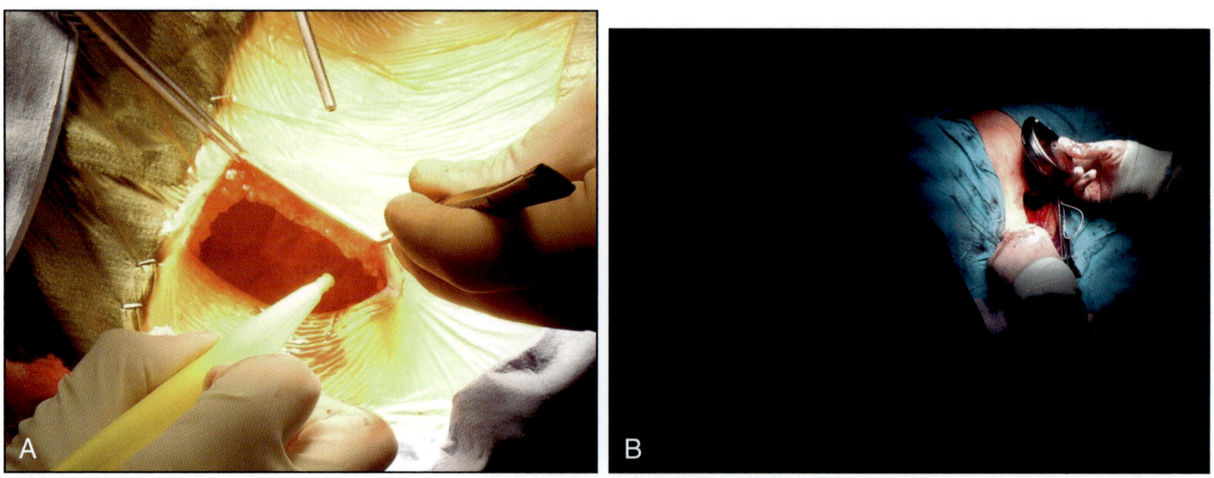

Fig. 23.14 (A, B) The size of the pocket must be adjusted to the size of the implantable device, in this case, the intrathecal pump. The implant must always be bigger than the impulse generator. (23.15A courtesy Dr. Robert Plunkett, Department of Neurosurgery, SUNY at Buffalo, Buffalo General Hospital, Buffalo, NY; 23.15B courtesy Dra. Canos, Department of Anesthesiology, Hospital Universitario y Politécnico La Fe, Valencia, Spain.)

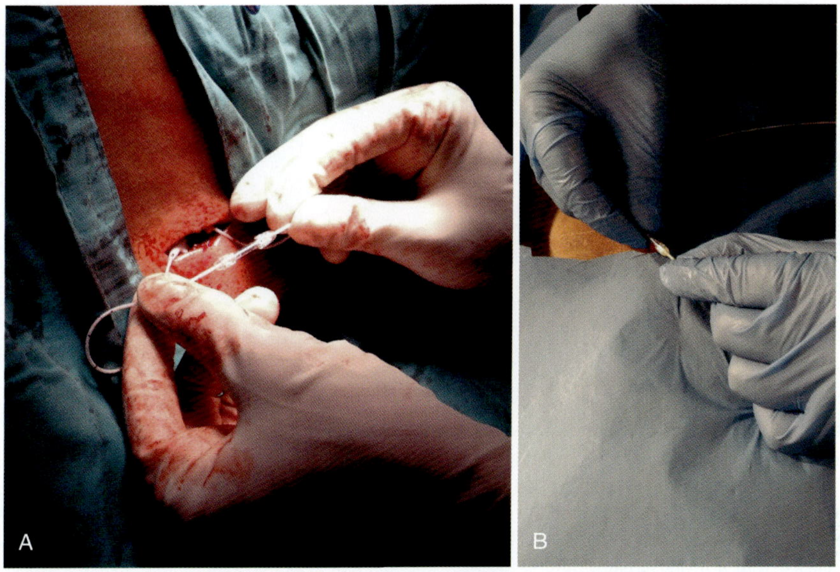

Fig. 23.15 (A, B) Connection of the tunneled catheter to the pump once the pocket has been constructed correctly and appropriately sized. The middle connection is used to connect the intrathecal catheter to the pump, as seen in both A and B.

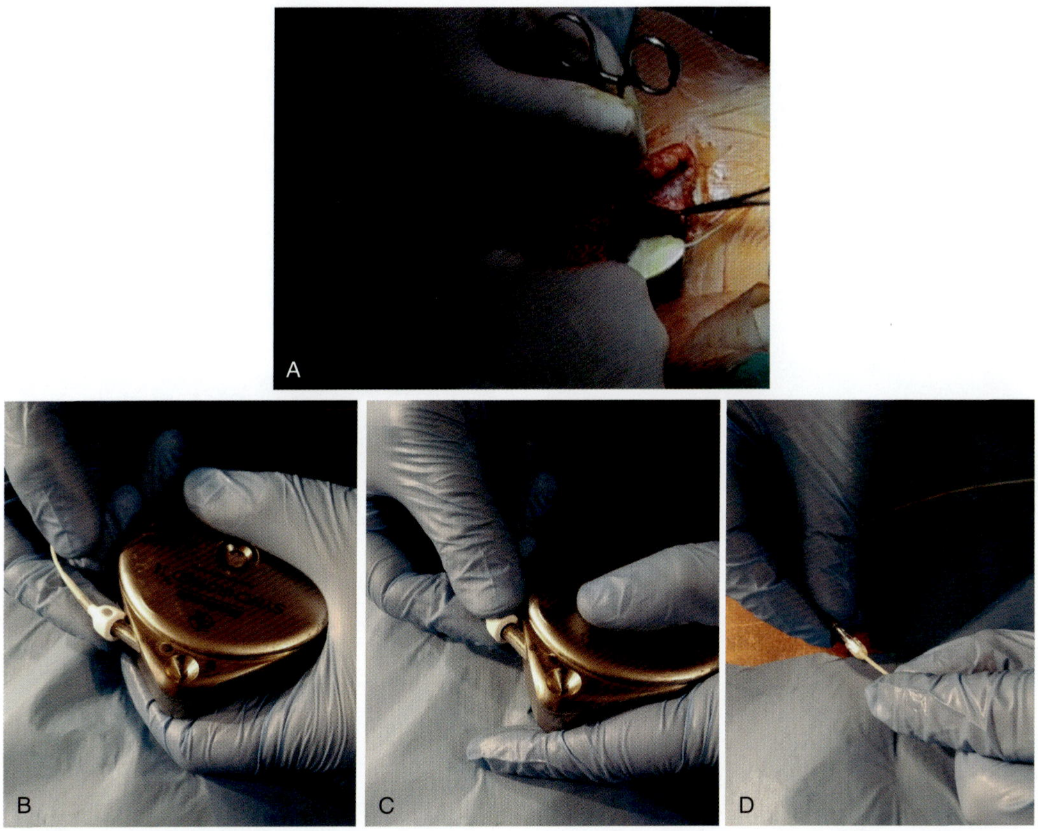

Fig. 23.16 (A–D) Once the catheter is connected to the pump, it is placed inside the pocket. Some providers prefer to suture the pump or even suture the excess catheter to avoid movement or kinking.

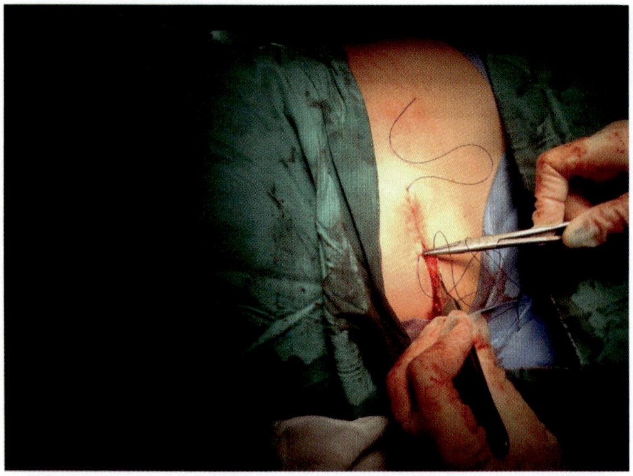

Fig. 23.17 Final closing after confirming proper functioning and connections of the pump. It is important to verify the state of all components for the pump as well as cerebrospinal leakage from the catheter before connecting it to the pump. Closing must be performed by plane and the skin must be closed with a nonabsorbable suture. (Courtesy Dra. Canos, Department of Anesthesiology, Hospital Universitario y Politécnico La Fe, Valencia, Spain.)

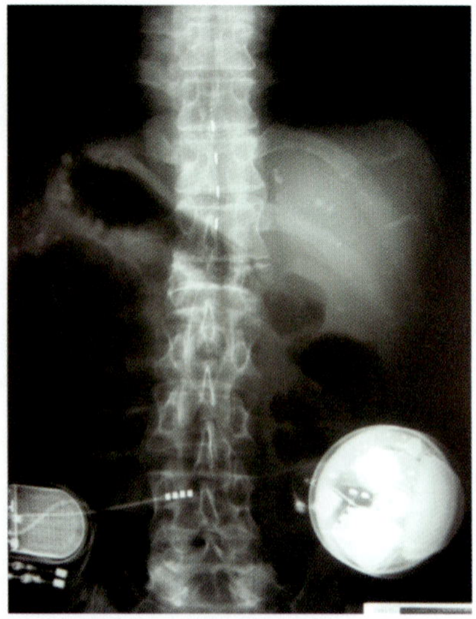

Fig. 23.19 Radiographic image of the pump and catheter connected at the end of the procedure. Anteroposterior view. (Courtesy Dr. Francisco Sánchez, Hospital Clinico Universitario Salamanca, Salamanca, Spain.)

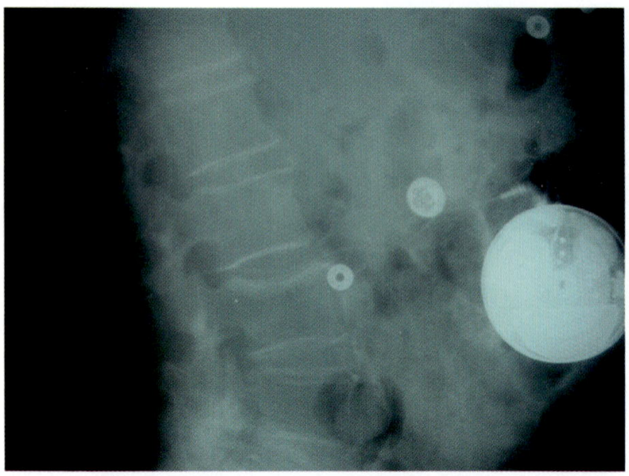

Fig. 23.18 Radiographic image of the pump and catheter connected at the end of the procedure. Lateral view. (Courtesy Dr. Francisco Sánchez, Hospital Clinico Universitario Salamanca, Salamanca, Spain.)

Drugs Used

Morphine and ziconotide are the only medications approved by the US Food and Drug Administration (FDA) for the intrathecal treatment of chronic pain. Baclofen is the only FDA-approved medication for treatment of spasticity using intrathecal drug delivery (IDD). Recommendations on drug choice, concentration limits, and starting doses were outlined in the PACC's 2012 publication.[11–14] A panel of experts on behalf of the International Neuromodulation Society (INS) convened on intrathecal therapy to promote safety and efficacy. The medication tiers were designed based on nociceptive or neuropathic pain. Tables 23.4 through 23.7 show the maximum daily dose, initial dosage, and the

TABLE 23.4 Drugs and Dosage for Intrathecal Use

Drug	Maximum Daily Dose	Maximum Concentration
Morphine	15 mg	20 mg/mL
Hydromorphone	10 mg	15 mg/mL
Bupivacaine	10 mg	30 mg/mL
Clonidine	40–600 μg	1,000 μg/mL
Fentanyl	Not determined	10 mg/mL
Sulfentanyl	Not determined	5 mg/mL
Ziconotide	19.2 μg	100 μg /mL
Baclofen	2 mg	2 mg/mL

algorithms for neuropathic and nociceptive pain, respectively.

Refilling the Pump

When the pump has been implanted, functions well, and the patient's pain has improved, the patient's care has just begun. Unlike other analgesic treatments used to treat pain, infusion is a treatment modality that involves a significant commitment from the medical and nursing teams in charge of the patient. A problem with the refills, or a miscalculation of the dose or concentration of the refill can have fatal consequences for the patient. Unlike this system,

TABLE 23.5 Recommended Initial Doses for Intrathecal Drugs (Bolus Test Phase)

Drug	Recommended bolus dose
Morphine	0.2–10 mg
Hydromorphone	0.04–0.2 mg
Ziconotide	1–5 μg
Fentanyl	25–75 μg
Bupivacaine	0.5–2.5 mg
Clonidine	5–20 μg
Sulfentanyl	5–20 μg

TABLE 23.6 Polyanalgesic Consensus Conference 2012 Intrathecal Algorithm for Neuropathic Pain

Line 1	Morphine	Ziconotide		Morphine + bupivacaine
Line 2	Hydromorphone	Hydromorphone + bupivacaine/hydromorphone + clonidine		Morphine + clonidine
Line 3	Clonidine	Ziconotide + opioid	Fentanyl	Fentanyl + bupivacaine/ Fentanyl + clonidine
Line 4	Opioid + clonidine + bupivacaine		Bupivacaine + clonidine	
Line 5	Baclofen			

TABLE 23.7 Polyanalgesic Consensus Conference 2012 Intrathecal Algorithm for Nociceptive Pain

Line 1	Morphine	Hydromorphone	Ziconotide	Fentanyl
Line 2	Morphine + bupivacaine	Ziconotide + opioid	Hydromorphone + bupivacaine	Fentanyl + bupivacaine
Line 3	Opioid (morphine, hydromorphone, fentanyl) + clonidine			Sulfentanyl
Line 4	Opioid + clonidine + bupivacaine		Sulfentanyl + bupivacaine/ sulfentanyl + clonidine	
Line 5	Sulfentanyl + bupivacaine + clonidine			

neurostimulation system issues do not usually lead to fatal consequences.[15]

The first pump refill is performed in the operating room, before drug infusion with the intrathecal pump is begun. First, providers must empty the pump as it comes from the manufacturer filled with saline. To ensure the proper functioning of the pump, the provider must check that the amount of saline extracted from the pump is the same as the amount specified by the manufacturer (Figs. 23.20 and 23.21).

To program the pump, the radiofrequency antenna is placed at the percutaneous level in the area where the pump is implanted (Fig. 23.22). This way, the pump communicates with the computer, which programs the pump and simultaneously obtains information on its status, including infused drugs, dose and mode of infusion, residual volume of the medication tank, and battery.

Different infusion modalities can be programmed according to the patient's needs:

1. Continuous infusion
2. Simple boluses at predetermined hours

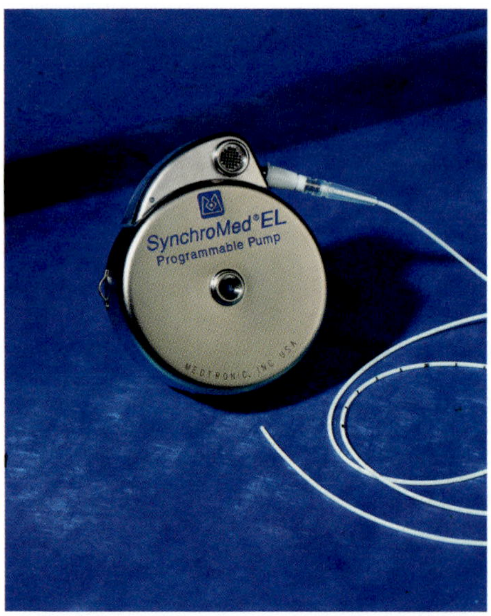

Fig. 23.20 **Intrathecal pump with the refill port in the middle of the pump and the lateral port to verify the correct functioning of the catheter. The provider must be precise and must be sure the needle is inside the port during the refill. Every time the lateral port is used, we recommend withdrawing the length of the catheter to avoid overdose.**

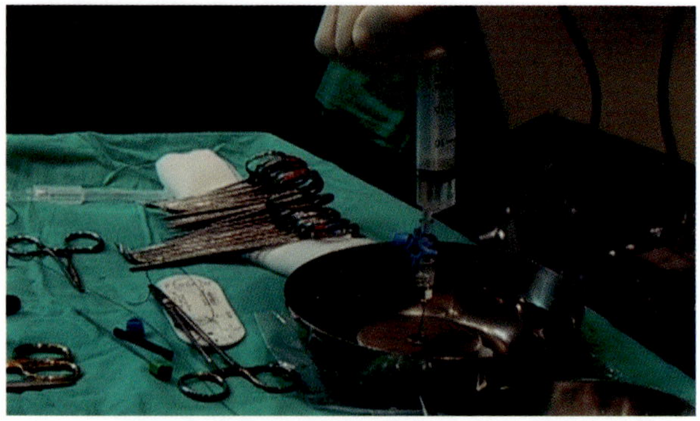

Fig. 23.21 **Before implanting the pump, the saline that comes precharged in the pump from the manufacturer must be extracted. This verifies that the system works correctly. Then, the first refill is performed before programming the desired dosage calculated for the patient.**

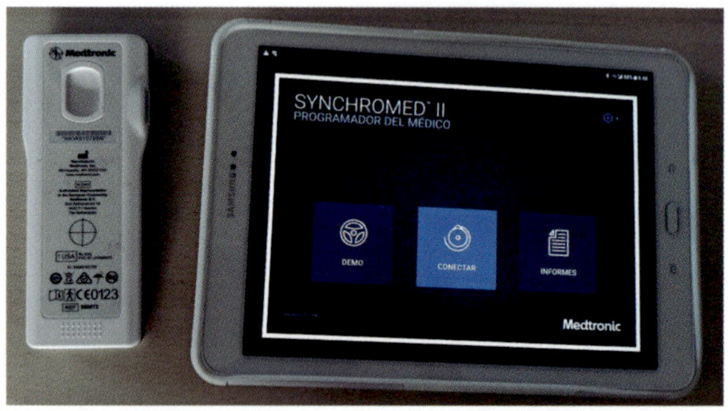

Fig. 23.22 **The Medtronic C900 Clinician Tablet.**

3. Continuous infusion with predetermined boluses
4. Continuous complex, allowing an increase or decrease in the flow throughout the day according to the determined needs of the patient
5. Personalized therapy—with a remote control, the patient can self-administered additional boluses This type of therapy must be programmed per the determined needs of the patient (dose/bolus, number of boluses/day, time-block interval).

Current pumps have a wide margin of infusion flow. Take for example the Medtronic SynchroMed II Infusion System programmable pump, which can administer between 0.048 mL/day and 24 mL/day with great precision in release of the dose. Once the most appropriate program for the patient has been decided, the patient must be scheduled for an appointment for the provider to check the pump to evaluate its configuration and volume deposit. The provider should establish an alarm date and program, check the level of analgesia and functionality the patient has obtained, and reschedule the patient for follow-up visits until reaching the desired analgesic level. Subsequently, the alarm date should be checked and the patient should be scheduled for a refill 1 week before that date to be completed before the pump medication runs out.

Refilling the pump is a process that has to be done either in the operating room or in a day hospital with trained staff. There are refill kits that include all of the necessary materials to perform the refill. However, providers occasionally use a gripper with a 3-step key that allows them to perform the refill without complications. Also, this method is more economical in clinical practice. Access to the central port of the pump and its handling must be done in a sterile field to avoid introducing pathogens from the skin into the port. As mentioned, there are plastic templates with the same shape and dimensions of the pump that can facilitate access to the central port. Sometimes, ultrasound[16] or fluoroscopy can be used to locate the port when factors obscure its location, such as obese patients with excessive subcutaneous fat, hypermobility of the pump inside the pocket, deep implantation of the pump, inclination or inversion of the pump, suboptimal position of the patient, or either the excessive movement of the pump when attempting to recharge it or the patient moving at the time of puncture. Usually, however, filling the pump does not require the use of any imaging technique if it is done by an experienced provider per protocol.

The technique itself consists of interrogating the pump with telemetry to calculate the remaining drug still inside the pump. The precise location of the pump must be determined by palpation with both hands to locate its center without pushing the pump from any of its corners so that, when found, the place calculated and marked as the center of the pump will not move. Once the needle has been introduced into the pump, the remaining drug in the pump must be withdrawn and must match the computer-calculated value.

Once the pump refill begins, the provider must aspirate approximately every 5 mL to check that the drug goes in and comes out correctly without any obstructions in the entry or problems in the extraction. This is done so that providers can verify that the drugs are in the pump and not in the subcutaneous tissue. The most important step when refilling the pump is to precisely calculate the concentration of the drug that has been planned to treat the patient. If an error is made in this step, the consequences can be devastating, resulting in death or severe cerebral injuries. If the drug is injected into the subcutaneous tissue, this can also lead to serious consequences for the patient. Finally, even when every step is performed correctly, providers must be very vigilant about programming the pump; a mistake in this step can have the same consequences as those just discussed. Refilling the pump is a simple step but can have dire consequences if providers believe that their job finishes with the completion of surgery.

REFERENCES

1. Sicard A. Les injeccions medicamenteuses extradural par voie sacrococcygienne. *C R Soc Biol. Paris.* 1901;53:396-399,3.
2. Cathelin F. A new route of spinal injection; a method of epidural injections by way of the Sacral Canal; application to man. *C R Soc Biol.* 1901;53:452.
3. Pagés F. Anestesia Metamérica. *Rev San Mil Madrid.* 1921;11: 351-364.
4. Wang JK, Nauss LA, Thomas JE. Pain relief by intrathecally applied morphine in man. *Anestesiology.* 1979;50(2):149-151.
5. Onofrio BM, Yaksh TL, Arnold PG. Continuous low-dose intrathecal morphine administration in the treatment of chronic pain of malignant origin. *Mayo Clinic Proc.* 1981;56(8):516-520.
6. Deer T, Winkelmuller W, Erdine S, Bedder M, Burchiel K. Intrathecal therapy for cancer and nonmalignant pain: patient selection and patient management. *Neuromodulation.* 1999;2(2): 55-66.
7. Paulino M, Kim PS, Shaw E. Practical considerations and patient selection for intrathecal drug delivery in the management of chronic pain. *J Pain Res.* 2014;7:627-638.
8. Haddadan K, Krames ES. Technique that better localizes the dura mater during intrathecal catheterization should reduce inadvertent multiple dural punctures and reduce complications. *Neuromodulation.* 2007;10(2):164-166. doi:10.1111/j.1525-1403.2007.00105.x.
9. Follett KA, Naumann CP. A prospective study of catheter-related complications of intrathecal drug delivery systems. *J Pain Symptom Manage.* 2000;19(3):209-215.

10. Follett KA, Burchiel K, Deer T, et al. Prevention of intrathecal drug delivery catheter-related complications. *Neuromodulation*. 2003;6(1):32-41. doi:10.1046/j.1525-1403.2003.03005.x.
11. Deer TR, Prager J, Levy R, et al. Polyanalgesic Consensus Conference 2012: Recommendations for the Management of Pain by Intrathecal (Intraspinal) Drug Delivery: Report of an Interdisciplinary Expert Panel. *Neuromodulation*. 2012;15(5):436-464.
12. Deer TR, Pope JE, Hayek SM, et al. The Polyanalgesic Consensus Conference (PACC): Recommendations on Intrathecal Drug Infusion Systems Best Practices and Guidelines. *Neuromodulation*. 2017;20(2):96-132. doi:10.1111/ner.12538.
13. Deer TR, Prager J, Levy R, et al. Polyanalgesic Consensus Conference—2012: Recommendations on Trialing for Intrathecal (Intraspinal) Drug Delivery: Report of an Interdisciplinary Expert Panel. *Neuromodulation*. 2012;15(5):420-435; discussion 435. doi:10.1111/j.1525-1403.2012.00450.x.
14. Hassenbusch SJ, Portenoy RK, Cousins M, et al. Polyanalgesic Consensus Conference 2003: An Update on the Management of Pain by Intraspinal Drug Delivery—Report of an Expert Panel. *J Pain Symptom Manage*. 2004;27(6):540-563. doi:10.1016/j.jpainsymman.2004.03.001.
15. Krames E. Implantable devices for pain control: spinal cord stimulation and intrathecal therapies. *Best Pract Re. Clin Anaesthesiol*. 2002;16(4):619-649.
16. Maino P, van Kuijk SMJ, Perez RSGM, Koetsier E. Ease of fill port access during the ultrasound-guided vs. the blind refill technique of intrathecal drug delivery systems with a raised septum, a prospective comparison study. *Neuromodulation*. 2018;21(7):641-647. doi:10.1111/ner.12736.

Chapter 24

Interrogation and Refill

Tariq Malik

Chapter Outline

Introduction

Intrathecal drug delivery is an effective method to manage severe chronic and cancer pain.[1] It has been used for over 30 years, ever since it was first approved for clinical use in the 1980s. Currently, several devices are commercially available. However, the Synchromed-II (Medtronic; Minneapolis, MN) and Prometra-II (Flowonix Medical; Mount Olive, NJ) intrathecal drug delivery systems are most often used in the United States. The devices have the same basic construct: a hard metal shell, a reservoir for the medications, and a battery along with an electronic system to deliver precise amounts of drug to the cerebral spinal fluid (CSF) via an intrathecally placed catheter. The devices come in two sizes: a 20-mL and 40-mL reservoir system. The finite drug volume along with the limitation imposed by the US Food and Drug Administration (FDA) on the stability of the drugs in the device means that the device reservoir needs to be replaced or refilled every few months. Failure to do so will affect device functionality and can result in life-threatening complications if the pump runs dry. The patient's inability to reliably keep refill appointments would make the individual a poor candidate for this mode of therapy. Thus, the pump refill process is an important part of patient management. *Pocket refill*, in which medication is deposited outside the device reservoir, is a known and dreaded complication of the pump refill process. Its exact incidence is unknown and often underreported. According to an international pump registry involving a total of 77,584 pump refills done for 6179 implanted pumps over an 8-year period (2010–2018), 9 pocket refill events were reported, with another 17 events having post-refill symptoms possibly related to a pocket refill.[2] Medtronic sent a letter to members of the health care community in 2011 to remind them of this complication during the refill process after 8 deaths and 270 life-threatening adverse events related to pocket refills requiring medical intervention came to light.[3]

Technical Considerations

The intrathecal drug delivery device is surgically placed in the subcutaneous plane 2 to 3 cm below the skin. The site is selected based on patient comfort and ease of access to refill the device reservoir. If placed too deep, it would be hard to locate the device and to access its refill port; placed too shallow, it will stick out and cause skin breakdown. For safety and ease of locating the refill port, it is important to document orientation of the device in the medical record. The refill port should always be accessed with an approved needle, preferably using the manufacturer's provided refill kit and manufacturer-provided protocol. The device has a metallic shell that houses drug in a reservoir. The reservoir is accessed by a refill port covered with a silicone rubber septum. The septum is specially designed to prevent drug leakage from the reservoir after it has been punctured by a noncoring needle during the pump refill. Failure to follow the manufacturer guidelines in refilling can damage the device and result in life-threatening complications.

Step-by-Step Description of the Procedure

EVALUATE THE PATIENT

All patients should be evaluated before refilling their intrathecal pump. Review the previous refill notes to look for any potential complication or difficulty with the refill procedure. Drug formulation, including concentration, and dose should be reviewed. Orientation of the device should be checked. Targeted history is essential for detecting a pump malfunction. Review history looking for any signs or symptoms suggesting loss of therapeutic benefits or drug withdrawal (underdosing) or presence of medication-related side effects (overdosing). Examine the pump site for presence of skin disease or device flipping if significant weight gain or loss has occurred.

1. Device Interrogation: The pump should be interrogated before any refill. The interrogation will reveal pump model and capacity, drug name and concentration, expected drug volume, infusion mode, alarm status, and battery life (elective replacement interval [ERI] or end of service [EOS]). The information is not only important for safe refilling but also to plan for pump replacement in a timely fashion when battery life is nearing the EOS date.
2. Pump refill is technically a very simple procedure; however, patient habitus can make it very challenging. Accidental overdose is always a potential risk—therefore, proper training of personnel is important. Currently, there are no defined criteria as to what constitutes proper training or in-service for personnel who can manage the refill independently.
3. The refill should be performed by trained personnel with access to resuscitative drugs and equipment. Ensure that the manufacturer refill kit is available, the correct drug is available for the correct patient, and that the drug is not expired or contaminated in any way before emptying the reservoir.
4. Ergonomics and comfort of the patient are important. They will minimize accidental needle slippage during the refill. Supine position is comfortable and preferred by most patients. Devices implanted in wheelchair-bound patients can be refilled with the patient in the wheelchair as long as sterile conditions are maintained and proper access to the pump is possible. Use of imaging to refill the pump should be clearly documented to plan optimal positioning for the next refill.

Procedural Steps

The SynchroMed II system (Medtronic) and Prometra II system (Flowonix) are not refilled in the same way. Steps for each are provided next.

SYNCHROMED II MEDTRONIC PUMP[4]

The manufacturer's refill kit is a single-use kit that contains the following:

- Extension tubing and clamp
- 0.2-μ filter
- 22-gauge noncoring needle
- 20-mL empty syringe
- Fenestrated drape
- Template

Sterile gloves and antiseptic skin cleaning solution are not included in the kit but must be used for the procedure.

1. Place the patient supine.
2. Interrogate the pump with the programmer and collect necessary data.
3. Clean the pump area carefully using the same precautions and care as if performing a neuraxial block on a patient. Give appropriate time for the solution to kill skin bacteria.
4. Open the manufacturer refill kit (Fig. 24.1) and have the drug to be refilled available in the room.

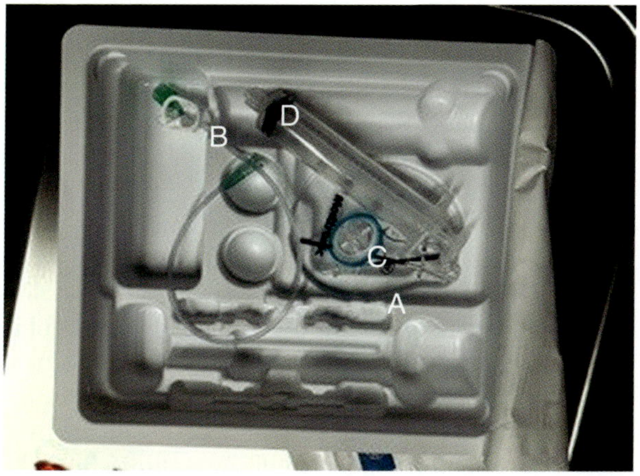

Fig. 24.1 Medtronic refill kit. *(A)* Template. *(B)* Extension tubing with clamp. *(C)* Filter. *(D)* Syringe.

5. Wear a surgical mask, wash your hands, and don sterile gloves.
6. Place a fenestrated drape on the patient and remind the patient to keep hands away from the sterile field.
7. Securely connect the needle and the 20-mL syringe to the extension tubing. Close the clamp on the extension tubing (see Fig. 24.1B).
8. Place the template onto the pump, aligning it with the outline of the pump. Then, insert the needle through the center hole of the template to enter the reservoir fill port (Fig. 24.2).

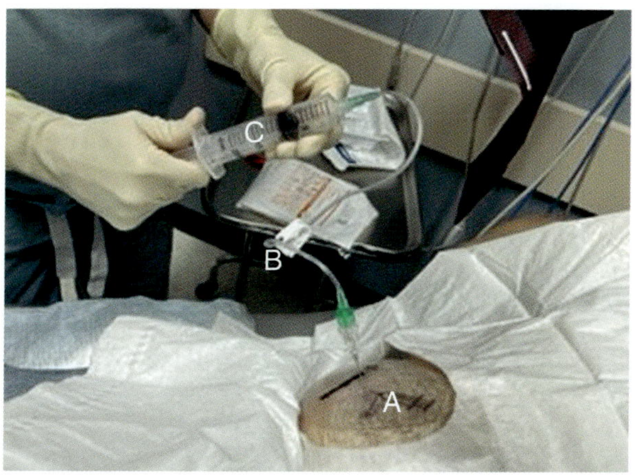

Fig. 24.2 Emptying the pump using the template. *(A)* Template. *(B)* Extension tubing. *(C)* Syringe

9. It is important that the needle enter the fill port perpendicularly and not at an angle. Entering the silicone septum of the fill port at an angle or rocking the needle will damage the septum, which can result in overdose from a drug leak.[5]
10. Use the template to hold the pump down steadily. The needle passes through the skin and subcutaneous tissue on its way to the silicone septum and comes to a hard stop as it touches the metal at the base of the reservoir fill port. The septum has a rubbery feeling when the needle goes through it. Do not use excessive force if resistance is met when locating the fill port. The needle is hitting the outside of the pump. Forceful bumping would damage the needle tip; this, in turn, would damage the silicone septum.
11. Once proper access to the fill port is established, open the clamp and aspirate the drug to empty the reservoir. When the reservoir is empty, a bubble will stop forming in the syringe and negative pressure on the syringe will be felt. Maintain the negative pressure on the syringe and close the clamp on the extension tube. Measure the aspirated drug volume; it should be the same as the calculated volume seen on device interrogation. Any discrepancy should be carefully documented and monitored for future refill. Increasing volume discrepancy with subsequent refills and/or signs and symptoms of drug overdose or underdose should merit interrogation of proper device and/or catheter functioning. In general, less than 5% volume discrepancy (<1 mL for a 20-mL pump and <2 mL for a 40-mL pump) is clinically insignificant if unaccompanied by any other symptoms.[6]
12. Once the reservoir is empty, close the clamp before disconnecting the syringe to dispose of the removed drug. This prevents air from entering the reservoir. If the syringe is full and more drug is still in the reservoir, reconnect the syringe after discarding the drug and aspirate the reservoir again. It is important that the needle does not slip out of the fill port and that the drug volume withdrawn is accurately measured. If a patient has missed the scheduled

refill appointment and the reservoir is empty, inject 10 mL of preservative free (PF) normal saline into the reservoir and aspirate all of it out to confirm proper needle placement before refilling the reservoir, especially if the fill port location is hard to find.

13. Once the reservoir is empty, the extension tubing clamp is closed and the syringe is disconnected. The new drug is drawn into a syringe if not already in a syringe. The 0.2-μ filter is connected to the syringe containing the new drug and the filter is carefully primed to remove air from it and then connected to the extension tubing (Fig. 24.3).
14. Ensure that the needle is still firmly against the hard metal within the fill port of the pump. Once the extension tubing is unclamped, negative pressure within the reservoir will suck in some of the medication from the syringe by itself, confirming proper placement of the needle within the fill port of the reservoir.
15. Inject the medication slowly. It is important to make sure that the needle does not slip out of the port during drug injection. It may require an extra set of hands to hold the needle into the port if patient habitus necessitates it. The medication is intermittently aspirated and reinjected back throughout the refill process as a safety check that the needle is still within the fill port.
16. Once refill is done, clamp the extension tubing, and remove the needle straight out to prevent lacerating the septum, avoiding any wiggling or angulation. Put a bandage over the needle hole and dispose of the removed drug and the refill fit appropriately.
17. Update the device with the new drug formulation and volume. The programmer will generate a new refill date. Print out the report and give a copy to the patient. Document the new information, along with any volume discrepancy and/or ERI/EOS in the patient medical record and schedule a refill appointment date. Observe the patient for at least 30 minutes before discharging from the clinic for any sign of drug overdose.

PROMETRA II PUMP

This pump refill comes with a manufacturer kit and a different refill approach from the SynchroMed II device. The kit has the following:

- Adhesive bandages
- Calibrated syringe barrel, 12 mL

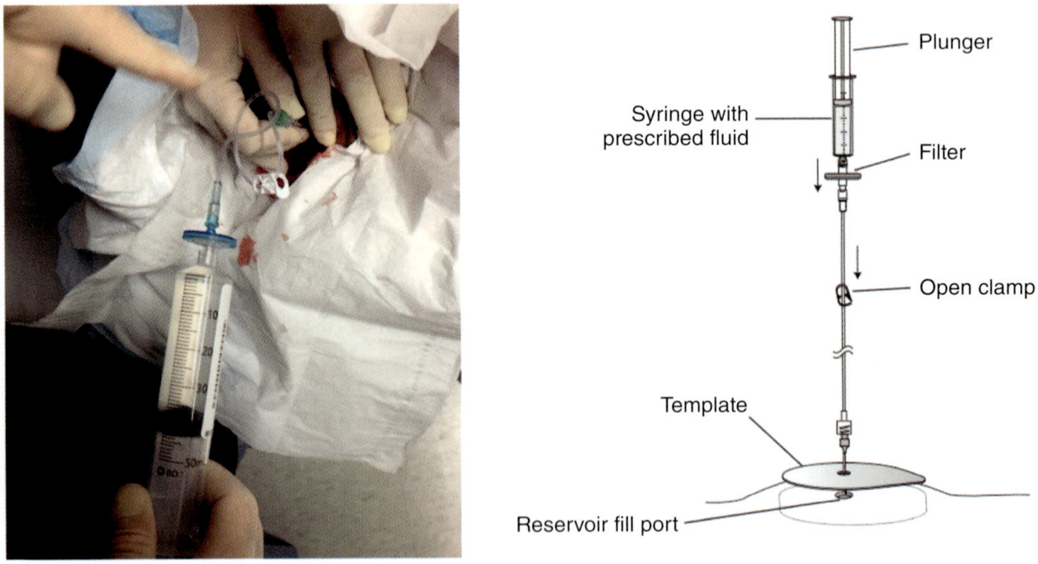

Fig. 24.3 Refilling the pump, holding the needle securely within the refill port.

- Syringe cap
- Stopcock
- CSR wrap
- Extension tubing with clamp
- Fenestrated drape
- Filter (0.22 μ)
- Gauze pads
- Noncoring needles, 0.7 mm (22-gauge) × 38 mm (1.5 in)
- Refill template

The overall principles of refill are the same.[7] The pump is interrogated, the reservoir is emptied using the kit and then refilled with the new medication. It is a sterile procedure. The same ergonomic principles apply with regard to patient position, access to the kit, and other supplies. After cleaning the skin, place the drape, and place the template over the pump to locate the pump refill port located in the middle of the pump. Unlike the SynchroMed II pump, the refill port has raised edges that are easily palpable (Fig. 24.4).

The pump is emptied of its contents before filling it up. The needle, extension tubing with clamp, and stopcock are connected. The syringe barrel is connected to the stopcock and the open end of the barrel syringe is covered with the cap (Fig. 24.5). Ensure that all connections are tight and secure. Close the clamp on the extension tubing and turn the stopcock off (stopcock wings perpendicular to the extension tubing).

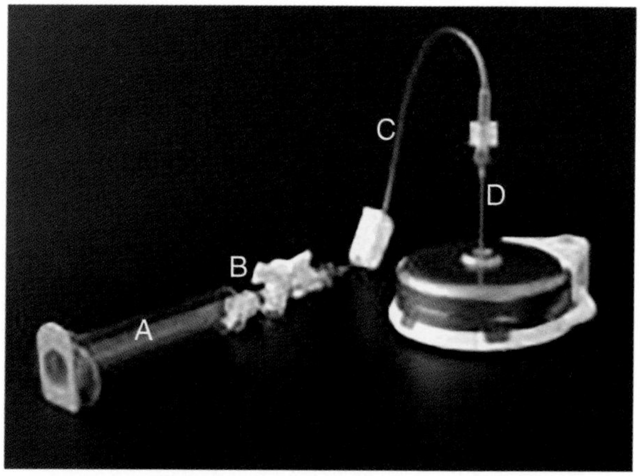

Fig. 24.5 *(A)* **Barrel syringe,** *(B)* **stopcock,** *(C)* **connection tubing, and** *(D)* **needle setup for emptying the pump.**

Access the refill port using the noncoring needle, unclamp the tubing, and turn the stopcock to the open position. The drug will collect in the calibrated barrel syringe. If less than 10 mL of drug is expected, then clamp the tubing once the entire drug is in the syringe and disconnect the syringe with the stopcock from the extension tube. The syringe is held at eye level vertically to measure the volume. The bottom of the meniscus is read to the nearest 0.2-mL calibration on the syringe. The drug is drained out of the syringe

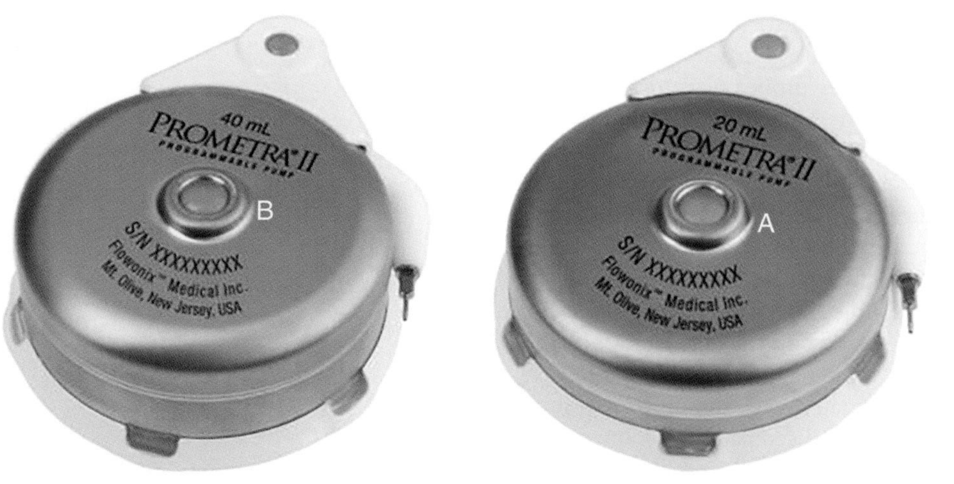

Fig. 24.4 **Prometra II pump; see the raised edges of refill port in the center.** *(A)* **Raised edge very distinctive of Prometra pumps.** *(B)* **Raised edge.**

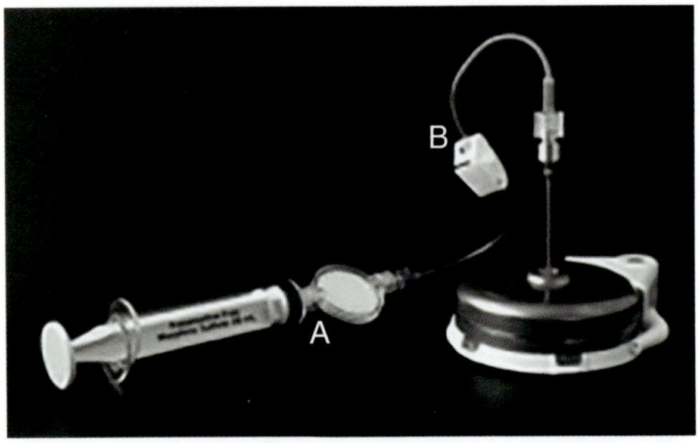

Fig. 24.6 The setup for refilling the pump; stopcock is replaced with the filter *(A)*, to which is added the tubing *(B)* for refilling the pump.

using the stopcock, and the syringe with the stopcock is reconnected to the tubing if more volume needs to be drained.

Once the entire drug reservoir is empty, the barrel syringe with stopcock is disposed of. The 0.22-μ filter is connected to the syringe with the new medication (Fig. 24.6).

The air is purged out of the filter and then connected to the extension tubing. Maintaining firm pressure on the syringe plunger, unclamp the extension tubing and inject 1 mL into the pump. Ease up the pressure off the plunger; proper needle placement in the refill port is confirmed if the drug comes back into the syringe. Repeat the process by injecting 2 mL into the reservoir and then allowing 1 mL to seep back into the syringe once pressure on the plunder is eased up. This ensures proper placement of the needle in the refill port. Thereafter, the pump is filled with the 20 or 40 mL depending on the pump capacity, allowing 1 mL of the medication to seep back into the syringe once the pressure is eased off the plunger after every 5 mL that has been injected, thus confirming proper needle placement in the refill port. Once all the volume is injected, maintain downward pressure on the plunger, clamp the extension tubing, and then remove the needle straight out.

The pump is updated with the new program. The new program with any discrepancy in volume is documented in the medical record. The patient is given a printout and, depending on the refill due date, is given a follow-up appointment.

Image-Guided Refill

The device is usually implanted 2 to 3 cm under the skin, its outline is easily felt, and refill is not an issue using the template. However, the pump refill can be an issue for a number of reasons (Box 24.1) and the possibility of depositing the medicine in any place other than the pump reservoir will cause a fatal overdose. Therefore, if the refill port access is difficult, image guidance is used. Fluoroscopy is used to visualize the reservoir refill port (Fig. 24.7).

Lately, ultrasound guidance has proved to be very useful. The refill port can be clearly visualized and marked using an ultrasound machine.[8] The pump is

BOX 24.1 Factors Contributing to Difficulty in Refill Port Access

- The pump is flipped in the pocket
- Deep implant
- Patient position (e.g., a seated patient)
- Patient movement (e.g., spasticity, difficulty holding still)
- Localized muscle spasms at the pump implant site
- Scar tissue at the pump implant site
- Seroma
- The pump is tilted in the pocket
- Obesity
- Pump movement within the pocket
- Weight gain after implant
- Weight loss after implant

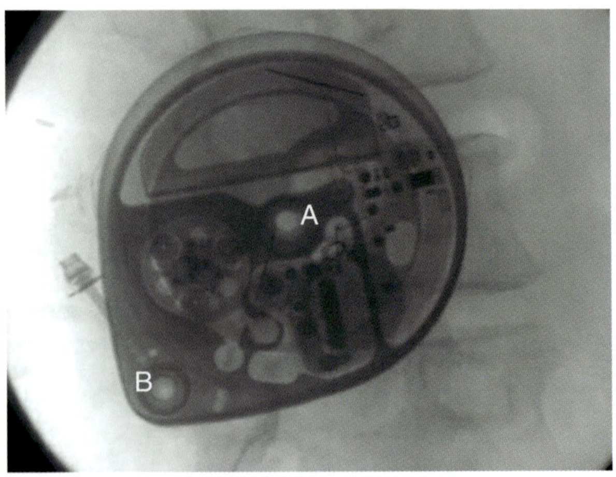

Fig. 24.7 Fluoroscopic view of Synchromed II pump. *(A)* Refill port. *(B)* Catheter access port.

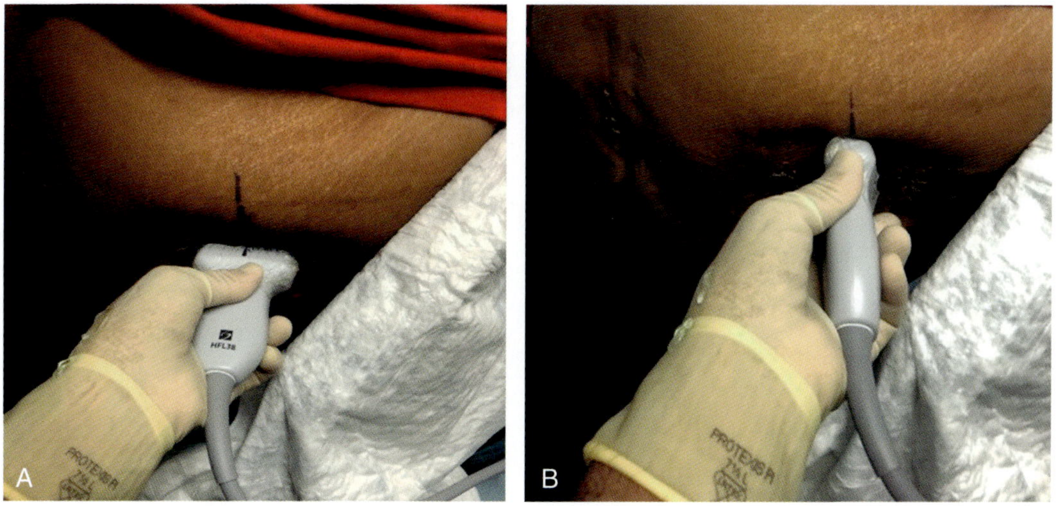

Fig. 24.8 Scanning the pump to localize the refill port in an obese patient. Pump is scanned in two axis: vertcal axis *(A)* and horizontal axis *(B)*

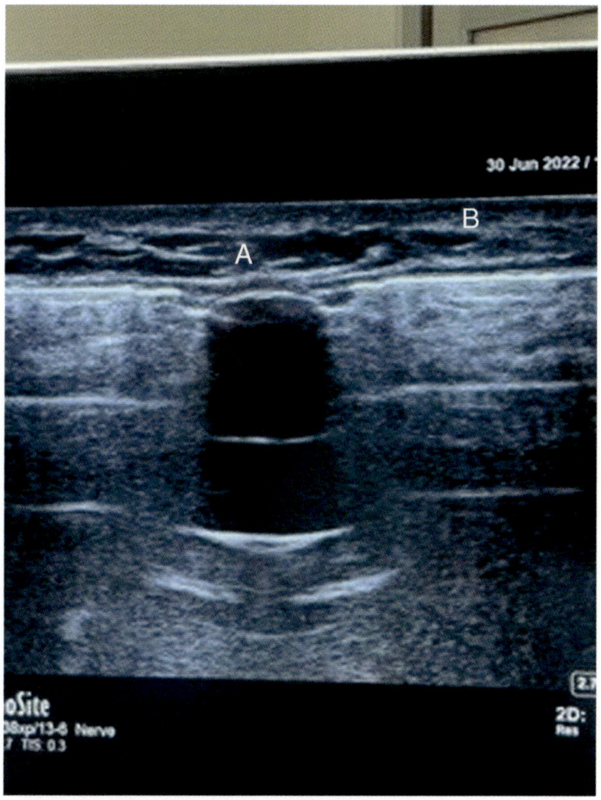

Fig. 24.9 *(A)* The central hypo-echogenic structure is the refill port. *(B)* The white line is pump metallic case.

scanned using a liner probe to visualize the refill port. The refill port is easily visualized and can be marked for easy and safe refilling in a hard-to-feel pump (Fig. 24.8). The refill port is seen as a hypoechoic rectangular well in the middle of the pump (Fig. 24.9). Ultrasound imaging has been used to drain pocket refill and to evaluate any drug deposition outside the pump if suspected.

Documentation

Each refill procedure should be well documented. A check list note will ensure that all information is captured (Box 24.2).

Complications

The pump refill is a simple but potentially high-risk procedure. The common complications are contamination or infection leading to meningitis, deposition of the medication outside the pump (also called *pocket refill*), over-pressurization of the pump due to reservoir valve activation, programming error, and damage to the silicon septum if a nonrecommended needle is used to access the refill port. Accidental access of the catheter access port during refill is possible but not probable if proper precautions are taken.

BOX 24.2 Checklist for Refill Procedure

- Make, model and pump capacity
- Previous refill date
- Sign/symptom of drug underdose or overdose
- Vital signs
- Drug name and its concentration
- Infusion mode
- 24-hour basal dose, bolus dose size, frequency, and maximum 24 hours possible
- Refill due date
- Any discrepancy between estimated vs. drained drug volume
- Pump battery life—ERI/EOS
- Low-volume alarm
- Discharge vital sign 30-minute post refill
- Scheduled next refill appointment date
- Clinic contact number for any questions

Maintaining full sterile conditions will prevent any infectious complication. Avoiding injection of any air, limiting volume to pump capacity, and avoiding rapid injection will prevent activation of the reservoir valve. When activated, it prevents injection of any more medicine into the reservoir. If that happens, the reservoir is completely emptied. This will lower the pressure with the reservoir, opening up the valve. The reservoir can then be filled.

It is imperative that the needle position is confirmed repeatedly during the refill process.[9,10] Any spill of the medication outside the pump will lead to drug overdose. If suspected, then an ultrasound should be carried out to check for fluid collection outside the pump; any fluid that is found should be drained. The patient should be admitted and observed for any drug-related side effects and managed accordingly. If an overdose is an intrathecal overdose, then 30 to 40 mL of CSF should be immediately removed in the absence of any contraindication to remove drug from the CSF. Monitor the patient in the hospital setting and treat with appropriate antidotes as the signs and symptoms of drug overdose appear. The pump can be stopped temporarily, dialed to minimum infusion rate, or the drug in the reservoir can be replaced with PF normal saline.

Silicone Septum Damage

The refill port is covered with silicone septum. The septum is pierced by the noncoring needle during refill. The SynchroMed II septum can withstand 500 puncture attempts and Prometra II can withstand 1000 puncture attempts without being damaged. Attempting to access the refill port with a nonapproved needle can damage the septum, creating a hole that can cause leakage of the drug from the reservoir into the surrounding tissue, which can cause drug overdose.[5] Forceful bumping of an approved access needle will result in a damaged needle tip. This, in turn, can shear the silicone septum. The needle should always be inserted and removed from the septum at a perpendicular angle without any rocking movement when it is within the septum.

Reservoir rinse: The pump reservoir is rinsed whenever the concentration of the new drug is significantly different from the previous drug formulation. After emptying the reservoir, 10 mL PF normal saline is injected and then removed twice to eliminate any left over drug in the reservoir before filling the reservoir with the new drug. Flowonix recommends rinsing the reservoir with 40 mL or 80 mL normal saline for the 20-or 40-mL pump, respectively.

Device Interrogation

The device interrogation is done using the manufacturer-provided portable programmer. The wireless device connects with the pump and retrieves data. The programmer will display patient information, device information, drug formulation, and the infusion mode. The programmer is used to edit the information regarding the drug, volume, alarm setup, and infusion mode. It can also interrogate the device log for any device errors stored in the log such as motor stall or other malfunctions. Incorrect programming may be introduced by human error—a team member entering incorrect information on drug concentration or units. This may lead to serious underdosing or overdosing. It is best practice to have a team member witness data entry for the new program to check the dose and concentration being entered and print out the new program to double check it to avoid any programming or dosing error.

General Considerations

Pain medication pump refill is technically an easy procedure to learn but is fraught with potential complications. Complications can be drug related, procedure

TABLE 24.1 SynchroMed II System—Approved Drugs and Refill Intervals

Morphine PF (up to 25 mg/mL)	180 days
Baclofen PF (500–2000 μ/mL)	180 days
Ziconotide PF (25–100 μ/mL)	14 days first initial refill, then 84 days

TABLE 24.2 Prometra II System—Approved Drugs and Refill Intervals

Morphine PF	90 days
Baclofen PF	60 days

related, and program related. These can be avoided by having a system in place. There should be a dedicated person ensuring timely pump refill. A pump refill appointment is a multistep process; the time slot should be long enough to ensure that all steps take place safely. The steps include evaluating the patient for any pump malfunction, interrogating the pump, refilling the pump, reprograming the pump, then printing out a hard copy of the new program for the medical record. Stay focused and do not get distracted when reprogramming. Stay vigilant to prevent pocket refill and document the whole procedure well. Have a low threshold for using image guidance for safe refill of the pump. The refill time period is governed by the FDA and manufacturer guidelines (Tables 24.1 and 24.2).

REFERENCES

1. Prager J, Deer T, Levy R, et al. Best practices for intrathecal drug delivery for pain. *Neuromodulation*. 2014;17(4):354-372; discussion 372. doi:10.1111/ner.12146.
2. Abd-Elsayed A. Pocket fill during intrathecal pump refill: is it a frequent occurrence? *Neuromodulation*. 2019;22(6):761. doi:10.1111/ner.13029.
3. Maino P, Koetsier E, Perez RSGM. The accuracy of template-guided refill technique of intrathecal pumps controlled by fluoroscopy: an observational study. *Neuromodulation*. 2015;18(5):428-432. doi:10.1111/ner.12212.
4. Medtronic. *Refill kit for Use with Medtronic Implantable Programmable Infusion Pumps*. Available at: https://manuals.medtronic.com/content/dam/emanuals/neuro/M964645A_c_001_view.pdf. Accessed May 19, 2021.
5. Perruchoud C, Bovy M, Rutschmann B, Durrer A, Buchser E. Silicone septum leakage at the origin of a drug overdose in a patient implanted with an intrathecal pump. *Neuromodulation*. 2013;16(5):467-470;discussion469-470.doi:10.1111/j.1525-1403.2012.00523.x.
6. Maino P, Perez RSGM, Koetsier E. Intrathecal pump refills, pocket fills, and symptoms of drug overdose: a prospective, observational study comparing the injected drug volume vs. the drug volume effectively measured inside the pump. *Neuromodulation*. 2017;20(7):733-739. doi:10.1111/ner.12597.
7. Prometra. *Refill Kit (REF 11825) for Use with Prometra® Programmable Infusion Systems*. Available at: https://flowonix.com/sites/default/files/pl-21794-03_-_prometra_infusion_systems_refill_kit_ifu_us_commercial.pdf. Accessed May 19, 2021.
8. Saulino M, Gofeld M. "Sonology" of programmable intrathecal pumps. *Neuromodulation*. 2014;17(7):696-698; discussion 698. doi:10.1111/ner.12159.
9. Gofeld M, McQueen CK. Ultrasound-guided intrathecal pump access and prevention of the pocket fill. *Pain Med*. 2011;12(4):607-611. doi:10.1111/j.1526-4637.2011.01090.x.
10. Johnson ML, Visser EJ, Goucke CR. Massive clonidine overdose during refill of an implanted drug delivery device for intrathecal analgesia: a review of inadvertent soft-tissue injection during implantable drug delivery device refills and its management. *Pain Med*. 2011;12(7):1032-1040. doi:10.1111/j.1526-4637.2011.01146.x.

Chapter **25**

Important Topics in Neuromodulation—Understanding of Imaging, Location of Pump or Generator Placement, and Anesthesia Need During Trial and Implants

Weston Nadherny, Behnum Habibi, and Chong Kim

Chapter Outline

Introduction

With the plethora of indications for a neuromodulating implant and numerous other possible indications, there is an ever-growing number of individuals with these implants. Given the broad degree of underlying pathology necessitating such devices, there is often a need for further imaging once these devices are implanted. The purpose of this chapter is to consolidate information regarding the intersection between magnetic resonance imaging (MRI), computed tomography (CT), and neuromodulating devices.

Overview of Magnetic Resonance Imaging

MRI is an indispensable imaging modality in modern medicine. It uses strong magnetic fields to produce images. When compared with CT, it has the advantage of being capable of producing high-resolution images of soft-tissue structures from deep within the body, whereas CT is limited in this capacity. It also avoids the use of ionizing radiation; however, magnetic fields are of concern when used in the setting of an implanted electrical device, thus, must be given special consideration in these circumstances.

MRI has a role in a wide range of applications. It is one of the preferred imaging modalities in neuroimaging for its ability to detail gray and white matter, identify demyelinating disease, and provide valuable information in the setting of stroke, dementia, and infectious processes of the central nervous system. In addition, MRI has significant utility in imaging the liver, gastrointestinal tract, and numerous other body systems. The American College of Radiology provides recommendations for appropriate imaging modalities. It indicates innumerable conditions for which MRI is the preferred modality.[1] For certain indications within the spine, CT or CT myelography is an option;

however, MRI is often the preferred modality. For non-spinal pathologies, X-ray, CT, and ultrasound may be alternatives. However, MRI is often the preferred modality when there is suspicion of cancer, infection, or immunosuppression.

Functionally, MRI uses highly powerful magnets to align protons within the object being studied. A radiofrequency (RF) current is applied that disrupts the orientation of the protons. When this radiofrequency field is turned off, the protons realign, thereby releasing energy to be detected. Based on the environment in which these protons are found and the chemical make-up, a proton tends to take a different amount of time to realign. Because of this, body tissues with different composition can be differentiated, even if they are of similar density. Most MRI scanners in clinical use are either 1.5 or 3 Tesla. The specific absorption rate is a measure of the rate of energy transfer to a material and is important because it has a direct impact on the rate of heating of the target. It primarily depends on the strength of the magnetic field, frequency of the RF pulses, and the size and conductivity of the target.

Focused Review of Devices

A brief review of the critical components of the devices discussed in this chapter is needed in order to understand their behaviors in various clinical scenarios. Neuromodulation includes various types of stimulators and intrathecal drug delivery devices. The implanted devices to be discussed within this chapter have varying degrees of similarities. Although the focus will be on intrathecal pump (ITP) devices, it is estimated that more than 82% of patients implanted with a spinal cord stimulation (SCS) device will require an MRI within 5 years of implantation.[2]

An intrathecal drug delivery system (IDDS) consists of several components. The most commonly implanted device is the Medtronic SynchroMed II.[3] It consists of a metal housing, which contains the drug and catheter that is tunneled through the skin with the tip placed at the appropriate level in the intrathecal space. The system uses pressurized gas as the driver for the drug. A variety of medications can be delivered intrathecally; the consequences of overdosing or underdosing due to pump malfunction are dependent on the specific drug. The only medications currently approved by the US Food and Drug Administration (FDA) for intrathecal delivery are baclofen, morphine, and ziconotide, though others may be used.[4,5] Because of the risk of the pump stalling during MRI, it is important to consider whether the drug delivery can be suspended for the duration of an MRI scan.

Intersection of Magnetic Resonance Imaging with Neuromodulation

Devices implanted into patients generally fall into one of three categories: *MR unsafe*, *MR conditional*, and *MR safe*. MR safe items pose no known risk in the setting of MRI and may be deemed safe based on scientific reasoning as opposed to specific testing. At the other end of the spectrum, MR unsafe items have the potential to be hazardous in all MRI environments. The area between these is labeled MR conditional. This label is obtained through sufficient testing of the devices in the setting of MRI. Noteworthy behaviors must be characterized, including displacement force on the device, torque, and heating. Further characterization based on the specific device may be warranted, for example, damage to the device, device malfunction, and neurostimulation.

Most devices are labeled either unsafe or conditional. Low specific absorption rate (SAR) sequences and less powerful magnets can be used to comply with manufacturer recommendations. Performing the scan over a longer period of time with reduced slices and echoes per acquisition can also decrease the SAR, causing less heating of the target. Induced currents occur when a conducting material is exposed to a changing magnetic field and the size of the produced voltage depends on the rate of change of magnetic flux as dictated by Faraday's law. Some of the key features of the devices covered in this chapter are summarized in Table 25.1.

Magnetic Resonance Imaging and Intrathecal Drug Delivery Systems

Potential risks when using MRI with an IDDS involve the magnetic forces on the device, alteration of settings, implanted device damage, and thermal injury.

TABLE 25.1 Intrathecal Drug Delivery System Devices, Manufacturers, Magnetic Field Strength, and Scan Regions

Manufacturer	Pump Model	Static Magnet Strength	Scan Region
Medtronic	SynchroMed II	1.5 and 3 T	Full body
Flowonix	Prometra I, Prometra II	1.5 T	Full body

Adapted from Sayed D, Chakravarthy K, Amirdelfan K, et al. A comprehensive practice guideline for magnetic resonance imaging compatibility in implanted neuromodulation devices. *Neuromodulation*. 2020;23(7):893–911.[6]

In terms of the force, it has been shown that stronger magnets produce greater forces on the device, as would be intuitively expected.[7] Complications are rare when appropriate precautions are taken, but may include mechanical forces causing structural failure, catheter disconnection, motor stalls, memory or programming issues, heating of adjacent tissue, and discharge of an inappropriate volume of drug.[6] Because of the use of pressurized gas, alteration in the temperature or pressure of the gas may change the amount of drug delivered; thus, care must be taken as the MRI can cause the device to become heated. The MRI may also cause the pump to stall or other failures, which can be discovered after the scan is complete by interrogating the device. One study in which 43 patients received MRI with an implanted SynchroMed device (Medtronic; Minneapolis, MN) found virtually no technical or medical complications. However, the providers did take the extra precaution of emptying the pump.[8] The Prometra device (Flowonix Medical; Mount Olive, NJ) was FDA approved in 2012. It uses a dosing chamber that mitigates the dosing variability caused by changes in pressure and temperature, but does not eliminate it entirely.[3] This theoretically decreases the risk of over-infusion from the device heating due to the SAR while in the MRI.

Basic Overview of Computed Tomography in Neuromodulation

CT is often the preferred imaging modality in individuals with implanted neuromodulation devices, though there are still concerns about potential complications as a result of radiation causing device lead malfunction.[9] In general, CT is safer for individuals with implants of unclear MRI safety profiles, and the probability of an adverse event is very low. When the CT scanner directly irradiates the circuitry, it may impact the function of the device; when not directly irradiated, interference is completely avoided. Adverse effects that have been reported include pain, shocks, dizziness, loss of therapy, tingling or burning sensations, and spontaneously turning on/off during the scan. It is advisable to use the lowest dose of radiation for the shortest possible time, turn the device off, and interrogate the device after the scan is complete to ensure correct functioning of the device.

Locations for Intrathecal Drug Delivery System Placement

With respect to intrathecal drug pumps, the implant location of the device must be carefully considered. Both are typically placed in a subcutaneous pocket. Lack of interference with daily activities and comfort are two of the primary considerations when choosing a placement in the patient of either device. For example, revision rates due to pocket pain from a neuromodulation device are about 12% and should be avoided when possible. Thus, establishing a comfortable location for the device is critical.[10] Rubbing against bony structures should be avoided.

IDDS devices are most commonly implanted in the abdomen, taking care to avoid the belt line. Consideration must also be given to placing the device away from the patient's preferred sleeping side so that it does not cause discomfort when the patient lies on that side. The abdomen is a particularly strong option in individuals who are wheelchair bound or immobile since implants on the posterior aspect of the body may rub against the chair and cause skin irritation and breakdown. Important nerves in the area include cutaneous branches of the subcostal, thoracoabdominal, and ilio-hypogastric nerves. Irritation of these nerves can cause allodynia or hyperalgesia in the region. The abdominal region is also dynamic in movements such as bending and twisting, which may further exacerbate pain or irritation in the region. The abdomen should be avoided, when possible, in people with scars from prior surgery, stoma, underlying pathology that may require abdominal surgery, and women of childbearing age. It may also be problematic in patients who lose weight after implantation due to risk of migration.

IDDS devices can be implanted in the buttock as well as the flank and even the posterior chest wall.[10,11] Patient body habitus, preferences, activity level, and common positioning need to be supportive of the buttock and posterior placement. Important structures to avoid include the T12 rib and the bra line in women. As with the placement on the abdomen, the belt line should also be avoided. Posterior chest wall placement has shown promise as a strong option for placement and in some centers is the preferred option.[10] Cutaneous divisions of the upper thoracic nerves are present and must be considered when implanting a device in the region. The superior cluneal nerves innervate the region of the buttock—compression of these nerves may cause pain or numbness in the corresponding areas of innervation.[12] Irritation of bony prominences is also a concern, particularly in patients with a lower body mass index or who are wheelchair bound.

Other implant locations have been reported when implantation in more typical sites is impossible. Narang et al. detail nine cases of implantation in the upper antero-medial thigh. For these patients the typical implantation locations were impossible for a variety of reasons, including multiple surgical scars on the abdomen, colostomy, ileostomy, urostomy, skin erosion, and abdominal hernias.[13]

Intrathecal Drug Delivery System Trialing and Implantations and the Implications for Anesthesia

IDDS trialing can be a single intrathecal bolus injection, multiple intrathecal bolus injections, continuous intrathecal infusion, or continuous epidural infusion. The injection or catheter placement is commonly done under local anesthesia. However, it is not uncommon for very light sedation, using intravenous benzodiazepines such as midazolam along with an opioid, or fentanyl, to be used in ambulatory surgery centers or in hospital operating rooms. One potential benefit of local anesthetic only is that it can allow the patient to report pain that may indicate nerve or spinal cord trauma. For implantation, monitored anesthesia care (MAC) with local anesthesia or general anesthesia can be used. Use of MAC depends on the level of consciousness/sedation required for the procedure as well as accessibility of the airway in the event that general anesthesia is required. Procedures that necessitate deeper sedation, limit access to the airway, or in patients at high risk for aspiration are better suited for general anesthesia.

Conclusion

IDDS devices are now well established in treating chronic pain. As such, clinicians must be aware of the interactions that these devices have, particularly with advanced imaging modalities, particularly MRI but also CT. A working knowledge of the device components and the function of the technology is important to keep patients safe while maximizing access to necessary imaging. Therefore, it is critical to keep up with the continued advancements in technologies, their clinical application, and key areas of concern that may harm the patient. Additionally, the techniques that are used, including location of the component and the type of anesthesia, need to be continually reevaluated to ensure optimal patient care.

REFERENCES

1. American College of Radiology. *ACR Appropriateness Criteria*. Available at: https://acsearch.acr.org/list. Accessed March 7, 2021.
2. Desai MJ, Hargens LM, Breitenfeldt MD, et al. The rate of magnetic resonance imaging in patients with spinal cord stimulation. *Spine (Phila Pa 1976)*. 2015;40(9):E531-E537. doi:10.1097/brs.0000000000000805.
3. Wilkes D. Programmable intrathecal pumps for the management of chronic pain: recommendations for improved efficiency. *J Pain Res*. 2014;7:571-577. doi:10.2147/JPR.S46929.
4. Deer T, Krames ES, Hassenbusch SJ, et al. Polyanalgesic Consensus Conference 2007: recommendations for the management of pain by intrathecal (intraspinal) drug delivery: report of an interdisciplinary expert panel. *Neuromodulation*. 2007;10(4):300-328. doi:10.1111/j.1525-1403.2007.00128.x.
5. Bottros MM, Christo PJ. Current perspectives on intrathecal drug delivery. *J Pain Res*. 2014;7:615-626. doi:10.2147/JPR.S37591.

6. Sayed D, Chakravarthy K, Amirdelfan K, et al. A comprehensive practice guideline for magnetic resonance imaging compatibility in implanted neuromodulation devices. *Neuromodulation*. 2020;23(7):893-911. doi:10.1111/ner.13233.
7. Baker KB, Nyenhuis JA, Hrdlicka G, Rezai AR, Tkach JA, Shellock FG. Neurostimulation systems: assessment of magnetic field interactions associated with 1.5- and 3-Tesla MR systems. *J Magn Reson Imaging*. 2005;21(1):72-77. doi:10.1002/jmri.20224.
8. De Andres J, Villanueva V, Palmisani S, et al. The safety of magnetic resonance imaging in patients with programmable implanted intrathecal drug delivery systems: a 3-year prospective study. *Anesth Analg*. 2011;112(5):1124-1129. doi:10.1213/ANE.0b013e318210d017.
9. U.S. Food & Drug Administration. *Electromagnetic Compatibility (EMC)*. Available at: Available at: https://www.fda.gov/radiation-emitting-products/radiation-safety/electromagnetic-compatibility-emc. Accessed March 7, 2021.
10. Baranidharan G, Bretherton B, Richert G, et al. Pocket pain, does location matter: a single-centre retrospective study of patients implanted with a spinal cord stimulator. *Reg Anesth Pain Med*. 2020;45:891-897. doi:10.1136/rapm-2020-101752.
11. Schultz DM, Orhurhu V, Khan F, Hagedorn JM, Abd-Elsayed A. Patient satisfaction following intrathecal targeted drug delivery for benign chronic pain: results of a single-center survey study. *Neuromodulation*. 2020;23(7):1009-1017. doi:10.1111/ner.13167.
12. Isu T, Kim K, Morimoto D, Iwamoto N. Superior and middle cluneal nerve entrapment as a cause of low back pain. *Neurospine*. 2018;15(1):25-32. doi:10.14245/ns.1836024.012.
13. Narang S, Srinivasan SK, Zinboonyahgoon N, Sampson CE. Upper antero-medial thigh as an alternative site for implantation of intrathecal pumps: a case series. *Neuromodulation*. 2016;19(6):655-663. doi:10.1111/ner.12469.

Chapter 26

Measuring Outcomes for Neuromodulation

Xiaoying Zhu

Chapter Outline

Introduction

Chronic pain is a common health problem. In the United States, between 20% and 30% of the population has chronic pain, with prevalence higher in females than males and increasing with age.[1,2] Chronic pain has a substantial negative impact on a patient's mood, quality of life, and relationships. It can affect a patient's ability to work, leading to financial implications for the patient and society. According to the National Pain Advocacy Center, chronic pain is the number one cause of disability in America, affecting more Americans than any other disease, including cancer, heart disease, or diabetes.[3]

Successful management of chronic pain is crucial in decreasing suffering and improving function and quality of life. With the population aging, an increasing percentage of people will suffer from chronic pain and, therefore, need pain treatments. The need for proper outcome measures is high because of the increasing demand for scientifically valid demonstrations of treatment efficacy. Neuromodulation is an effective treatment modality for chronic pain[4-8] through modulation of various structures of the nervous system to achieve analgesia. It includes electrical stimulation and chemical modulation. Common types of electrical stimulation therapies are stimulation of the spinal cord, dorsal root ganglion, peripheral nerves, and others. Chemical modulation includes intrathecal drug therapy. Neuromodulation is usually the last resort for pain treatment after patients fail other less invasive therapies such as physical therapy, medications, and injections. How do we assess the success of neuromodulation therapies?

Measuring Outcomes for Neuromodulation

Pain has been redefined by the International Association for the Study of Pain as "an unpleasant sensory and emotional experience associated with, or resembling that associated with, actual or potential tissue damage."[9] Since pain is a complex subjective experience, there is no direct measurement tool to objectively quantify its intensity and associated stress. Currently, we rely mainly on self-report measures to determine the impact of pain. Pain is influenced to varying degrees by biological, psychological, and social factors.[9] The effects of chronic pain may include decreased activity, poor sleep and mood, greater use of medications, and more health practitioner visits. All of these factors make pain assessment and outcomes measurement of pain treatments challenging.

Due to the complex and subjective nature of pain, multidimensional tools and approaches should be employed to assess pain and the outcomes of pain treatments such as neuromodulation. These dimensions include pain relief, physical function, sleep, mood, medication use, medical visits, side effects/complications, and patient satisfaction,[10,11] with pain relief as the primary outcome.

PAIN RELIEF

Pain intensity can be measured with various pain scales. The Numerical Pain Rating Scale (NPRS) is commonly used to assess the subjective intensity of pain (0 is no pain and 10 is extreme pain/worst possible pain). This scale can help guide the diagnostic process, track the progression of pain, and assess the effect of pain treatments.

A reduction of approximately 2 points or a reduction of approximately 30% in the NPRS was considered a clinically significant difference.[12] This level corresponds with a "much improved" or "very much improved" response from patients on a global impression of change. However, a later study indicated that chronic pain patients considered larger reductions in their pain, a mean pain reduction of 3.4 points on the 11-point NPRS (56%), to represent treatment success.[13]

In addition to pain intensity, the temporal aspects of pain should be evaluated, including variability in pain intensity, time to onset of meaningful pain relief, durability of pain relief, and frequency, duration, and intensity of pain episodes.[14]

At least 50% overall pain reduction has been the standard used to define a successful neuromodulation trial and to gauge the efficacy of a permanent implant of a neuromodulation device, such as a spinal cord stimulator, dorsal root ganglion stimulator,[4,15] or intrathecal pump.[8]

PHYSICAL ACTIVITIES

Chronic pain interferes with physical activities. Improvement in physical functions is expected with pain relief. Therefore, physical activity levels are considered an important factor in pain assessment and could indicate functional outcomes.[14,16] Activities of daily living—such as self-care, household chores, walking, working, or travel—are included in various pain evaluation questionnaires and inventories.[11,14] Studies have shown that significant pain relief was associated with functional improvements in patients after treatments.[17,18] A mean reduction in activity interference of 68% represents treatment success.[13]

SLEEP

Ample evidence suggests that sleep and pain are reciprocally related.[19-21] While sleep impairments reliably predict exacerbations of chronic pain, objective polysomnographic measures indicate that individuals with chronic pain experience significant sleep disturbances, particularly sleep initiation and maintenance. The exact mechanisms underlying the relationship between chronic pain and disturbed sleep are unclear and appear to be very complicated.[21] For improvement in chronic pain to be inferred, pain-related sleep issues need to be measured and improved.

MOOD

Mood is a state of mind or emotion. Chronic pain is often accompanied by symptoms of psychological distress and psychiatric disorders, including depression, anxiety, and anger.[14] Studies have shown that the prevalence of major depression in patients with chronic pain ranges from 18% in general population, 27% in primary care, and 52% in pain clinics.[22] Up to 50% of pain patients have been reported to suffer from anxiety, with particularly high rates of generalized anxiety disorder.[23] Patients with multiple pain symptoms such as back pain, headache, abdominal pain, and facial pain are 3 to 5 times more likely to be depressed than patients without pain. In addition, as pain severity increases, depressive symptoms and depression diagnoses become more prevalent. According to a study by Robinson et al., a reduction of 65% in emotional distress is considered treatment success by chronic pain patients.[13]

MEDICATION USE

The change in the use of pain medications can be considered as an outcome measure for pain treatments.[14] Decreased frequency of medication, especially short-acting opioids, would logically follow decreased pain intensity and decreased frequency of pain flares as a result of successful pain management. Historically, success in neuromodulation has been indicated by decreased medication use.

PHYSICIAN/EMERGENCY DEPARTMENT VISITS

Similar to medication use, meaningful pain relief results in less frequent pain-related physician or emergency department visits. Therefore, a patient's frequency of physician and/or emergency department visits for pain relief should also be one of the factors in assessing the effectiveness of chronic pain management.

SIDE EFFECTS AND COMPLICATIONS

Interventions aiming for pain relief can cause side effects and complications. Both electrical stimulation and intrathecal drug therapy can produce complications from the surgical procedures and the devices.[7,8,15] In addition, intrathecal drug therapy may have adverse events from the medications infused intrathecally.[7] After initiation of these pain treatments, patients ought to be monitored closely for side effects and complications. In addition, management needs to be provided in a timely fashion should any complications and side effects occur. All adverse events should be taken into consideration when assessing the success of these pain interventions.

PATIENT SATISFACTION

Given the subjective nature of the pain experience and potential discrepancy between patients' and health care providers' conclusions about treatment success, decisions about what constitutes treatment success ought to consider the patient perspective. Patients' satisfaction with chronic pain management is an important indicator of clinical outcomes. It can be seen as the final result of the match between expectations and subsequent experiences.[24] Each chronic pain patient has different expectations, needs, and goals. Therefore, pain management should be customized and realistic expectations should be set up prior to initiation of treatments, particularly neuromodulation therapies, which are more invasive than medications and injections.

Over the past decades, numerous pain assessment tools have been developed to measure the outcomes of pain treatments[10,11,25] (Table 26.1). Even though no single one of these tools includes everything discussed here, the outcomes of neuromodulation can be fairly accurately measured by combining some of them.

TABLE 26.1 List of Pain Questionnaires

Domain	Questionnaires	Assess	Link
Pain	Numerical rating scale (NRS)	Pain intensity	—
	Visual analogue scale (VAS)	Pain intensity	—
	Verbal rating scale (VRS)	Pain intensity	—
	McGill Pain Questionnaire (MPQ)	Sensory and affective components of pain	https://www.sralab.org/sites/default/files/2017-07/McGill Pain Questionnaire (1).pdf
Functional	Brief Pain Inventory (BPI)	Severity of pain and impact of pain on daily functions	https://www.mdanderson.org/research/departments-labs-institutes/departments-divisions/symptom-research/symptom-assessment-tools/brief-pain-inventory.html
	Pain Disability Index (PDI)	Impact of pain on the ability to participate in essential life activities	www.med.umich.edu/1info/FHP/practiceguides/pain/detpdi.pdf
	Roland-Morris Disability Questionnaire (RMDQ)	Functional disability from low back pain	http://www.rmdq.org
	Oswestry Disability Questionnaire (ODI)	Functional disability from low back pain	https://eprovide.mapi-trust.org/instruments/oswestry-disability-index

Continued

TABLE 26.1 List of Pain Questionnaires—cont'd

Domain	Questionnaires	Assess	Link
	West Haven–Yale Multidimensional Pain Inventory (WHYMPI)	Impact of pain on daily life and functions	https://www.va.gov/PAINMANAGEMENT/docs/WHYMPI.pdf
Psychosocial	Beck Depression Inventory (BDI)	Depressive symptoms and complaints	https://www.pearsonclinical.com/psychology/products/100000159/beck-depression-inventoryii-bdi-ii.html
	Centre for Epidemiologic Studies—Depression Scale	Depression	www.chcr.brown.edu/pcoc/cesdscale.pdf
	Short Form Medical Outcomes Scale (SF-MOS)	Vitality, social functioning, role-emotional, and mental health	https://www.rand.org/health/surveys_tools/mos/36-item-short-form.html
	Pain Catastrophizing Scale	Emotional response to pain	https://eprovide.mapi-trust.org/instruments/pain-catastrophizing-scale
	Pain Self-Efficacy Questionnaire	Confidence of people with chronic pain in engaging in activity despite pain	https://novopsych.com.au/assessments/health/pain-self-efficacy-questionnaire-pseq/
	Tampa Scale of Kinesiophobia	Pain-related fear of movement	https://www.physio-pedia.com/Tampa_Scale_of_Kinesiophobia
Quality of life	Sickness Impact Profile (SIP)	Pain interference with physical and emotional functioning	https://www.sralab.org/rehabilitation-measures/sickness-impact-profile
	EuroQol 5D	Health-related quality of life: mobility, self-care, usual activities, pain/discomfort, and anxiety/depression	https://euroqol.org/
Multidimensional	Pain Outcomes Questionnaire—For Veterans (POQ-VA)	Comprehensive assessment of pain	www.midss.org/content/pain-outcomes-questionnaire-veterans-poq-va

Conclusion

Due to the complex and subjective nature of pain, the outcomes of pain treatments need to be measured using multidimensional approaches and combining various pain assessment tools. Neuromodulation therapies such as spinal cord stimulation, dorsal root ganglion stimulation, and intrathecal drug infusion have been shown to be efficacious treatment options for various types of chronic pain. The success criteria of neuromodulation should include at least 50% pain relief; improvement in physical function, sleep, and mood; reduction in pain medication use; decrease in pain-related medical visits; no significant side effects/complications; and the patient's overall satisfaction. If these criteria are met during a neuromodulation trial, a permanent implant of the neuromodulation device is indicated. If these criteria are met following a permanent implant, then success of neuromodulation can be inferred.

REFERENCES

1. Johannes CB, Le TK, Zhou X, Johnston JA, Dworkin RH. The prevalence of chronic pain in United States adults: results of an Internet-based survey. *J Pain*. 2010;11(11):1230-1239.
2. Dahlhamer J, Lucas J, Zelaya C, et al. Prevalence of chronic pain and high-impact chronic pain among adults—United States, 2016. *MMWR Morb Mortal Wkly Rep*. 2018;67(36):1001-1006.
3. National Pain Advocacy Center. *Fast Facts about Chronic Pain*. 2021. Available at: https://nationalpain.org/fast-facts-about-pain. Accessed April 30, 2021.

4. Sdrulla AD, Guan Y, Raja SN. Spinal cord stimulation: clinical efficacy and potential mechanisms. *Pain Pract*. 2018;18(8): 1048-1067.
5. Stelter B, Karri J, Marathe A, Abd-Elsayed A. Dorsal root ganglion stimulation for the treatment of non-complex regional pain syndrome related chronic pain syndromes: a systematic review. *Neuromodulation*. 2021;24(4):622-633.
6. Deer TR, Pope JE, Lamer TJ, et al. The Neuromodulation Appropriateness Consensus Committee on best practices for dorsal root ganglion stimulation. *Neuromodulation*. 2019;22(1):1-35.
7. Deer TR, Pope JE, Hayek SM, et al. The Polyanalgesic Consensus Conference (PACC): recommendations for intrathecal drug delivery: guidance for improving safety and mitigating risks. *Neuromodulation*. 2017;20(2):155-176.
8. Deer TR, Pope JE, Hayek SM, et al. The Polyanalgesic Consensus Conference (PACC): recommendations on intrathecal drug infusion systems best practices and guidelines. *Neuromodulation*. 2017;20(2):96-132.
9. Raja SN, Carr DB, Cohen M, et al. The revised International Association for the Study of Pain definition of pain: concepts, challenges, and compromises. *Pain*. 2020;161(9):1976-1982.
10. Younger J, McCue R, Mackey S. Pain outcomes: a brief review of instruments and techniques. *Curr Pain Headache Rep*. 2009; 13(1):39-43.
11. The British Pain Society and Faculty of Pain Medicine of the Royal College of Anaesthetists. *Outcome Measures*. January 2019. Available at: https://www.britishpainsociety.org/media-centre/news/bps-launches-joint-outcome-measures-document/. Accessed May 8, 2021.
12. Farrar JT, Young JP, LaMoreaux L, Werth JL, Poole MR. Clinical importance of changes in chronic pain intensity measured on an 11-point numerical pain rating scale. *Pain*. 2001;94(2):149-158.
13. Robinson ME, Brown JL, George SZ, et al. Multidimensional success criteria and expectations for treatment of chronic pain: the patient perspective. *Pain Med*. 2005;6(5):336-345.
14. Dworkin RH, Turk DC, Farrar JT, et al. Core outcome measures for chronic pain clinical trials: IMMPACT recommendations. *Pain*. 2005;113(1-2):9-19.
15. Deer TR, Mekhail N, Provenzano D, et al. The appropriate use of neurostimulation of the spinal cord and peripheral nervous system for the treatment of chronic pain and ischemic diseases: the Neuromodulation Appropriateness Consensus Committee. *Neuromodulation*. 2014;17(6):515-550; discussion 550.
16. Wæhrens EE, Amris K, Fisher AG. Performance-based assessment of activities of daily living (ADL) ability among women with chronic widespread pain. *Pain*. 2010;150(3):535-541.
17. Barthel HR, Peniston JH, Clark MB, Gold MS, Altman RD. Correlation of pain relief with physical function in hand osteoarthritis: randomized controlled trial post hoc analysis. *Arthritis Res Ther*. 2010;12(1):R7.
18. Argoff C, Arnstein P, Stanos S, et al. Relationship between change in pain intensity and functional outcomes in patients with chronic pain receiving twice daily extended-release hydrocodone bitartrate. *J Opioid Manag*. 2015;11(5):417-424.
19. Finan PH, Goodin BR, Smith MT. The association of sleep and pain: an update and a path forward. *J Pain*. 2013;14(12): 1539-1552.
20. Fishbain DA, Cole B, Lewis JE, Gao J. What is the evidence for chronic pain being etiologically associated with the DSM-IV category of sleep disorder due to a general medical condition? A structured evidence-based review. *Pain Med*. 2010;11(2): 158-179.
21. Mathias JL, Cant ML, Burke ALJ. Sleep disturbances and sleep disorders in adults living with chronic pain: a meta-analysis. *Sleep Med*. 2018;52:198-210.
22. Gambassi G. Pain and depression: the egg and the chicken story revisited. *Arch Gerontol Geriatr*. 2009;49(suppl 1):S103-S112.
23. Feingold D, Brill S, Goor-Aryeh I. Depression and anxiety among chronic pain patients receiving prescription opioids and medical marijuana. *J Affect Disord*. 2017;218:1-7.
24. Geurts JW, Willems PC, Lockwood C, et al. Patient expectations for management of chronic non-cancer pain: a systematic review. *Health Expect*. 2017;20(6):1201-1217.
25. Clark ME, Gironda RJ, Young RW. Development and validation of the Pain Outcomes Questionnaire-VA. *J Rehabil Res Dev*. 2003;40(5):381-395.

Index

Page numbers followed by *b, t,* and *f* indicate boxes, tables, and figures, respectively.